Working in the Operating Department

To Corrinne

For Churchill Livingstone:

Commissioning editor: Inta Ozols
Project manager: Valerie Burgess
Project development editor: Dinah Thom
Design direction: Judith Wright
Sales promotion executive: Hilary Brown

Working in the Operating Department

Bakul Kumar MBBS DA FFARCSI
Consultant in Anaesthesia and Pain Management and
Honorary Senior Clinical Lecturer in Anaesthesia City Hospital NHS Trust, Birmingham

Foreword to the First Edition by
Peter Hutton BSc PhD MBChB FRCA
Professor of Anaesthesia, University of Birmingham

SECOND EDITION

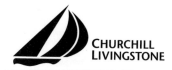
CHURCHILL
LIVINGSTONE

NEW YORK EDINBURGH LONDON MADRID MELBOURNE SAN FRANCISCO AND TOKYO 1998

CHURCHILL LIVINGSTONE
Medical Division of Pearson Professional Limited

Distributed in the United States of America by Churchill
Livingstone Inc., 650 Avenue of the Americas, New York,
N.Y. 10011, and by associated companies, branches and
representatives throughout the world.

First Edition 1990
Second Edition 1998

ISBN 0 443 05573 4

British Library of Cataloguing in Publication Data
A catalogue record for this book is available from the British
Library.

Library of Congress Cataloging in Publication Data
A catalog record for this book is available from the Library
of Congress.

Medical knowledge is constantly changing. As new
information becomes available, changes in treatment,
procedures, equipment and the use of drugs become
necessary. The author and the publishers have, as far as it is
possible, taken care to ensure that the information given in
this text is accurate and up to date. However, readers are
strongly advised to confirm that the information, especially
with regard to drug usage, complies with latest legislation
and standards of practice.

Produced by Longman Singapore Publishers (Pte) Ltd
Printed in Singapore

Contents

Foreword to the First Edition

I was delighted to be asked to write a Foreword introducing this book. Not only does its subject area fill a very real gap in the literature, but also the selection and standard of content are ideal for its purpose.

Working in the operating theatre and its associated environments are topics which have been relatively neglected by authors. Until now, they have been covered piecemeal in a variety of texts with the consequence that a student's knowledge has often been determined more by chance than by judgement.

This problem has now been solved with the publication of Dr Kumar's book. There is much within it which will be of great value to student nurses, trainee ODAs and anaesthetic and recovery nurses. It is particularly useful because it covers a wide field to a depth which is both appropriate and sufficient for the practical and examination requirements of its intended audience. It also combines together the relevant factors of traditionally diverse subjects so as to build up an integrated picture of patient care. The MCQs at the end of each chapter allow a convenient form of self-assessment.

Recent publications on 'The Efficiency of Theatre Services' and 'Assistance for the Anaesthetist' from the Association of Anaesthetists of Great Britain and Ireland and 'The Management and Utilisation of Operating Departments' from the NHS Management Executive have emphasized the need for an up-to-date and well-informed theatre staff. This book is therefore very timely and I wish it every success.

P.H.

Preface to the Second Edition

Since the first edition of this book was published in 1990, a number of positive comments have been made by operating department nurses and operating department personnel (ODPs). With the changes in the field of surgical technology and research-based education for nurses and ODPs, I have, to a large extent, changed the format of this book.

The chapters on anatomy and physiology have been retained as a revision guide for those who wish to use the book for examination purposes. Other chapters, such as those on theatre technique and preparation, have been expanded. Following changes to the cardiopulmonary resuscitation guidelines, a part of the relevant chapter has been rewritten. The chapter on the National Health Service found in the previous edition has been omitted as the structure of the NHS is evolving daily. There has also been a dramatic shift in the amount of research-based education for theatre nurses and ODPs, so two new chapters (Nursing research and statistics, and Audit and computers) have been added.

I have placed special emphasis on the references and suggestions for further reading to enable nurses and ODPs to carry out further research into individual subjects.

In preparing this revised edition, I have once again spent a number of hours discussing the format of the syllabus with nurses and ODPs.

I hope you find as much joy in reading this book as I have found in revising it.

B.K. 1998

Anatomy and physiology

CELLS AND TISSUES

Anatomy is defined as the study of the form of the body, whereas physiology is defined as the study of the functions of the body.

The cell (Fig. 1.1) is the unit from which tissues are made up. Cells vary in size, shape and content based on the functions they carry out.

A cell consists of:

- a cell membrane, a thin membrane made up of protein and lipid, which encloses the cell;
- cytoplasm, the substance of which most of the cell is made up; it contains a fine network and granules;
- a nucleus, a thick structure that lies within the cytoplasm; it contains chromatin and is surrounded by a membrane;
- the nucleolus, a small circular body that lies within the nucleus and is made up of ribonucleoprotein.

Each group of cells has a different function. For example, cells in the thyroid gland produce thyroid hormone, and cells of cardiac muscle (in the heart)

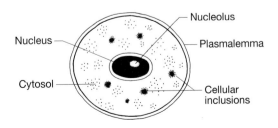

Figure 1.1   The cell.

bring about contraction and relaxation of the heart. The cells are separated by a thin space occupied by interstitial fluid, which allows water and certain chemical substances to pass from fluid to cell and cell to fluid.

Cells:

- usually require oxygen and produce carbon dioxide;
- contain enzymes (those substances which bring about a chemical reaction without themselves being altered) having a specific action;
- break down food and release chemical energy.

TISSUES

There are five main types of tissue (Fig. 1.2): (1) epithelial, (2) connective, (3) nervous, (4) muscular, and (5) blood.

Epithelial tissue

This tissue covers the external and internal surfaces of the body and lines the ducts and glands that open onto these surfaces. The cells which make up the epithelial tissue are: squamous, or flat, cells; columnar, or tall, cells; and cuboidal, or cube-shaped, cells.

Squamous, or flat, cells are again divided into three groups:

1. Simple squamous epithelium (endothelium), made up of one layer of flat cells, for example the cells that line the inside of blood vessels, the alveoli (air sacs) of the lungs and the heart.
2. Stratified epithelium, made up of more than one layer of squamous cells, for example the skin.
3. Transitional epithelium made up of three, four or more layers of squamous epithelium, for example the inner lining of the uterus, the bladder and part of the female urethra.

Columnar epithelium lines the inner surface of the stomach and intestines. One of the groups included in this section is ciliated columnar epithelium, which has fine cilia (cilia are movable,

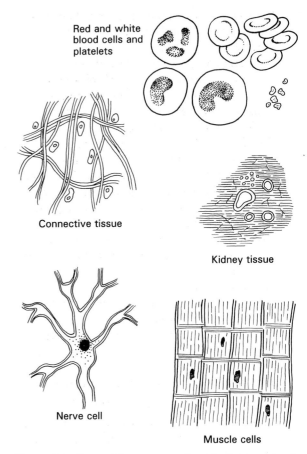

Red and white blood cells and platelets

Connective tissue

Kidney tissue

Nerve cell

Muscle cells

Figure 1.2 Types of tissue: connective, blood, nervous and muscle.

fibre-like structures). By their constant movement, cilia keep dust out of the lungs and move ova (eggs) along the fallopian tube.

Connective tissue

Connective tissue helps in binding together, supporting and protecting structures. It can be either dense or soft.

Dense connective tissue. This includes:

- Tendons. These are made up of closely packed fibres. One end of the tendon is attached to the end of a muscle and the other to bone.
- Bone, made up of bone cells and a matrix. Bone cells are again divided into two groups: osteocytes, which form new bone; and

osteoclasts, which remodel bone. Matrix is made up of ground substance, mineral deposits and fibres.

- Cartilage, made up of cells and fibres enclosed in a solid matrix. It is elastic in nature and has no blood vessels, lymph vessels or nerve supply. There are three different types of cartilage:
  - (i) hyaline cartilage, which is present in the larynx and rings of the trachea, the cartilage at the anterior ends of the ribs, the articular cartilage within the joints and the cartilage in which most bones are formed;
  - (ii) elastic cartilage, which is present in the epiglottis, pinna of the ear and auditory tube;
  - (iii) fibrocartilage, which contains many collagen fibres and is seen in the discs of the sternoclavicular and temporomandibular joints and in the pubic symphysis.

Soft connective tissue. This is made up of:

- ground substance (cells and fibres);
- fibres. Cells could be plasma cells, which are oval cells, fat cells, mast cells, fibroblasts or histocytes.

Soft connective tissue is divided into: (i) areolar tissue, a loose tissue with few fibres as seen under the mucous membranes, skin and surrounding blood vessels and nerves; and (ii) fat, consisting of a large number of fat cells, as seen below the skin and between the layers of the peritoneum in the abdomen.

Nervous tissue

This tissue type is made up of nerve cells with their attached fibres. It is found in the brain, spinal cord and all the nerves.

Muscular tissue

Muscle cells and tissues take part in contraction and relaxation. There are three types of muscle: skeletal, smooth and cardiac (Fig. 1.3).

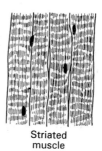 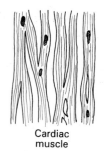

Striated muscle   Cardiac muscle

Figure 1.3 Types of muscle: striated (skeletal) and cardiac.

Skeletal muscle is also called striated, or voluntary, muscle. It assists in voluntary movements and forms about 40% of the total body weight. It is found in the muscles attached to bone, skin or cartilage. The fibres show cross-striations, and the movements are controlled by the central nervous system.

Smooth muscle is also called unstriated, or involuntary, muscle and does not show cross-striations. This type is found in the walls of blood vessels and viscera, for example stomach and bladder. Smooth muscle comes in two types:

1. Single unit. In muscle cells interconnected by gap junctions, as in the heart, some cells will depolarize spontaneously (pacemaker potential) and the wave of excitation will spread throughout the entire sheet of cells. Contraction is largely, but not completely, outside the control of the nervous system. An example is the muscle of smaller blood vessels.
2. Multi-unit. Gap junctions are fewer and therefore excitation, often from the autonomic nervous system, remains more localized. Most blood vessels and the iris of the eye have this type of muscle.

Cardiac muscle is found in the heart. Its cells are branched (unlike those of skeletal muscle) and the fibres appear striated.

Blood cells

There are three main types of blood cell:

- red blood cells (RBCs)

- white blood cells (WBCs)
- platelets.

BODY FLUIDS

In the human body, fluids and electrolytes are present in certain proportions in the various tissues, the quantity varying depending on the age of the individual.

Water makes up 70% of body weight in an adult man, a 70 kg man for example having 50 L of water in his body. Adult women have 10% less water than men because they have more fat, which has a lower water content. In an infant, water forms 75% of the body weight. In an old person, water forms 55% of the body weight.

This body water is maintained in two body 'compartments': extracellular fluid (ECF) and intracellular fluid (ICF). Extracellular fluid (ECF) is that water present outside the cells. It makes up 30% of the total body water and is seen in blood plasma, cerebrospinal fluid, fluids in cavities and joints, lymph and interstitial fluid (fluid present in the tissue spaces between cells). Intracellular fluid (ICF) is water present inside the cells. It makes up 70% of the total body water. ECF helps in the transport of chemical substances from one cell to another, whereas it is in the ICF that the cell's chemical changes take place.

A continuous exchange of chemical substances takes place between ECF and ICF to maintain a normal electrolyte and acid–base balance. The normal electrolytes in the body are shown in Box 1.1. The maintenance of acid–base balance is described on page 251.

Box 1.1 Electrolytes in the body	
Electrolytes	*Symbol*
Sodium	Na
Potassium	K
Calcium	Ca
Magnesium	Mg
Chloride	Cl
Bicarbonate	HCO_3
Phosphate	PO_4
Sulphate	SO_4

RESPIRATORY SYSTEM

ANATOMY

The respiratory system begins at the nose and ends at the alveoli of the lungs. For simplicity, the respiratory system can be divided into:

- nose
- pharynx
- nasopharynx
- oropharynx
- larynx
- trachea
- bronchi (right and left)
- lungs (right and left)
- pleura (covering both lungs).

Nose

The nose is made up of the external nose and the nasal cavities behind the external nose.

The external nose is made up of cartilage below and the nasal bones above, covered inside by mucous membrane and outside by skin. The nose has nostrils, or external openings.

The nasal cavities begin at the nostrils in front and extend to the posterior openings of the nose, which open into the nasopharynx. They are lined by mucous membrane.

The nasal septum is a thin structure made up of bone and cartilage, lined by mucous membrane, which separates the two nasal cavities. The lateral wall of the nasal cavity is formed by the parts of the sphenoid, palatine and maxillary bones. The floor of the nasal cavity is formed by the palatine and maxillary bones. The roof of the nasal cavity is formed by the sphenoid and frontal bones.

Paranasal sinuses

The paranasal sinuses, lined with mucous membrane, are those spaces in the cranial bones which open into the nasal cavity:

- sphenoid sinus
- ethmoid sinus
- frontal sinus
- maxillary antrum.

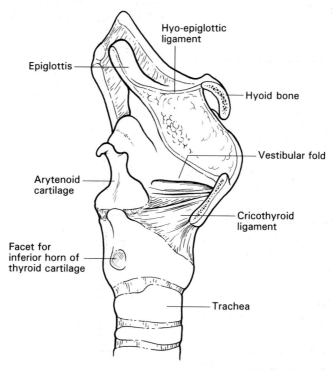

Epiglottis

Hyo-epiglottic ligament

Hyoid bone

Vestibular fold

Arytenoid cartilage

Cricothyroid ligament

Facet for inferior horn of thyroid cartilage

Trachea

Figure 1.4   The larynx.

Other structures which open into the nasal cavity are the nostrils and the nasolacrimal duct.

Pharynx

The pharynx is divided into the nasopharynx and oropharynx. The nasopharynx opens into the nasal cavities in front and into the oral pharynx below. The eustachian (auditory) tubes open into its lateral wall on each side.

The oropharynx is common to the respiratory and alimentary systems, as air enters it from the nasopharynx and lungs, and food from the mouth.

Larynx

The larynx (Fig. 1.4) is made up of cartilage, membrane, mucous membrane, muscles and vocal cords.

1. The *cartilage* is made up of:
    *   The thyroid cartilage, a V-shaped cartilage with the 'V' projecting prominently into the neck as the Adam's apple.

*   The cricoid cartilage, a signet ring-shaped piece of cartilage that is rigid both anteriorly and posteriorly. It lies below the thyroid cartilage and is connected to it by the cricothyroid membrane. The presence of this complete ring is made use of in cricoid pressure (Sellick's manoeuvre). Here, pressure on the cricoid cartilage causes the posterior part of the cartilage to compress the softer oesophagus, thus preventing food from being regurgitated upwards. The cricothyroid membrane can be punctured to form an alternative route into the trachea.
*   The epiglottis is a leaf-shaped piece of cartilage which extends upwards behind the base of the tongue. It is attached to the back of the hyoid bone and the thyroid cartilage. It is very floppy in small children, and infection by *Haemophilus influenzae* can cause swelling of the epiglottis (acute epiglottitis), which makes breathing very difficult and in an emergency needs endotracheal intubation.

- The aryepiglottic folds stretch from the side of the epiglottis to the arytenoid cartilages.
  - The arytenoid cartilages are two small, pyramid-shaped pieces of cartilage that sit on the cricoid cartilage.

2. *Membrane.* This connects the cartilages to each other.

3. *Mucous membrane.* The larynx is lined by ciliated columnar epithelium.

4. *Muscles.* Small muscles attached to the thyroid, cricoid and arytenoid cartilages assist in opening and closing the vocal cords by their contraction and relaxation. All the muscles are supplied by branches of the vagus nerve (10th cranial nerve).

5. *Vocal cords.* These are two thin sheets of mucous membrane lying over the vocal ligaments. The vocal ligaments are attached to the inside of the thyroid cartilage in front and the arytenoid cartilages behind. The vocal cords assist in making sound by vibrating during expiration. There are two folds of mucous membrane just above the true vocal cords. These are called the false vocal cords and are not involved in making sound.

Trachea

The trachea is a cylindrical tube, which in adults is about 10 cm long and 2.5 cm in diameter. It lies in the front of the neck, starting at the cricoid cartilage and ending behind the manubrium sterni by dividing into right and left bronchi at the carina. In the neck, the isthmus of the thyroid gland and veins lie in front of the trachea.

Bronchi

The right and left bronchi run outwards and downwards from the trachea to their respective lungs. In adults, the right bronchus is wider, shorter and straighter than the left. For this reason, during endotracheal intubation, if the tube is pushed pass the carina it will usually lodge in the right main bronchus, loss of ventilation through the blocked-off left main bronchus leading to collapse of the left lung and to one-lung ventilation.

Lungs

Each lung is cone-shaped and is covered by a closed sac of pleura. The right lung consists of upper, middle and lower lobes; the left lung consists of an upper and a lower lobe. At the root of the lung, each main bronchus, arising from the trachea, enters its respective lung.

A bronchiole is one of the smaller branches of the bronchi, which further divides into smaller branches. The smallest of these branches is the alveolar duct, each one of which ends in a cluster of alveoli. An alveolus is a thin-walled air-containing sac through whose walls gaseous exchange occurs.

The structures that enter or leave the lung at its root are:

- the bronchus and its main branches;
- the pulmonary artery;
- the pulmonary veins;
- the lymph drainage;
- nerves.

Blood supply. Each lung receives a branch of the pulmonary artery, which brings deoxygenated blood (from the right ventricle of the heart). The terminal branches of this artery end in a network of capillaries on the surface of each alveolus. Here, gaseous exchange occurs, and the capillaries then drain into the pulmonary veins, which carry the newly oxygenated blood back to the left atrium.

Nerve supply. The sympathetic nerve supply is derived from the sympathetic chain, while the parasympathetic nerve supply arises from the vagus nerve.

PHYSIOLOGY

Respiration is the transfer of gases between body cells and the environment.

Mechanics of breathing

Air moves into the lungs during inspiration and out during expiration owing to changes in pressure within the chest.

During inspiration, the diaphragmatic muscle contracts and the dome of the diaphragm descends. At the same time, external intercostal muscles (present in the chest wall) contract, thus increasing the space in the chest, expanding the lungs and allowing air to enter them. During expiration, the diaphragm and external intercostal muscles relax, the diaphragm rises and the air moves out of the lungs passively.

An adult breathes between 12 and 16 times per minute, whilst a newborn baby can breathe up to 40 times per minute.

During respiration, oxygen diffuses into the blood from the alveoli whereas carbon dioxide diffuses from the blood into the alveoli, i.e. in the opposite direction. Ventilation (breathing in and out) allows the exchange of alveolar gas with fresh atmospheric gas and the excretion of carbon dioxide into the atmosphere. The composition of gases in the atmosphere is shown in Box 1.2.

Box 1.2 Percentages of gases in the atmosphere	
Oxygen	20.98%
Carbon dioxide	0.04%
Nitrogen	78.06%

Gas exchange in the lungs. Oxygen diffuses out of the breathed air into the alveoli and from there enters the bloodstream, carbon dioxide diffusing out into the alveoli from the blood. The volume of gases transferred depends on the surface area of the alveoli and the thickness of the alveolar wall.

Transport of gases in the blood. Oxygen combines with haemoglobin in the red blood cells to form oxyhaemoglobin. Each gram of haemoglobin carries between 1.34 and 1.39 ml of oxygen. Plasma carries oxygen in a dissolved form (0.003 ml/100 ml of blood per mmHg Po_2). The fully oxygenated arterial blood thus contains 19.8 ml of oxygen (in a person with a haemoglobin concentration of 15.0 g/100 ml).

Oxyhaemoglobin dissociation curve. This is a curve relating the percentage saturation of the haemoglobin with oxygen to the oxygen-carrying potential of the haemoglobin. It has a characteristic sigmoid shape.

Carbon dioxide is transported by plasma proteins, haemoglobin and bicarbonate.

Gas exchange in the tissues. When oxygenated blood reaches the tissue fluid, oxygen, which is at a higher partial pressure, diffuses out into the tissues. From the tissue fluid, oxygen passes into the cells according to requirements. Because carbon dioxide is produced by the cells, it is present at a higher concentration, so diffuses down the concentration gradient into the tissue fluid and from there into the blood.

Control of respiration

Respiration is controlled by the nervous system and by chemical factors.

1. *Nervous system.* Respiration is regulated by a respiratory centre located in the medulla oblongata of the brain.

2. *Chemical factors.* The carotid bodies (which are present at the bifurcation of each common carotid artery) and the aortic bodies (which lie on the arch of the aorta) are tiny organs made up of nerve cells and blood vessels. They send messages to the respiratory centre in the medulla oblongata. The carotid and aortic bodies sense changes in the carbon dioxide tension and hydrogen ion concentration in the blood passing through them. An increase in carbon dioxide level and a fall in pH causes the respiratory centre to send impulses to the respiratory muscles, which in turn contract with greater frequency (increased breathing), thus expelling carbon dioxide from the lungs and restoring the pH to normal.

Tests of lung function

The *tidal volume* is the amount of air that moves into the lungs with each inspiration. The normal value is 7 ml/kg body weight, so a 70 kg man has a tidal volume of 490 ml, of which 2 ml/kg body weight is the dead space, i.e. the gas that does not take part in gas exchange.

The *residual volume* is the air left in the lungs after a maximal expiration, the normal value being 1.2 L in a 70 kg man.

The *vital capacity* is the greatest amount of air that can be expired after a maximal inspiration (normally 4.8 L in a 70 kg man).

The *forced expiratory* volume at 1 second (FEV1) is the fraction of the vital capacity expired in 1 second.

CARDIOVASCULAR SYSTEM

ANATOMY

The cardiovascular system is made up of the heart, arteries and arterioles, capillaries, venules and veins.

Heart (Fig. 1.5)

The heart lies in the chest and is the size of a clenched fist. Its relations are:

- above, the aorta and pulmonary trunk;
- below, the diaphragm;

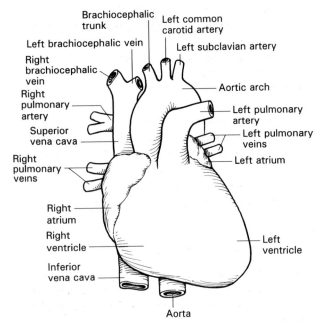

Figure 1.5 The heart.

- behind, the descending aorta, oesophagus and spinal column;
- on either side, the lungs.

The heart has four chambers – right atrium, right ventricle, left atrium and left ventricle – and four valves – tricuspid and pulmonary valves on the right, and mitral and aortic on the left.

Right atrium. This lies on the right side of the heart, behind the sternum. The deoxygenated blood enters it via the superior vena cava at the upper end, the inferior vena cava at the lower end, the coronary sinus (a small vein through which blood comes from the heart) and the right auricle (a small projection from the atrium that lies in front of the aorta and pulmonary artery).

Right ventricle. This forms a major portion of the front of the heart and has a thick-walled chamber. It consists of:

- The right atrioventricular valve (also called the tricuspid valve), which guards the opening between the right atrium and the ventricle (right atrioventricular opening). This valve is made up of three flaps. The base of each flap is attached to the atrioventricular opening, and its free border is held in place by the chordae tendinae. These are small, cone-like projections of muscle arising from myocardium and projecting into the ventricle.
- The pulmonary outflow tract and pulmonary valve.

Left atrium. This is a thin-walled cavity that lies at the back of the heart. Two pulmonary veins bringing oxygenated blood from the lungs enter the left atrium on each side. The atrium opens below into the left ventricle via the left atrioventricular opening.

The left ventricle. The left ventricle is situated at the left and back of the heart, and is thick walled compared with the right ventricle. It consists of: (1) the left atrioventricular valve (also called mitral valve); this surrounds the left atrioventricular opening and has two flaps, which are attached to the chordae tendinae; and

(2) an opening into the aorta at the upper end of the ventricle with the aortic valve.

The heart is made up of three types of tissue: pericardium, myocardium and endocardium. The pericardium is a fibrous bag in which the heart is enclosed. It is a double-layered fibrous sac with a small amount of fluid between the layers. The myocardium forms the muscular wall of the heart. Myocardium is made up of cardiac muscle fibres that are striated and connected to each another by cellular branches. The endo-cardium lines the inside of the chambers of the heart and covers the valves on both sides.

Blood supply to the heart

The wall of the heart is supplied by two coronary arteries (right and left), arising from the aorta immediately above the aortic valve. They supply the respective sides of the heart.

Arteries (Fig. 1.6)

The arteries are hollow tubes through which blood flows to the tissues and organs. They are made up of an outer layer of connective tissue, a middle layer of smooth muscle and an inner layer of intima (or endothelium).

The major arteries in the body are outlined below.

Aorta. The aorta is the major artery of the body. It is divided into the thoracic aorta, which lies in the chest, and the abdominal aorta, which lies in the abdomen.

The thoracic aorta begins at the aortic valve of the left ventricle. It consists of three parts: the ascending aorta, the arch of the aorta and the descending thoracic aorta.

The abdominal aorta begins at the termination of the descending thoracic aorta; this occurs where the vessel passes through the diaphragmatic opening.

The main branches of aorta are:

- In the thorax:
  - right and left coronary arteries;

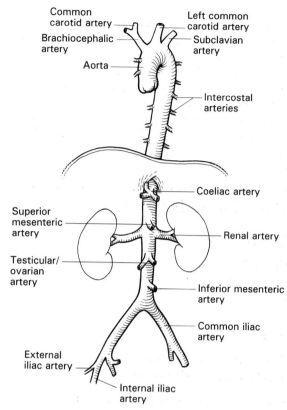

Figure 1.6   Principal arteries of the body.

  - brachiocephalic artery (dividing into the right common carotid and right subclavian arteries);
  - left common carotid artery;
  - left subclavian artery.
- In the abdomen:
  - celiac artery;
  - right and left renal arteries;
  - right and left testicular arteries (in males);
  - right and left ovarian arteries (in females);
  - superior and inferior mesenteric arteries;
  - right and left lumbar arteries;
  - right and left common iliac arteries.

Blood supply to the organs

The head and neck are supplied by the common carotid arteries. The common carotid artery on the right side arises from the brachiocephalic artery.

The common carotid artery divides into external and internal carotid arteries. The external carotid artery supplies various organs in the head and neck through its branches:

- the lingual artery to the tongue;
- the facial artery to the face;
- the superior thyroid artery to the thyroid gland.

The eye is supplied by the ophthalmic artery, a branch of the internal carotid artery.

The brain is supplied by the right and left internal carotid arteries and right and left vertebral arteries.

The upper extremity is supplied by the subclavian artery and its branches. The right subclavian artery is a branch of the brachiocephalic artery, whereas the left subclavian artery is a branch of the aorta. The subclavian artery continues into the axilla as the axillary artery. The axillary artery runs in the arm as the brachial artery, which then divides into radial and ulnar arteries at the wrist.

In the abdomen, the arteries supply the various organs as listed in Box 1.3.

Box 1.3 Blood supply to organs	
Organ	*Artery*
Stomach	Splenic artery, hepatic artery and the left gastric artery
Spleen	Splenic artery
Liver	Hepatic artery
Kidneys	Renal arteries
Testes	Testicular artery on each side
Small intestine	Superior mesenteric artery
Large intestine	Superior and inferior mesenteric arteries
Rectum	Inferior mesenteric artery and internal iliac artery
Uterus	Uterine artery
Ovary	Ovarian artery

Pelvic organs and lower extremity. The common iliac arteries are the right and left terminal branches of the abdominal aorta, each common iliac artery also dividing into an external and an internal branch. Each internal iliac artery supplies blood to the bladder, the lower end of the rectum, uterus and vagina, and the gluteal muscles on its par-

ticular side of the body. The external iliac artery continues into the thigh as the femoral artery, which gives off branches to the muscles of the thigh and femur. The femoral artery continues as the popliteal artery below the knee and divides into the anterior and posterior tibial arteries, which supply the ankle and foot.

Arterioles are smaller than arteries. Like arteries, they have walls made of smooth muscle, which can contract and relax. Arterioles are present everywhere as the smaller branches of major arteries. Arteriolar dilatation (also called vasodilatation) is facilitated by carbon dioxide, adenosine monophosphate (AMP), and bradykinin. Arteriolar contraction (vasoconstriction) is facilitated by adrenaline, noradrenaline and angiotensin.

Veins and venules are shown in Figure 1.7. Venules are small veins formed by the union of capillaries. Veins are formed by the union of venules. They are made up of three layers: an outer layer of collagen fibres, a thin middle layer of smooth muscle and elastic fibres, and an inner smooth layer of endothelial cells (the intima).

Valves are present in many veins, to direct blood back towards the heart and to prevent back flow of blood away from the heart.

Venous drainage of organs

Brain. Veins in the brain form valveless venous sinuses, which drain into the internal jugular vein.

Head and neck. The veins of the head and neck drain into the right and left internal jugular veins. The two internal jugular veins start at the inferior surface of the skull. They join the subclavian vein from the respective arm to form the right and left brachiocephalic veins. The two brachiocephalic veins unite to form the superior vena cava, which empties into the right atrium.

Upper extremity. Veins from the hand travel upwards in the forearm as the cephalic and basilic veins. The basilic vein continues in the axilla as the axillary vein, which in the neck becomes the subclavian vein. The superior vena cava is formed

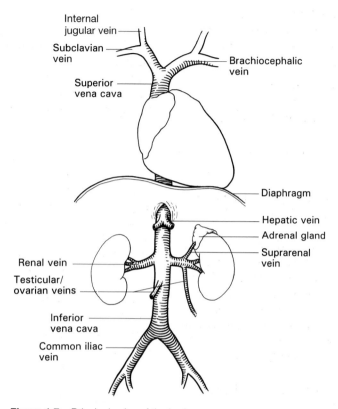

Figure 1.7 Principal veins of the body.

by the union of the right and left brachiocephalic veins and therefore drains blood from the head, neck, arms and upper thorax.

Lower extremity. The long saphenous vein begins on the dorsum of the foot and passes upwards to join the femoral vein. The short saphenous vein starts at the back of the calf and ascends upwards to join the popliteal vein. The popliteal vein passes upwards to the front of the thigh to become the femoral vein, which continues as the external iliac vein. The internal iliac vein, which drains blood from the pelvic organs (bladder and rectum), joins the external iliac vein to form the common iliac vein. The right and left common iliac veins in turn unite to form the inferior vena cava.

PHYSIOLOGY

The chambers of the heart normally beat in an orderly manner. Atrial contraction (also called atrial systole) is followed by the contraction of ventricles (also called ventricular systole). During diastole, all four chambers of the heart are relaxed. The heart beat is coordinated by a specialized conduction system beginning at the sinoatrial (SA) node and continuing on to the atrioventricular (AV), the bundle of His and the Purkinje system.

Heart beat

The SA node is the normal cardiac pacemaker, whose rate determines the heart beat. At the beginning of systole, a wave of excitation starts in the SA node, spreads through the walls of both atria, causing atrial contraction, and reaches and stimulates the AV node, which lies in the wall between the right atrium and the right ventricle. The bundle of His is a band of muscle running in the septum between the two ventricles and reaching the apex of the heart, where it divides into two main branches, one for each ventricle. The wave of excitation that begins in the SA node causes atrial contraction and from there reaches the two ventricles via the AV node, to cause ventricular contraction.

The cardiac cycle is the sequence of events during one heart beat. It occurs in two phases: diastole and systole. Each cycle lasts for 0.8 s when the heart rate is about 75 beats/min.

Diastole is the period of relaxation that follows the contraction and lasts for 0.5 s. During this period, the following events take place:

1. Initially, venous blood enters the right atrium from the superior and inferior vena cavae, and oxygenated blood enters the left atrium from the pulmonary veins.

2. Blood is prevented from entering the ventricle from the atrium by the closure of the two atrioventricular valves (tricuspid and mitral; see p. 8).

3. Similarly, blood is prevented from flowing back into the ventricles from the aorta and the pulmonary artery by closure of the pulmonary and aortic valves.

4. Later, as the blood enters the atria, the pressure rises. When it exceeds that in the ventricles, the atrioventricular valves open and blood flows from the atria into the ventricles.

Systole is the period of muscular contraction and lasts for 0.3 s. During this period, the following events take place:

1. The walls of the atria contract, following stimulation by the SA node, thus expelling blood into the ventricles.

2. As the pressure in the ventricles exceeds that in the atria, the atrioventricular valves close, the aortic and pulmonary valves open and ventricular contraction occurs.

3. Blood from the right ventricle is expelled into the pulmonary artery, and from the left ventricle into the aorta.

4. When the blood is fully expelled, the muscular contraction stops and the relaxation phase (diastole) begins.

Cardiac output. The blood expelled from the heart during each minute depends upon stroke volume and heart rate.

1. *Stroke volume.* This is the amount of blood expelled from a ventricle at each beat. At rest, it is about 70 ml; this can increase to 125 ml with mild exercise. The stroke volume is controlled by changes in the force of contraction. The greater the length of the muscle fibres, the greater the contraction.

2. *Heart rate.* At rest, this is usually about 70 beats/min. It can be increased by (i) a reduction in stimulation of vagus nerve fibres (parasympathetic), and (ii) to some extent, stimulation of the sympathetic fibres.

Cardiac output is the product of heart rate and stroke volume, as shown below.

Heart rate × Stroke volume
70 beats × 75 ml
= approx. 5 L/min

Nerve supply to the heart

Although the heart can beat on its own, it is normally influenced by two sets of nerve fibres:

- parasympathetic fibres, which arise from the vagus (10th cranial) nerve. When these fibres are stimulated, they slow down the heart rate and decrease the force of contraction;
- sympathetic fibres, which arise from the ganglia on the cervical part of the sympathetic trunk (see p. 17). When the fibres are stimulated, they increase the heart rate and force of contraction.

Heart sounds. The heart, when it is contracting, produces sounds that can be heard with the help of a stethoscope. Usually, two heart sounds are heard, but on some occasions a total of four heart sounds can be detected.

The first heart sound is produced by the closure of the mitral and tricuspid valves at the beginning of the ventricular systole. It sounds like 'lub' when spoken softly.

The second heart sound is produced by the vibrations caused by the closure of the aortic and pulmonary valves. It sounds like 'dub'.

The third heart sound is due to sudden tightening of the mitral valve cusps. It is a low, soft thud, normal in the young (less than 30 years old).

The fourth heart sound is produced when either atrium (right or left) contracts against an abnormally stiff ventricle. It is a low, soft sound that precedes the first heart sound.

Electrocardiograph

The electrocardiograph (ECG) is a recording of the electrical changes that occur in the heart during each beat. A normal ECG shows:

- a P wave, produced by the contraction of the atria and lasting for 0.10 s;
- a QRS complex, produced by contraction of the ventricles and lasting for up to 0.09 s;
- a T wave, produced by ventricular relaxation;
- a PR interval, which is the time taken for the impulse to pass down the bundle of His.

The ECG is recorded using 12 different electrode positions.

Arterial pulse

This is a wave transmitted through the arteries as a response to the ejection of blood from the heart into the aorta. It is best felt when an artery is compressed lightly against a bone. Sites at which pulses can be felt easily are:

- the wrist – radial artery and ulnar artery;
- the antecubital fossa – brachial artery;
- in front of the ear – superficial temporal artery;
- on the dorsum of the foot – dorsalis pedis artery.

Pulse rate

A decreased pulse rate (also called bradycardia) occurs in:
- heart block
- rest

and an increased one (also called tachycardia) in:
- exercise

- hyperthyroidism
- anxiety
- anaemia.

The pulse is weak in:
- shock

strong in:
- excitement
- hyperthyroidism
- raised blood pressure

and absent in:
- cardiac arrest
- complete obstruction of an artery.

Arterial blood pressure

Blood pressure (BP) is the pressure exerted by blood within a blood vessel. It depends upon cardiac output and the resistance to flow caused by the diameter of the arterioles. There are two measurements: systolic pressure (the pressure at cardiac systole) and diastolic pressure (the pressure at cardiac diastole).

Blood pressure is measured in millimetres of mercury (mmHg) or kilopascals (kPa). The normal pressures are given in Box 1.4.

Box 1.4 Normal blood pressures	
In aorta and large vessels	
Systolic	120 mmHg
Diastolic	80 mmHg
In small arteries	
Systolic	110 mmHg
Diastolic	70 mmHg
In arterioles	
Systolic	40 mmHg
Diastolic	insignificant

Pressures in various chambers of the heart are shown in Box 1.5.

Box 1.5 Pressure in chambers of the heart		
	Systolic (mmHg)	Diastolic (mmHg)
Right atrium	5	0
Right ventricle	25	0
Left ventricle	121	0
Aorta	120	80
Pulmonary artery	25	12

The blood pressure is normally raised by emotion and exercise and tends to fall during sleep. Hypertension is a sustained rise in blood pressure for which there may or may not be a cause.

Circulation through special organs

Box 1.6 illustrates the blood flow to various organs in the body.

Box 1.6 Blood flow to organs	
	Blood flow (ml/min)
Brain	750
Heart muscle	250
Liver	1500
Skin	460
Kidneys	1260
Whole body	5400

Cerebral circulation. The blood flow to the brain is kept fairly constant by the process of auto-regulation. Cerebral blood flow is affected by:

- arterial blood pressure
- intracranial pressure
- viscosity of the blood
- constriction or dilatation of cerebral blood vessels.

Coronary circulation. The two coronary arteries that supply the myocardium arise from the sinuses at the root of the aorta. Blood flow in the coronary arteries occurs principally during diastole of the heart. Coronary blood flow at rest in man is 250 ml/min, or 5% of the cardiac output.

Pulmonary circulation. Deoxygenated blood from the right ventricle passes via the pulmonary arteries to the capillaries that surround the alveoli in the lungs, and back to the left atrium of the heart. The pulmonary artery arises at the upper end of the right ventricle.

CENTRAL NERVOUS SYSTEM

ANATOMY

The nervous system is made up of neurons (nerve cells and fibres) and neuroglia (cells that support the neurons).

The neuron is the basic unit of the nervous system. Each neuron consists of a nerve cell and its fibres. Each cell has a nucleus and a number of granules and fibrils in its cytoplasm.

Dendrites are short, brush-like fibres that furnish a large area for contact with other neurons. They receive signals from other neurons.

The axon is a fibre through which nerve impulses leave the cell to be transmitted to other cells. Most axons are covered with a sheath of the lipid material myelin; such axons are called myelinated. This myelin sheath is interrupted at the nodes of Ranvier.

Transmission of nerve impulse

Transmission occurs in one direction: into the cell through the dendrites and out through the axon. The nerve impulse is an electrochemical change. As a wave of impulse passes along the axon, potassium (K^+) ions leave the axon and sodium (Na^+) ions enter. The nerve impulse occurs as a result of the difference in *electrical* potential between potassium and sodium. After the wave has passed along the axon, potassium and sodium ions slowly return to their original position.

A synapse is the point of contact between one neuron and another. At this point, transmission of the nerve impulse from the first cell to the second occurs *chemically*, the chemicals liberated being acetylcholine, noradrenaline and dopamine.

Neuromuscular junction (Fig. 1.8)

Transmission of an impulse from a nerve to a muscle occurs at the neuromuscular junction. At this point, the nerve axon loses its myelin sheath and divides into a number of terminal buttons, or end-feet. The end-feet contain small clear vesicles that store acetylcholine, the chemical transmitter. These end-feet fit into the thickened muscle membrane (also called the motor end-plate). This whole structure is collectively called the neuromuscular junction. The nerve impulses arriving at the neuron's end-feet cause the liberation of acetylcholine from vesicles in the

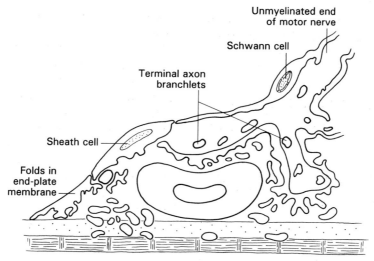

Figure 1.8 The neuromuscular junction.

nerve terminals. The acetylcholine increases the permeability of the underlying muscle cell membrane, and the entry of sodium produces a potential which in turn stimulates the muscle cell to contract.

The function of the neuromuscular junction is to transfer nerve impulses from small motor neurons to a large muscle fibre and cause it to contract.

Parts of the nervous system

The nervous system is divided into:

- the central nervous system, which includes the brain and spinal cord;
- the peripheral nervous system, which includes the cranial and spinal nerves;
- the autonomic nervous system, which includes the parasympathetic and sympathetic systems.

White matter is the nervous tissue in which there is a high proportion of nerve axons, whereas grey matter is that nervous tissue in which there is a high proportion of nerve cell bodies.

Central nervous system

This consists of the brain and the spinal cord.

Brain. The brain is made up of the cerebral hemispheres (right and left), midbrain, pons, cerebellum and medulla oblongata (which is continuous with the spinal cord).

The cerebral hemispheres together make up the largest part of the brain. They consist of:

- cortex (outer layer)
- thalamus and basal ganglia
- corpus callosum.

The surface of the cerebral hemispheres is marked by gyri (ridges) and sulci (fissures). Each cerebral hemisphere is divided into four lobes: frontal, parietal, occipital and temporal.

The midbrain is a small structure that lies between the cerebral hemispheres above and the pons below. It is made up of nerve fibres, which pass up and down it.

The pons is a thick mass of nervous tissue situated between the midbrain above and the medulla oblongata below.

The cerebellum consists of a small central lobe and large right and left lobes. It is connected by nerve fibres (in bundles called peduncles) to the midbrain, pons and medulla oblongata.

The medulla oblongata is a narrow piece of nervous tissue lying between the pons above and the spinal cord below. It contains the cardiac and respiratory centres through which the heart action and breathing are controlled.

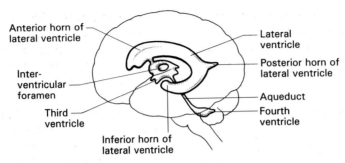

Figure 1.9 The ventricular system of the brain.

Ventricular system of the brain (Fig 1.9). This is a series of interconnected chambers in the brain containing cerebrospinal fluid (CSF). They are:

- the lateral ventricles, which are present in each cerebral hemisphere;
- the third ventricle, present in the midbrain and connected to the lateral ventricles above and via a narrow tube called an aqueduct to the fourth ventricle below;
- the fourth ventricle, a lozenge-shaped space that lies between the pons and medulla oblongata in front and the cerebellum behind.

The ventricles are filled with CSF, formed from the blood plasma in the choroid plexuses, whorls of capillaries lying in the ventricles. About 500 ml of CSF are secreted daily. Normal values for the constituents of CSF are listed in Box 1.7.

Box 1.7	Constituents of CSF	
Volume	120–135 ml	
Pressure	70–150 mmHg	
Glucose	50–85 mg/100 ml	(2.2–3.4 mmol/L)
Protein	20–45 mg/100 ml	(20–45 g/L)
Sodium	147 mEq/L	(147 mmol/L)
Potassium	2.9 mEq/L	(2.9 mmol/L)
Chloride	113 mEq/L	(113 mmol/L)

Spinal cord. The spinal cord is about 45 cm long and occupies the upper two-thirds of the vertebral column. It is continuous above with the medulla oblongata and ends at the level of the 1st or 2nd lumbar vertebra by tapering into a cone called the conus medullaris. The conus medullaris is connected to the coccyx by the filum terminale, a thin strand of connective tissue.

The spinal cord is made up of nerve fibres on the outside (white matter) and an H-shaped group of nerve cells (grey matter) in the middle. A central canal runs through the grey matter (Fig. 1.10).

The nerve fibres are organized in three groups: anterior columns, lateral columns and posterior columns. Within the cord:

- sensory fibres run upwards in the posterior and lateral columns;
- motor fibres run downwards in the anterior and lateral columns;
- short nerve fibres interconnect at different levels of the cord.

Spinal nerves are attached by anterior and posterior roots to the whole length of the spinal cord. They are numbered in relation to their vertebral level.

The meninges are the coverings of the brain and spinal cord. They consist of the:

- dura mater, a thick, white membrane that encloses the whole of the brain and the spinal cord;
- arachnoid membrane, a thin membrane that in places fuses with the pia mater and in

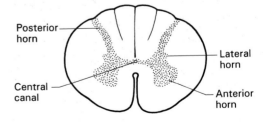

Figure 1.10 Cross-section of the spinal cord.

others is separated from it by a subarachnoid space filled with cerebrospinal fluid;

- pia mater, a very thin membrane attached to the surface of the brain and spinal cord.

Peripheral nervous system

Cranial nerves. There are 12 pairs of cranial nerves, which are nerves connected to the brain. They are numbered as in Box 1.8.

Box 1.8 Cranial nerves

1. Olfactory nerve
2. Optic nerve
3. Oculomotor nerve
4. Trochlear nerve
5. Trigeminal nerve
6. Abducent nerve
7. Facial nerve
8. Auditory nerve
9. Glossopharyngeal nerve
10. Vagus nerve
11. Accessory nerve
12. Hypoglossal nerve

Brachial plexus (Fig. 1.11). This plexus is formed by the anterior branches of cervical nerves C5 to T1. It arises in the lower part of the neck and passes behind the clavicle into the axilla. The major nerves arising from this plexus are the:

- radial nerve
- median nerve
- ulnar nerve
- musculocutaneous nerve
- circumflex nerve.

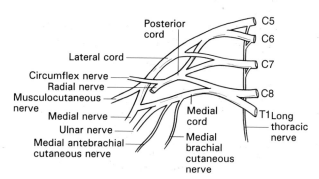

Figure 1.11 The brachial plexus.

Lumbar plexus. This plexus is formed by the anterior branches of the 12th thoracic nerve and the first and second lumbar nerves (T12, L1–L2). The nerves that arise from this plexus are the femoral and the obturator nerves.

Sacral plexus. The sacral plexus is formed by the anterior branches of the nerves from L4, L5 and S1–S4. From this arises the sciatic nerve, which further divides into lateral and medial popliteal nerves, supplying the hamstring muscles at the back of the thigh and all the muscles below the knee.

Autonomic nervous system (Fig. 1.12)

The autonomic nervous system (ANS) is made up of two parts: the parasympathetic system and the sympathetic system. The ANS supplies the nerves to blood vessels, internal organs (stomach and oesophagus) and endocrine glands. Its functions are integrated with the central nervous system. The actions of parasympathetic and sympathetic systems are opposite in nature (Table 1.1).

Parasympathetic system. This is made up of the following parts:

- The cranial part, which has connections with the cerebral cortex and the hypothalamus. Fibres from these connections are distributed to the oculomotor, facial, glossopharyngeal, vagus and accessory nerves.
- The sacral part, from which the pelvic organs such as the bladder and rectum get their nerve supply.

Sympathetic system. This system is made up of:

- controlling centres in the cortex, hypothalamus and medulla and lateral horn of the grey matter in the spinal cord;
- a number of ganglia that run down from the neck to the abdomen. Fibres which arise from these ganglia supply arteries and other organs.

There are three major groups of ganglia:

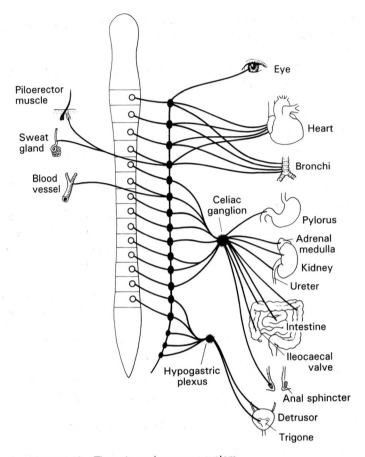

Figure 1.12 The autonomic nervous system.

Table 1.1 Summary of the functions of the autonomic nervous system

Body organ	Parasympathetic	Sympathetic
Skin	–	Stimulates sweat glands Erection of hair
Heart	Heart rate and cardiac output decreased	Heart rate and cardiac output increased
Coronary arteries	–	Dilated
Blood pressure	Lowered	Raised
Respiratory bronchioles	Constricted	Dilated
Gastrointestinal tract	Increased peristalsis Sphincters relaxed	Decreased peristalsis Sphincters closed
Liver	Converts glucose to glycogen	Converts glycogen to glucose
Urinary bladder	Sphincters relaxed Muscle tone decreased	Sphincters closed Muscle tone increased

1. cervical ganglia, which distribute the nerve supply to the carotid arteries, larynx, trachea, thyroid gland and heart;
2. thoracic ganglia, which distribute the nerve supply to the heart, lungs, aorta and its branches, and the abdominal organs;
3. lumbar and sacral ganglia, which distribute the nerve supply to the iliac arteries and to pelvic organs such as the rectum and urinary bladder.

The sympathetic system comes into action during an emergency. For example, during shock or fright, the heart rate and cardiac output are increased, as is the level of adrenaline, whereas bowel and bladder movements are decreased.

PHYSIOLOGY

The main functions of the nervous system are to:

- receive impulses from inside and outside the body and act accordingly. For example, if a person touches a hot object, the cerebral cortex receives the sensations via temperature receptors in the skin, which ascend the spinal cord and promptly send messages down to the hand to withdraw it;
- store memories and express emotions such as anger or depression;
- coordinate the activity of various parts of the body.

Sensory pathways to the brain. Receptors in the skin for temperature, touch, pain and pressure relay their signals via the tracts in the spinal cord to the postcentral gyrus of the cerebral cortex.

Cerebral cortex. Large areas of the cerebral hemispheres are concerned with sensory motor functions, some parts being concerned with hearing and vision. The right cerebral hemisphere recognizes various objects, expresses emotions and controls the left side of the body, whereas the left cerebral hemisphere controls the activities of the right side of the body.

There are two major systems by which signals are transmitted from the brain to the spinal cord to produce movement: the pyramidal (cortico-spinal system) and the extrapyramidal (extra-cortical system).

Cerebellum. The cerebellum is involved in the production of coordinated movements.

Reticular activating system. This is made up of large interconnected neurons in the brainstem. The reticular system is involved in setting the level of consciousness and in the regulation of respiration, heart rate and blood pressure.

Limbic system. This is made up of cortical tissues in the cerebral cortex encircling parts of the hypothalamus, thalamus, amygdaloid nucleus and hippocampus.

Hypothalamus. The hypothalamus is an extremely important brain centre, controlling body temperature, appetite and the release of a number of hormones from the pituitary gland.

SPECIAL SENSES

EAR AND HEARING

The ear is made up of the external, middle and inner ear.

External ear

The external ear is composed of the auricle (pinna) and the external auditory meatus. The auricle (pinna) is made up of elastic cartilage covered with skin. The external auditory meatus is the tube leading from the auricle to the tympanic membrane. The outer third of this meatus is cartilaginous, and the inner two-thirds made up of bone. Wax is formed by ceruminous glands in the cartilaginous part of the meatus.

Middle ear (tympanic cavity)

This a small, oblong-shaped cavity in the temporal bone, comprising the tympanic membrane and the ossicles. The tympanic membrane (eardrum) occupies most of the lateral part of the middle ear and is tightly stretched except in the upper segment. The ossicles are three small bones – malleus, incus and stapes – which occupy much of the tympanic cavity.

Inner ear (Fig. 1.13)

Situated in the petrous portion of the temporal bone, the inner ear consists of two organs: the organ of hearing and the organ of balance.

The *labyrinth* is made up of the vestibule, cochlea and three semicircular canals. It is divided into the bony labyrinth, which is a series of interconnected cavities, and the membranous labyrinth, a closed sac within the bony labyrinth.

The *perilymph* is a clear fluid occupying the space between the bony and membranous labyrinths, while the endolymph is a fluid lying within the membranous labyrinth.

The *vestibule* is a small chamber that communicates anteriorly with the cochlea, posteriorly with the semicircular canals and laterally with the middle ear by two openings, the oval window and the round window.

The *cochlea* is shaped like the shell of a snail. It is hollow, with a cochlear canal running inside the tube. The ascending tube begins at the oval window and is called the scala vestibuli; the descending tube is called the scala tympani and ends at the round window.

The *organ of Corti* is a complicated structure that runs spirally up the cochlea and contains about 15 000 hair cells.

The *semicircular canals* – superior, lateral and posterior – are set at right angles to each other.

They contain endolymph and open into the posterior wall of the vestibule. Nerve endings of the vestibular branch of the 8th cranial nerve (see below) are connected to hair cells projecting into the endolymph. The utricle and the saccule are parts of the membranous vestibule.

The *8th cranial (auditory)* nerve is the cranial nerve of the internal ear, comprising a vestibular and a cochlear part.

Hearing is the ability of the ear to detect pressure vibrations in the air and to interpret them as sound. The ear converts the energy of the pressure waves into nerve impulses, which are carried to the cerebral cortex and interpreted. The human ear can pick up frequencies ranging from 20 to 16 000 Hz, 1 Hz being equal to one cycle per second.

Sound transmission in the ear. Sound waves are received by the auricle and transmitted to the tympanic membrane via the external auditory meatus. The tympanic membrane vibrates with an amplitude proportional to the intensity of sound. From here, the vibration is transmitted by the ossicles, from the malleus through the incus and to the stapes. The stapes then transmits this vibration to the oval window. The sound vibrations within the cochlea stimulate the hair cells in the organ of Corti, which send impulses into the nerve fibres of the cochlear nerve. The cochlear nerve then transmits these impulses to the brain.

Balance. The semicircular canals, saccule and utricle are responsible for maintaining balance.

EYE AND VISION

The eye consists of a transparent cornea, lens, retina, pupil, iris and aqueous and vitreous humour.

Perception of light (Fig. 1.14)

The light enters the eye through the transparent cornea and the lens inverts the image. The amount of light entering the eye is regulated by the iris, which acts as a diaphragm. The size of the pupil

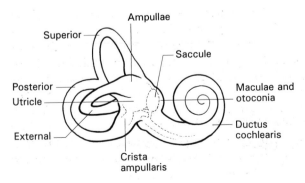

Figure 1.13 The inner ear.

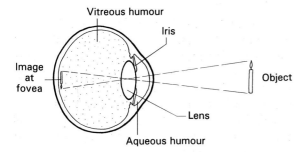

Figure 1.14 Perception of light.

is controlled by the circular and radial muscles of the iris, the pupil enlarging in darkness and constricting in bright light.

The rods and cones are light-sensitive cells in the retina. Rods are used for seeing in dark or dim light, whereas cones are used in bright light and to appreciate colours.

ALIMENTARY SYSTEM

ANATOMY

The alimentary system (Fig. 1.15) begins at the mouth and ends at the anus. The structures that lie between these two organs are the pharynx, the oesophagus, the stomach, the small intestine and the large intestine.

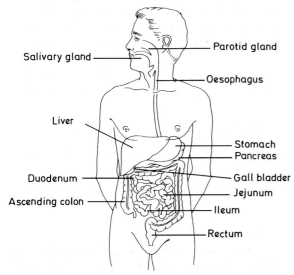

Figure 1.15 The alimentary system.

The mouth is surrounded by the hard and soft palate above, by the cheeks laterally, by the mandible and tongue below and by the opening into the pharynx behind.

The tongue is made up of muscle enclosed by a mucous membrane. The taste buds are specialized cells that lie at the junction of the anterior two-thirds and the posterior third of the tongue. The blood supply to the tongue is from the lingual artery (a branch of the external carotid artery).

The motor nerve supply to the tongue is derived from the hypoglossal (12th cranial) nerve. The sensory nerve supply to the anterior two-thirds of the tongue is derived from the lingual nerve (a branch of the 5th cranial nerve) and the facial (7th cranial) nerve. The 5th cranial nerve identifies the touch sensation, whilst the 7th identifies taste. The posterior third of the tongue is supplied by the glossopharyngeal (9th cranial) nerve, which identifies touch and taste.

Salivary glands are made up of specialized secretory cells. The human salivary glands are the right and left parotid glands, the right and left submandibular glands and the right and left sublingual glands.

The pharynx is a fibromuscular tube attached to the base of the skull above and continuous with the oesophagus below. It is made up of three parts: the nasopharynx, the oropharynx, and the laryngeal pharynx, that part of the pharynx which lies behind the epiglottis and larynx. Food passes through the oropharynx and laryngeal pharynx to enter the oesophagus.

The oesophagus is a muscular tube, about 25 cm long, which begins in the neck as a continuation of the pharynx, travels down the neck and thorax, and then passes through the left crus of the diaphragm to enter the stomach. The oesophagus is surrounded in front by trachea and heart, on either side by lungs and pleurae, and behind by the vertebral column. It is slightly narrower at its upper end, where the left bronchus crosses it and also where it passes through the diaphragm.

The stomach (Fig. 1.16) is a wide, dilatable part of the alimentary tract, whose position and shape vary according to the amount of food in it, the presence of peristaltic waves and respiration.

The stomach is a J-shaped organ lying in the upper left quadrant of the abdomen. It has an anterior and a posterior surface, a greater curvature on the left side and a lesser curvature on the right side, a cardiac orifice where the oesophagus joins it, a dome-like fundus, which lies above the level of the cardiac orifice, a body, which forms a large part of the stomach, a pyloric canal (a narrow tube below the body of the stomach) and a pyloric opening into the first part of the duodenum.

The pyloric opening is surrounded by the pyloric sphincter, formed by a thickening of the circular muscles of the stomach. The cardiac orifice has no special sphincter but is closed by the mucous membrane and muscle fibres at the bottom of the oesophagus.

From inside out, the stomach is made up of a mucous membrane containing the ducts of millions of glands, a submucous coat of loose areolar tissue, muscular coats of circular, oblique and longitudinal muscle fibres, and a peritoneal covering.

The blood supply to the stomach is from the gastric and celiac arteries. Venous drainage is into the portal system, and lymph drainage is into the lymph nodes along the lesser and greater curvatures. The nerve supply is from parasympathetic (vagus) and sympathetic nerves.

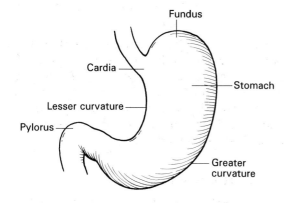

Figure 1.16 The stomach.

Small intestine

This is the part of the alimentary system that lies between the stomach and large intestine. It is made up of the duodenum, jejunum and ileum.

The duodenum is a C-shaped tube, about 25 cm long, which lies at the back of the abdomen, curved around the head of pancreas. It is divided into four parts, the pancreatic and bile ducts opening into the second part by a common opening. This opening is controlled by a sphincter called the sphincter of Oddi.

Jejunum and ileum. The combined length of the jejunum and ileum varies from 300 to 900 cm. The jejunum is slightly bigger, with a thicker wall, more folds of mucous membrane and fewer Peyer's patches than the ileum.

The blood supply to the small intestine is from the branches of the superior mesenteric artery. Venous drainage is into the superior mesenteric vein, which drains into the portal vein, and lymph drainage is into the nodes in the mesentery. The nerve supply is from the parasympathetic (vagus) and sympathetic nerves.

From inside out, the layers of small intestine are:

- Mucous membrane, which is coiled into a number of circular or spiral folds. The surface of the mucous membrane is covered by a large number of villi, tiny projections covered with a single layer of cells. This layer surrounds blood vessels, nerves and lymph vessels. Peyer's patches are patches of lymph tissue in the mucous membrane; they are more common in the ileum than in the jejunum.
- Submucous coat.
- Muscular coats of circular and longitudinal fibres.
- Peritoneal coat.

Large intestine

The large intestine has an average length of 150 cm. It is differentiated from the small intestine by its larger diameter and the presence of taeniae

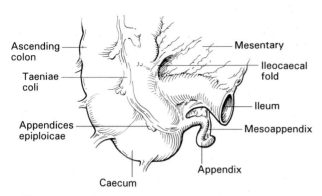

Figure 1.17   The caecum.

coli and appendices epiploicae (Fig. 1.17). The taeniae coli are three bands of longitudinal fibres on the outside of the colon but absent from the appendix and rectum, which gives the bowel a puckered appearance. The appendices epiploicae are tags of fat-containing peritoneum that lie on the surface of the caecum.

The large intestine is made up of the caecum, appendix, ascending colon, transverse colon, descending colon, sigmoid colon (pelvic colon), rectum and anal canal.

The caecum is a wide sac lying in the right iliac fossa. The ileum enters into the caecum at the ileocaecal opening, and the appendix opens into it below the ileocaecal opening. The caecum is continuous above with the ascending colon (Fig. 1.17).

The appendix is a worm-like diverticulum up to 18 cm long that opens into the caecum about 2.5 cm below the ileocaecal valve. It has a narrow lumen and its position is variable, either lying behind the caecum, hanging into the pelvis or being found in front of the caecum.

The ascending colon extends from the caecum, in the right iliac fossa, up the right side of the abdomen and to the right colic flexure under the right lobe of the liver.

Transverse colon. At the right colic flexure, the colon bends sharply to the left and passes, as the transverse colon, across the abdomen. It continues

to the left side to end in the left colic flexure under the spleen.

Descending colon. At the left colic flexure, the colon bends to pass downwards on the left side of the abdomen to the brim of the pelvis, where it continues as the sigmoid colon.

The sigmoid (pelvic) colon has several loops within the pelvis and becomes continuous with the rectum opposite the middle of the sacrum.

The rectum is about 12 cm long, beginning at the middle of the sacrum and ending at the anal canal.

The anal canal, about 3 cm long, runs downwards and backwards and ends at the anus. On either side of this canal are the ischiorectal fossae. An internal and an external sphincter muscle control the opening and closing of the anus.

The blood supply to the large intestine is from the branches of the superior mesenteric artery up to the left colic flexure, and then from the branches of the inferior mesenteric artery. Venous drainage is into the superior and inferior mesenteric veins.

Lymph drainage is into lymph nodes in the peritoneum and finally into the aortic glands. The nerve supply is from the parasympathetic and sympathetic nerves.

From the inside out, the layers of the large intestine are mucous membrane, submucous coat, muscular coat and peritoneum.

Pancreas

The pancreas is a long organ situated at the back of the upper part of the abdomen. It consists of a head (which lies in the curve of the duodenum), neck, body and tail (which reaches the spleen). The pancreas is made up of (1) cells that secrete pancreatic juice and (2) intra-alveolar islets, also called islets of Langerhans.

Liver and biliary system

The liver is the largest gland in the body, weighing about 1300–1500 g. It is soft, vascular and wedge shaped, with its base to the right and its apex to the left. It lies in the right upper quadrant of the abdomen, protected by the ribs. Its smooth, rounded upper surface lies below the diaphragm. Its visceral (postero-inferior) surface lies above the stomach, duodenum, colon and right kidney.

The liver is divided into a large right lobe, a small left lobe, quadrate and caudate lobes, and smaller lobes.

Structures that enter or leave the liver are the right and left branches of the portal vein, the right and left branches of the hepatic vein, the right and left hepatic ducts, lymph vessels and nerves.

About 80% of the blood to the liver is supplied by the portal vein, about 20% coming from the hepatic artery, which is a branch of the celiac artery. Venous drainage from the liver is via two large hepatic veins, which enter the inferior vena cava at the back of the liver.

Structure of the liver. The liver is made up of:

1. *Lobules.* There are a large number of very small lobules, each composed of hepatic cells arranged in columns.
2. *Sinusoids.* These are channels between the columns of cells through which blood passes from the portal vein and the hepatic artery. They are lined by endothelial cells and the cells of the reticulo-endothelial system (see p. 29).
3. A *central vein* in the middle of each lobule.
4. *Canaliculi*, which run between adjacent columns of hepatic cells and unite to form the hepatic ducts.

The biliary system is made up of the common hepatic ducts, right and left hepatic ducts, cystic duct, gall bladder and bile duct. The right and left hepatic ducts arise from the visceral surface of the liver and unite to form the common hepatic duct. The cystic duct runs from the end of the common hepatic duct to the gall bladder. The bile duct, which is formed by the union of the common hepatic and cystic ducts, joins the pancreatic duct and opens into the second part of the duodenum, the opening being controlled by the sphincter of Oddi.

The gall bladder is a pear-shaped sac that can hold up to 50 ml of bile. It lies in the groove between the right lobe and the quadrate lobe of the liver. It consists of a fundus (rounded end), a body and a neck. The neck of the gall bladder is continuous with the cystic duct.

PHYSIOLOGY

Food is digested to smaller molecules at different points in the intestinal tract, especially in the small intestine. Enzymes, the substances involved in the breakdown of food molecules, are found in the secretions of the salivary glands of the mouth, gastric juice, bile from the liver, pancreatic juice and secretions from the mucous membrane of the small intestine.

The salivary glands secrete an enzyme called ptyalin, which digests carbohydrates. Saliva also moistens the food, enhances chewing and allows food to be swallowed easily.

Swallowing

After the food has been chewed and mixed with saliva, it is formed into a small bolus, which is then swallowed. During swallowing, contraction and relaxation of voluntary and involuntary muscles takes place. As the tongue pushes the bolus of food backwards, respiration is inhibited, the larynx raised and the glottis closed to prevent food entering the trachea.

The process of swallowing relaxes the oesophageal sphincters, allowing the food bolus to pass down into the oesophagus. As the bolus enters the oesophagus, a wave of contraction passes along the oesophageal wall. This wave of contraction is immediately followed by a wave of relaxation, resulting in the food bolus being pushed through the cardiac sphincter into the stomach. This process is called peristalsis.

Function of the stomach

The stomach acts as a receptacle, collecting food that is then passed on to the duodenum at a controlled rate for digestion and absorption. The stomach helps in mixing the swallowed food with gastric secretions, forming a semi-liquid substance called chyme. The mixing process is associated with rhythmic contractions of the gastric smooth muscle. The peristaltic waves push the liquid contents through the pylorus into the duodenum.

Gastric secretions

Gastric secretions consist of mucus, pepsinogen, hydrochloric acid and intrinsic factor, all of which arise from cells in the gastric mucosa. The main enzyme in gastric juice, pepsin, is secreted as inactive pepsinogen from serous, or chief, cells. Hydrochloric acid is secreted by the parietal, or oxyntic, cells. The neck cells of the gastric glands secrete both mucus and intrinsic factor. The mucus protects the gastric mucosa from digestion by gastric juice. The pepsin digests protein.

Control of gastric secretion

Gastric secretions are produced continuously and increase markedly during a meal. The first phase of increased secretion is called the cephalic phase because it is regulated from the brain via the vagus nerve. The second phase of increased secretion, called the gastric phase, occurs when the food arrives in the stomach. The presence of proteins in food in the stomach causes the release of a local hormone, gastrin, from the antral mucosa. The presence of proteins (polypeptides) and alcohol acts as a stimulus for the secretion of gastrin.

Intestinal absorption

The small intestine is the main site of digestion and absorption. Enzymes that break down carbohydrate and protein are located in the brush border of the epithelial cells. In the duodenum, further breakdown of carbohydrates occurs. Proteins in the duodenum are broken down by the pancreatic enzymes, trypsin and chymotrypsin, into dipeptides and amino acids. The amino acids are absorbed into the bloodstream from the lumen of the gut. The fat is digested and absorbed in the small intestine.

Bile salts break down large fat droplets, which arrive from the stomach, into smaller size. These small-sized fat droplets are broken down by the enzyme lipase into free fatty acids and glycerol.

Free fatty acids and glycerol, in combination with bile salts, result in the formation of even smaller droplets, called micelles. These come into contact with intestinal mucosa, allowing the free fatty acids and monoglycerides to pass into the epithelial cells. Within these epithelial cells, triglycerides are formed from fatty acids and glycerol by the activity of the endoplasmic reticulum. These triglycerides form chylomicrons, which are then released into the bloodstream.

Pancreatic secretion

The exocrine secretions of the pancreas are of two types: a watery solution with high bicarbonate content secreted by the cells lining the ducts of the glands, and a secretion rich in enzymes, which comes from the acinar cells at the base of the glands. The pancreatic secretions are increased by the presence of food in the stomach, and the main secretions from the glands occur when the gastric contents (chyme) enter the duodenum. If the chyme is acid, the pancreatic secretion is rich in bicarbonate, which neutralizes the acid. This response is mediated by the release of secretin from the duodenal mucosa. The presence of fatty acids and amino acids in the duodenum results in pancreatic juice rich in enzymes being released, the mediating hormone in this case being cholecystokinin-pancreozymin.

Biliary secretion

Bile is required for the digestion and absorption of fat, and is secreted by liver cells into small ducts that open into the duodenum via the common bile duct. Owing to the presence of the sphincter of Oddi, bile does not enter the duodenum regularly; it is diverted into the gall bladder. Here, sodium is absorbed and the concentrated bile is made up of: (1) bile salts, (2) bile pigments, (3) cholesterol, and (4) lecithin-A (a phospholipid). The bile pigment is yellow in colour but is chemically altered in the intestine, resulting in the brown colour of normal faeces. Approximately 1000 ml of bile are secreted daily and are stored in the gall bladder until required for the digestion of a meal.

Motility of small intestine

The aim of the movement of the small intestine is to mix the food contents with digestive secretions, allow the digested end-products (of proteins, fat, carbohydrates) to come into contact with the mucosa so they may be absorbed and to move the residue towards the large intestine. The mixing movement is called segmentation, in which rings of intestinal wall contract, dividing the contents into segments. These rings of wall then relax and adjacent rings contract, breaking up the first segments.

In addition to segmentation, peristaltic waves are seen in the small intestine proceeding towards the large intestine. This movement is controlled by parasympathetic nerves (which increase the movement) and sympathetic nerves (which decrease it).

Absorption of water, electrolytes and vitamins

The average intake of water is 1200 ml/day and the average content of water in the faeces is 100 ml/day. A large quantity of water is absorbed in the small intestine. Sodium ions are absorbed actively, and chloride and bicarbonate ions may be actively absorbed or follow other ions passively. Water-soluble vitamins are rapidly absorbed in the small intestine. Fat-soluble vitamins are absorbed along with fats in the jejunum.

The large intestine absorbs water and electrolytes from chyme and stores the resultant faeces until the time is convenient for excretion. Active absorption of sodium is associated with the absorption of water. The potassium content of the faeces is higher than the plasma level. Peristaltic waves travel for a greater distance than in the small intestine, propelling the contents into the sigmoid colon.

Defaecation

The contents of the sigmoid colon reach the rectum by peristalsis and distend the rectal walls, which act as a stimulus for defaecation. If conditions are suitable, further peristalsis occurs in the sigmoid colon, the rectal walls contract and both the internal and external anal sphincters relax, resulting in the elimination of faeces through the anus. Defaecation is assisted by the inhalation of a deep breath, closure of glottis and an increase in the intra-abdominal pressure owing to the forced contraction of abdominal muscles.

METABOLISM AND NUTRITION

Consumed food provides energy for the maintenance of vital functions, growth and for physical activity. When the food is converted into energy and heat, oxygen is utilized and carbon dioxide produced.

Energy requirements

The basal metabolic rate (BMR) is the energy requirement under basal conditions. The basal conditions are that a person must be resting and not have had a meal for at least 12 hours. Energy is measured in megajoules (MJ) (Table 1.2). The BMR is increased in hyperthyroidism and decreased in old age, in hypothyroidism and in women.

Food is made up of carbohydrates, proteins, fats, vitamins, minerals and water.

Carbohydrates

The average intake by an adult is 300–450 g. Carbohydrates are present in food as monosaccharides (glucose, fructose and galactose), disaccharides (sucrose, lactose and maltose) and polysaccharides (starches).

Sources: Wheat, barley, maize, rice and potatoes.

Table 1.2 Energy expenditure in the average man and woman

	Man	Woman
Sedentary work	10.5 MJ	8.7 MJ
Light work	12.5 MJ	9.6 MJ
Moderate work	–	10.5 MJ
Heavy work	17–20 MJ	14–16 MJ

Digestion: Disaccharides and polysaccharides are converted into monosaccharides, as only the mono-saccharides are absorbed by the small intestine.

Absorption and fate: Glucose is the end-product of the digestion and absorption of all carbohydrates. Glucose passes freely in and out of cells. It is converted to glycogen by insulin and stored in the cells of the liver. Glycogen is converted back to glucose by the action of glucagon (a pancreatic hormone) and adrenaline.

Proteins

The average daily intake of proteins is between 40 and 60 g.

Sources: Milk, fish, meat, peas, lentils and eggs.

Proteins are necessary for the growth and replacement of damaged tissues. A protein is a complex molecule made up of simpler substances called amino acids. Some amino acids are called essential because they cannot be synthesized in the body and must be made available in the diet. These are phenylalanine, valine, histidine, iso-leucine, leucine, threonine, methionine, arginine, lysine and tryptophan. The 'non-essential' amino acids are just as important, but they can be synthesized in the body.

Digestion: Proteins in the food are acted upon by pepsin in gastric juice, chymotrypsin and trypsin in pancreatic juice. By the action of these enzymes, proteins are broken down into amino acids.

Absorption and fate: Amino acids are absorbed through the wall of the small intestine into the bloodstream. Excess amino acids are converted into proteins by the liver, some being broken down into urea and excreted by the kidneys.

Fat

The average daily intake is between 90 and 120 g.

Sources: Butter, margarine, cream, cheese and fatty meat.

Fats are made up of glycerol and fatty acids; lipid is a term used to describe fats and sterol.

Digestion: As the fats are not soluble in water, bile salts convert them into small droplets. Lipase (an enzyme in pancreatic juice) helps the bile salts in their action and breaks down some of the fatty

acids into free fatty acids, monoglycerides and diglycerides.

Absorption and fate: The small fat droplets pass into the lymph vessels of the small intestine and reach the bloodstream via the thoracic duct. Some fats pass into the capillaries of the small intestine and through the portal vein into the liver. Fat is stored or converted into energy. The fat that is not required for energy is deposited in the fat depots of the body (which lie within the abdomen and under the skin). When the need arises, fat is converted into glycerol and fatty acids in the liver. The glycerol is converted into glycogen and used. The fatty acids are oxidized into heat and energy, or into water and carbon dioxide.

VITAMINS

Vitamins are substances necessary in small amounts for the health of the body. They are:

- water-soluble: vitamin B complex and vitamin C;
- fat-soluble: vitamins A, D, E and K.

Vitamin B complex. The most important of the B complex vitamins are thiamin, riboflavin (B_2), pyridoxine (B_6) and B_{12} (cobalamines).

Lack of *thiamin* produces beriberi (peripheral neuropathy and cardiac failure). It is found in liver, kidney, eggs, pork and beans.

Lack of *niacin* (now occasionally called vitamin H) produces pellagra (diarrhoea, dermatitis and dementia). It is found in cereals, meat, liver, yeast and fish.

A deficiency of *riboflavin* produces degeneration of the cornea and mucous membrane of the mouth, and dermatitis. It is found in milk, cheese, green vegetables, liver and eggs.

Vitamin B_{12} (cyanocobalamin) is necessary for red blood cell formation, and its deficiency leads to pernicious anaemia. It is found in liver, kidney, meat, fish, eggs and milk, and is absorbed in the small intestine in the presence of intrinsic factor (which is a constituent of gastric juice).

Folic acid is necessary for the formation of red blood cells. It is found in liver, yeast and green vegetables.

Vitamin C (also called ascorbic acid) is necessary for the health of capillary walls and for prompt wound healing. Lack of it causes scurvy (leading to haemorrhage and anaemia). It is found in fresh fruit and vegetables, especially tomatoes, grapefruit and blackcurrants.

Vitamin A is necessary for healthy epithelium and visual purple, and for the growth and development of new bone. It is present in fish liver oils (such as halibut liver oil and cod liver oil), butter, milk, cream, liver and eggs. Carotenes, which are present in green vegetables and carrots, are converted into vitamin A in the body.

Vitamin D is necessary for bone formation. Its deficiency leads to rickets in children and osteo-malacia in adults. It is found in liver, cheese, eggs, butter and fish liver oils.

Vitamin K is necessary for the formation of the clotting factors II (prothrombin), VII, IX and X by the liver and thus for the clotting of blood. It is found in green vegetables (e.g. spinach) and meat.

MINERALS

The essential minerals are:

Sodium	Iodine
Calcium	Magnesium
Potassium	Cobalt
Iron	Zinc
Phosphorus	Copper

Sodium is an important constituent of cells and tissue fluids. It is found in common salt (sodium chloride), fruits and vegetables. The amount required by the body is less than 1 g daily; require-ments increase during sweating and diarrhoea.

Calcium is necessary for the ossification of bone and teeth, coagulation of the blood, cardiac contraction and the transmission of nerve impulses. It is found in most foods, especially milk, butter and cheese.

Potassium is important in cell membrane activity and muscle contraction. It is present in most foods, especially fresh orange juice.

Iron is the essential part of the haemoglobin molecule and thus is necessary for the formation of red blood cells. It is found in liver, beef and spinach.

BLOOD

ANATOMY

Blood is an important transport system within the body. In a man weighing 70 kg, the total amount of blood is approximately 5 L. Blood is composed of red blood cells (RBCs), white blood cells (WBCs), platelets and plasma.

Red blood cells

Also called red corpuscles or erythrocytes, red blood cells are biconcave discs with a diameter of 8.5 μm. They do not have a nucleus, and consist of an outer membrane, haemoglobin (an iron-containing protein) and carbonic anhydrase, an enzyme involved in the transport of carbon dioxide.

The normal range of values for the red cell count is:

Male	$4.5–6.5 \times 10^{12}/L$
Female	$3.9–5.8 \times 10^{12}/L$

Red blood cells live for a period of on average 120 days. At the end of this period, they are destroyed by the cells of the reticulo-endothelial system. Haemoglobin is broken down into haem, which contains the iron and is used in the manu-facture of new red cells, and porphyrin, which is broken down into bilirubin. This bilirubin is removed by the cells of the liver.

White blood cells

Also called leukocytes, the types of white cells are granulocytes (neutrophils, eosinophils and basophils), lymphocytes, and monocytes. The average values for the levels of these in the blood are given in the Appendix.

Granulocytes have small granules in their protoplasm. Based on the staining properties of these granules, the cells are divided into three groups:

1. neutrophils – granules that do not stain;
2. eosinophils – granules that stain red with acid dyes;
3. basophils – granules that stain blue with basic dyes.

Granulocytes are about 10–12 μm in diameter. As the cell matures, the nucleus divides into several lobes, hence the name polymorphonuclear leukocytes (polymorphs). These develop in bone marrow and are discharged into the circulation as and when required.

Lymphocytes have a large, round and slightly indented nucleus that occupies most of the cell. Varying in size from 7 to 15 μm, they develop in lymph tissue.

Monocytes are large cells, up to 20 μm in diameter, with an oval or kidney-shaped nucleus. They are formed in the bone marrow.

Platelets

These are round or oval, biconvex, non-nucleated discs numbering between 150 000 and 400 000/μl. They form a part of some large cells in the bone marrow and have a life of about 10 days.

Plasma

Plasma is the fluid part of the blood, forming 5% of body weight. It provides the medium in which the formed elements of blood (red blood cells, white blood cells and platelets) circulate; it also transports organic and inorganic substances from one organ or tissue to another. Plasma is made up of:

- water: 91–92%;
- plasma proteins: albumin, globulin, fibrinogen and prothrombin;
- inorganic compounds such as sodium, potassium, calcium, magnesium, iron and iodine;
- organic compounds such as urea, uric acid, creatinine, glucose, lipids, amino acids, enzymes and hormones.

The functions of plasma proteins are:

1. They maintain the oncotic pressure of plasma, which is necessary for the formation and absorption of tissue fluid.
2. Prothrombin and fibrinogen are necessary for the clotting of blood.
3. They act as buffers and maintain the normal pH of the body.
4. They transport immunoglobulins, which help in the defence of the body against infection.

Reticulo-endothelial system

This system consists of a number of cells of similar structure with common functions, situated in various organs. The reticulo-endothelial cells are present in spleen, liver, thymus, lymph nodes, bone marrow, blood and vessel walls. A common function of all reticulo-endothelial cells is the removal of particles of foreign matter and the destruction of ageing red cells.

PHYSIOLOGY

Red blood cells

Haemoglobin present in the red blood cells carries oxygen. The rate of production of red blood cells depends on the level of the oxygen supply to the kidney. If it is low, as seen in hypovolaemia, production is increased owing to the release of the hormone erythropoietin.

Blood pigments

Haemoglobin, the pigment found in red blood cells and the carrier of oxygen, has a molecular weight of 65 000. It is made up of four subunits, each consisting of a pigment part (haem) joined to a polypeptide part (globin). The haem part is an iron-containing porphyrin, which combines reversibly with oxygen. Owing to differences in amino acid composition, haemoglobin can be classified as adult haemoglobin, fetal haemoglobin and sickle-cell haemoglobin.

Formation and destruction of haemoglobin

Haemoglobin is formed by the developing red blood cells within the bone marrow; the substances essential for its formation are amino acids, iron, vitamin B_{12} and folic acid. When the red blood cell is broken down, the haemoglobin is split into haem and globin. The haem molecule is split open and the iron removed for recycling. The remaining pigment is called biliverdin, which in man is converted to bilirubin and then transported to the liver where it is made water soluble and excreted via the bile. In the gut, the bile pigments are converted to stercobilinogen, which colours the faeces.

White blood cells

These are the main agents in the body's defence against infection. This is carried out by either: (1) scavenging (phagocytosis), in which a foreign body is ingested and retained; or (2) production and distribution of antibodies – molecules which combine with foreign bodies to inactivate them.

The *granulocytes* are produced in the bone marrow and remain there in store. They enter the circulation for a few hours and are destroyed while performing body defence functions.

Neutrophils are active phagocytes and remain the body's first line of defence against bacterial invasion.

Eosinophils increase in number with parasitic infection.

Monocytes act as scavengers and help in the immune response.

Haemostasis (Fig. 1.18)

If a small blood vessel is cut, repair processes are activated which seal off the vessel. A number of factors are involved in this mechanism of clotting, which converts fibrinogen to fibrin in the blood and forms a clot at the site of the injury. The clotting factors are shown in Box 1.9. The series of events leading to clotting is:

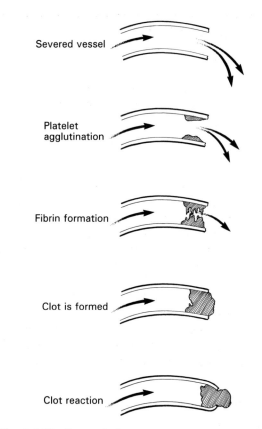

Severed vessel

Platelet agglutination

Fibrin formation

Clot is formed

Clot reaction

Figure 1.18   Haemostasis.

Box 1.9	Clotting factors
Factor	*Name*
I	Fibrinogen
II	Prothrombin
III	Thromboplastin
IV	Calcium
V	Proaccelerin
VI	–
VII	Proconvertin, stable factor
VIII	Antihaemophilic factor
IX	Christmas factor
X	Stuart–Prower factor
XI	Plasma thromboplastin antecedent
XII	Hageman factor
XIII	Fibrin stabilizing factor

1. constriction of the blood vessel to narrow the lumen;
2. formation of a plug of platelets;
3. conversion of this plug into a clot of fibrin.

URINARY SYSTEM

ANATOMY

The urinary system is made up of the right and left kidneys, the right and left ureters, the bladder and the urethra.

Kidneys

Each kidney, about 12 cm long, 7 cm wide and 2.5 cm thick, lies at the back of the abdomen in the gutter that runs alongside the vertebral bodies. The right kidney lies slightly lower than the left owing to the presence of the liver on the right side. An adrenal gland sits on top of each kidney.

The renal artery and vein, lymphatics, nerves and upper end of the ureter join the kidney at the hilum. Each kidney is supplied by a renal artery, which arises from the aorta. Venous drainage is by the renal vein into the inferior vena cava.

Structure of the kidney

The kidney is made up of:

- a fibrous capsule on the outside;
- a cortex, made up of glomeruli;
- a medulla, composed of a number of conical renal papillae that project into the pelvis.

Each kidney is made up of approximately one million nephrons, the functional units of the kidney. Each nephron comprises a renal tubule and a glomerulus (Fig. 1.19).

The renal tubule is a long, bent tube lined by a single layer of cuboidal cells. It begins at Bowman's capsule, which encloses the glomerulus, and then twists on itself to form the proximal convoluted tubule. The proximal convoluted tubule runs from the cortex to the medulla and back again, forming the loop of Henle. The loop of Henle leads into the distal convoluted tubule, which then ends as the collecting tubule. Each collecting tubule joins other tubules in the medulla of the kidney and opens on the surface of a renal papilla within the pelvis of the ureter.

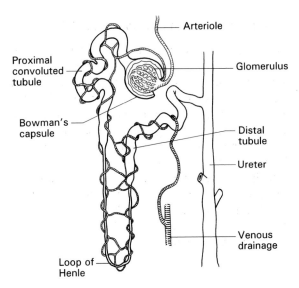

Figure 1.19   The nephron.

Blood supply. The glomerulus is a whorl of capillaries enclosed within the Bowman's capsule, receiving blood via an afferent arteriole. An efferent vessel passes from the glomerulus to the renal tubules and divides into capillaries on its surface. The capillaries drain into a vein, which joins other vein branches to form the renal vein.

Ureter

The ureter is a tube that connects the kidney to the bladder. It is about 25 cm long, starting as a dilated region (called the pelvis), which is attached to the hilum of the kidney. The ureter runs down behind the peritoneum in the posterior abdominal wall. In the pelvis, it turns forwards and inwards to enter the urinary bladder.

Urinary bladder

This is a muscular sac into which the ureters empty the urine. The relationship of the bladder to other organs is as follows:

- In front of the bladder lies the pubic symphysis.
- In the female, the uterus and vagina lie behind the bladder.
- In the male, the vas deferens, seminal vesicle and rectum lie behind the bladder.

- At the sides lie the pelvic fascia and ligaments and the levator ani muscles.
- Above the bladder lie the coils of the small intestine.
- In the female, the anterior vaginal wall lies below the bladder.
- In the male, the prostate gland lies below the

The ureters enter the bladder posteriorly, and the urethra leaves the bladder anteriorly.

From the outside in, the bladder consists of: (1) peritoneum or pelvic fascia on the outside; (2) a muscular coat, which forms the bladder wall; (3) a submucous coat; and (4) a mucous membrane, which is folded when the bladder is empty.

Female urethra

This is a small tube about 3 cm long, which extends from the bladder to an opening between the labia minora about 2 cm behind the clitoris. It runs in front of the vagina.

Male urethra

The male urethra is a tube about 20 cm long, which extends from the bladder to the end of the penis. It is made up of three parts: (1) the prostatic urethra, which passes through the prostate gland; (2) the membranous urethra, which is enclosed by a sphincter of muscle fibres; and (3) the spongy urethra, which is 15 cm long and passes through the corpus spongiosum of the penis to end near the tip.

PHYSIOLOGY
Formation of urine

The kidneys are the main excretory organs of the body. They receive about 25% of the cardiac output. The glomerulus and the tubules play an active part in the formation of urine.

Glomerular function

The initial stage in the formation of urine is the filtration of almost protein-free plasma through the glomerular capillaries into the Bowman's capsule. During urine's passage through the tubular system, its composition is altered by selective reabsorption of certain substances and selective secretion of others. In a healthy adult, about 120 ml urine/min are filtered out, i.e. approximately 170 L in 24 hours.

Tubular secretion

As the filtrate passes along the tubule and collecting duct, its composition is altered by exchanges between it and the blood in the capillaries. The substances that are reabsorbed into the blood are:

Sodium (90%)
Chloride (90%)
Glucose (100%)
Water (90%)
Amino acids, calcium and bicarbonate.

The substances that pass out of the blood into the filtrate to maintain a constant pH are ammonium salts, hydrogen ions, phosphates and potassium.

Antidiuretic hormone (ADH), which is secreted by the hypothalamus and stored in the posterior lobe of the pituitary gland, controls the reabsorption of water in the collecting duct. Of the 23 L of fluid that pass into the ducts, about 21.5–22.0 L are reabsorbed, 1.0–1.5 L being excreted as urine in 24 hours.

Excretion of end-products and drugs

End-products of protein metabolism, such as urea, uric acid and creatinine, are excreted in the urine. A number of drugs are excreted mainly through the kidneys. The constituents of urine are displayed in Box 1.10.

Physiology of micturition

Micturition is a reflex action controlled by higher centres in the nervous system. When the urine enters the bladder, it stretches the muscle fibres of the bladder wall. The afferent nerves in the bladder wall send impulses to the lumbar part

---

Box 1.10   Constituents of urine

Amount: 900–1500 ml/24 h
Specific gravity: 1002–1030
pH: Acid, pH 6.0
Uric acid: 0.6 g/per litre
Urea: 20–30 g/per litre
Water
Creatinine: 1–2 g/per litre
Ammonia, potassium, sodium, chloride, phosphates
and sulphates

---

of the spinal cord. From the spinal cord, the impulses are transmitted to the cerebral cortex, producing a desire to micturate.

The efferent nerves pass along the sacral parasympathetic nerves to the bladder, causing the muscle of the bladder wall to contract and the bladder sphincter to relax. The urine is expelled, assisted by the contraction of the muscles of the abdominal wall and the diaphragm, which collapse the bladder by raising the intra-abdominal pressure.

LYMPHATIC SYSTEM

ANATOMY

The lymphatic system is made up of lymph capillaries, lymph vessels and lymph nodes.

Lymph capillaries. These are thin-walled, blind-ended tubes that lie in the tissue spaces of various organs and tissues.

Lymph vessels. These are larger tubes, formed by the joining of lymph capillaries. They contain a number of valves, which give them a beaded appearance. Superficial lymph vessels drain the skin, whilst the deeper lymph vessels drain the deeper organs in the body. Lymph vessels drain into lymph nodes.

Lymph nodes. These are round or oval masses of lymph cells enclosed in a capsule. Lymph vessels enter or leave the glands, connecting one node to another.

Certain structures in the body, such as the tonsils, nasopharyngeal adenoids, thymus gland and Peyer's patches in the small intestine, are made up of lymph tissue.

Lymph is the fluid in the lymph vessels. It has a similar composition to blood plasma and contains lymphocytes.

Cisterna chyli and thoracic duct. The cisterna chyli is a large sac that lies in the upper part of the abdomen, behind the aorta and in front of the bodies of the upper two lumbar vertebrae. Lymph from the abdominal organs and legs passes to the cisterna chyli via the aortic glands. The thoracic duct, which is continuous with the cisterna chyli, passes into the thorax via the diaphragm and ends in the junction of the left subclavian vein and left internal jugular vein. It receives lymph vessels from the left arm, the left side of the head and neck, and the chest.

Box 1.11 outlines the drainage of lymph in the body.

Box 1.11   Lymph drainage

Organ	Drainage site
Head and neck	Nodes in the neck
Breast	Nodes in the axilla, neck and chest
Lungs	Nodes in the hilum of the lung, at the bifurcation of the trachea
Stomach	Nodes around the greater and lesser curvature of the stomach and at the lower end of the oesophagus
Small intestine	Nodes in front of the aorta, mesenteric nodes
Large intestine	Mesenteric nodes
Pelvic organs	Nodes in front of the lower end of the aorta
Genitalia	Nodes in the groin
Legs	Nodes in the popliteal fossa, in the groin and in front of the lower end of the aorta

---

PHYSIOLOGY

The functions of the lymphatic system are:

- Drainage of tissue spaces: fluids that pass out of the capillaries are removed by the lymphatics.

- Production of antibodies: the lymph nodes are sites of antibody production.
- Production of lymphocytes: lymphocytes that are produced in the lymph nodes reach the blood via the lymphatic system.
- Absorption of fat: approximately 60–70% of the fat absorbed from the small intestine enters the blood via the cisterna chyli and thoracic duct.

ENDOCRINE SYSTEM

The anatomy and physiology of the endocrine glands will be described simultaneously.

The endocrine system is made up of glands that secrete substances called hormones directly into the bloodstream. Some of the important endocrine glands are the pituitary, thyroid and parathyroids, adrenals, pancreas and pineal gland.

PITUITARY GLAND (Fig. 1.20)

The pituitary gland lies in a deep depression called the pituitary fossa in the upper surface of the body of the sphenoid bone in the skull. The stalk of the pituitary gland connects the hypothalamus with the gland. The gland is made up of two lobes, anterior and posterior.

Anterior lobe

This consists of three types of cell: (1) basophils, which stain blue; (2) acidophils, which stain red; and (3) chromophobes, which stain poorly.

The anterior lobe's activities are controlled by hormones secreted by the hypothalamus. The important hormones produced by the anterior pituitary are:

1. Growth hormone (GH), which is essential for growth and the storage of nitrogen.
2. Adrenocorticotrophic hormone (ACTH), which stimulates the cortex of the adrenal glands to produce glucocorticoids.
3. Thyroid-stimulating hormone (TSH), which stimulates the thyroid gland to produce triiodothyronine and thyroxine.

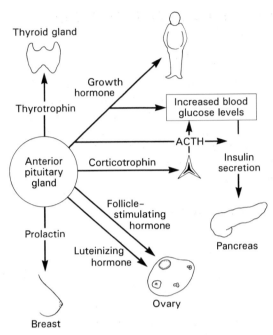

Figure 1.20 The pituitary gland and its relationship to other glands.

4. Gonadotrophic hormones such as interstitial cell-stimulating hormone (ICSH), which in men stimulates cells in the testes to produce androgens, follicle-stimulating hormone (FSH), which ripens the ovarian follicles in women, and luteinizing hormone (LH), which completes the ripening of the follicles and stimulates the development of the corpus luteum.

Posterior lobe

The hormones secreted by the posterior lobe of the pituitary gland are produced in the hypothalamus and pass down the nerve fibres to the posterior lobe. The important hormones are:

1. Oxytocin, which is involved in controlling uterine action during the birth of a baby and in contraction of the muscle of the ducts of the breast, causing the milk to be squeezed from the deeper to the superficial ducts.
2. Antidiuretic hormone, which stimulates the distal tubules of the kidney to reabsorb water from the fluid they contain.

THYROID AND PARATHYROID GLANDS

Thyroid gland

The thyroid gland is situated in the neck and consists of right and left lobes connected by a narrow isthmus. It secretes the iodine-containing hormones triiodothyronine and thyroxine, which are essential for oxidative processes in metabolism. Whenever the blood levels of thyroxine fall, its production is stimulated by the thyroid-stimulating hormone (TSH) of the anterior pituitary gland (Fig. 1.20).

Parathyroid glands

Four in number, the parathyroid glands lie behind the thyroid. They are made up of clumps of cells, separated by connective tissue with sinusoids for blood running around the cells.

The parathyroid glands secrete parathyroid hormone, which raises the amount of calcium in the blood plasma by:

- increasing the reabsorption of calcium by the tubules of the kidney;
- transferring calcium from bone to plasma;
- promoting the absorption of calcium by the intestines.

ADRENAL GLANDS

These glands lie at the back of the abdomen immediately above the kidneys. Each gland consists of a yellow cortex and an inner reddish-grey medulla.

Adrenal cortex

This has three zones of cells: an outer zone made up of cells in clusters, a middle one of cells in columns, and an inner layer of irregular columns. The adrenal cortex produces three types of hormone:

1. *Glucocorticoids*. Their secretion is regulated by ACTH from the pituitary gland. Cortisol (hydrocortisone), the most important hormone, breaks down tissue proteins which are converted in the liver into glycogen; it causes deposition of glycogen in the liver and raises the blood sugar level; it also controls the exchange of electrolytes and water between extracellular spaces and cells.

2. *Mineralocorticoids*. Aldosterone, an important hormone, controls the sodium balance in the body by acting on the tubules of the kidneys. It causes the retention of sodium and the excretion of potassium. Its secretion is regulated by the production of renin by the kidney, and by the level of plasma potassium.

3. *Androgens*. These are responsible for the development of secondary male sexual characteristics, such as the growth of hair on the face and deepening of the voice.

Adrenal medulla

The adrenal medulla, formed from the same tissues as the nervous tissue, is made up of irregular cells surrounded by blood sinuses and innervated by sympathetic nerves.

The adrenal medulla produces adrenaline and noradrenaline. These hormones are secreted in response to stress, allowing the body to adapt to a dangerous situation. The actions of noradrenaline and adrenaline are summarized in Table 1.3.

PANCREAS

The hormone-secreting groups of cells lying within the pancreas are called the islets of Langerhans. They contain two cell types: alpha cells, which produce glucagon, and beta cells, which produce insulin.

Glucagon

The chief function of this hormone is to convert glycogen in the liver into glucose. The production of glucagon is stimulated by a fall in the blood sugar, which could be due to either severe exercise or fasting.

Insulin

The function of insulin is to stimulate the transfer of glucose across cell walls and to facilitate the

Table 1.3 Action of noradrenaline and adrenaline

Organ	Noradrenaline	Adrenaline
Metabolism	Very little action	Increases oxygen consumption, raises blood sugar, converts glycogen to glucose
Heart	Initially, rate increased then decreased Very little action on cardiac output	Cardiac rate and output increased
Coronary arteries	Constricted	Dilated
Blood vessels in skin in voluntary muscle	Constricted Constricted	Constricted Dilated
Blood pressure	Increased	Increased initially, then decreased owing to dilatation of blood vessels in muscle
Involuntary muscles	Sphincters contracted. In the gut, tone and peristalsis decreased	Sphincters contracted. In the gut, tone and peristalsis decreased. Bronchi dilated

utilization of glucose by the cells. The production of insulin is stimulated by a rise in the blood sugar, which occurs after a meal containing carbohydrates. Normal blood sugar levels lie between 4.5 and 8.5 mmol/L. Factors that increase the blood sugar are adrenaline, cortisol, growth hormone and glucagon.

Insulin is the only hormone which lowers the blood sugar.

PINEAL GLAND

This a small oval structure, composed of epithelial cells, which lies near the midbrain. The pineal gland produces melatonin.

KIDNEY

In addition to controlling acid–base and water balance, the kidneys produce erythropoietin and renin.

- Erythropoietin is produced in response to hypoxia. It stimulates the formation of red blood cells in the bone marrow.
- Renin is produced by juxtaglomerular cells in the walls of the arterioles through which blood passes into the glomeruli. It is secreted in response to a fall in blood pressure, thus raising the pressure.

REPRODUCTIVE SYSTEM

ANATOMY

Female genital system (Fig. 1.21)

This consists of the right and left ovaries, the right and left fallopian tubes, the uterus, the vagina and the external genitalia.

Ovary

There are two ovaries, each being attached to the lateral wall of the pelvis by the broad ligament, a double fold of peritoneum. The fallopian tube arches over the ovary and ends on it.

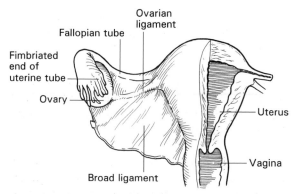

Figure 1.21 The female genital system: uterus, fallopian tube and ovary.

Fallopian tubes

These are two in number: right and left. Each tube is approximately 20 cm long, extending from the lateral angle of the uterus to the ovary. At the ovarian end, the tube opens by a small hole into the peritoneal cavity.

Uterus

This is a muscular, pear-shaped, thick-walled organ. It lies in the pelvis between the rectum behind, and the bladder in front. It consists of the fundus, which has a rounded upper end, and the body, which forms about two-thirds of the organ and is continuous with the cervix at an angle, so that the whole uterus bends forwards (anteversion). The uterus is hollow.

Cervix. The cervix is cylindrical in shape in its lower third and ends in the vagina. It has a cervical canal between the internal os (where the body of the uterus opens into the cervix) and the external os (where the cervix opens into the vagina).

Peritoneal attachments. The round ligament is a narrow, fibrous band that runs from the side of the uterus, through the broad ligament and down the inguinal canal to end in the labium majora.

The broad ligament runs on each side of the uterus to the lateral wall of the pelvis. The uterine blood vessels, nerves and lymph vessels run within this ligament.

The rectouterine pouch of Douglas is formed by the peritoneum between the rectum and the uterus.

Blood supply. The uterus is supplied by a uterine artery on each side, which is a branch of the internal iliac artery. Venous drainage is into the internal iliac vein.

Lymphatic drainage. From the fundus of the uterus, the lymph vessels drain into inguinal lymph nodes; from the cervix, they drain into the external iliac and internal iliac nodes.

Structure of the uterus. The uterus is made up of three layers: endometrium, which is the inner layer and is made up of columnar epithelial cells and glands (these undergo changes at various stages of the menstrual cycle); myometrium, which is the middle layer and is made up of smooth muscle fibres; and peritoneum, which covers the uterus externally.

Vagina

This is a tube-like structure that extends from the uterine cervix to the vulva, the cervix extending into the upper part of the vagina. The hymen is a thin, mucosal fold at the external opening of the vagina.

From inside out, the layers of the vagina are:

- mucosal membrane, made up of squamous epithelium;
- the muscular coat made up of smooth muscle;
- fibrous tissue.

The vagina is continuously kept moist by secretions from the cervix and transudate from the vaginal wall.

Vulva

This is the female external genitalia. It is made up of the following:

1. *Labia majora*: two layers of hair-bearing folds that begin at the mons pubis (the pad of fat in front of the pubic symphysis) and extend to the perineum in the midline behind.
2. *Labia minora*: two thin lips of skin that lie within the labia majora, enclosing the clitoris in front.
3. *Clitoris*: a small organ equivalent to the penis in the male.
4. *Vestibule*: the area enclosed by labia minora, containing the opening of the urethra and the opening of the vagina.
5. *Bartholin's glands*: a pair of oval, mucus-secreting glands that lie deep to the posterior parts of the labia majora; they open via a duct at the side of the labia minora.

Male genital system

This consists of the testes, epididymis and other ducts, prostate gland and penis.

Testes (Fig. 1.22)

The testes (singular testis) are oval bodies, each of which is suspended by the spermatic cord in its half of the scrotum. The tunica albuginea is the fibrous capsule of the testis, and the tunica vaginalis is a double-layered covering that encloses the testis.

Structure. Each testis is divided by septa (partitions) into 150–300 lobules, each lobule being made up of 1–3 seminiferous tubules. Spermatozoa are produced by the cells of these tubules. The seminiferous tubules open as efferent ducts at the back of the testis. Male hormone (testosterone) is produced by the interstitial cells.

Blood supply to the testes. Each testicular artery, which supplies the testis, arises from the abdominal aorta just below the renal arteries.

Venous blood draining from the testes is collected by the pampiniform plexus of veins in the spermatic cord. This plexus drains into the testicular vein. The right testicular vein drains into inferior vena cava and the left testicular vein into the left renal vein.

Lymph drainage. Lymphatic vessels from the testes drain into aortic lymph nodes.

Nerve supply. The testes are innervated by sympathetic nerves.

Epididymis and other ducts

The epididymis consists of a series of tubes through which the spermatozoa pass. The vas deferens is a thick-walled tube, beginning at the lower end of the epididymis, passing through the inguinal canal and opening at the back of the urinary bladder. The seminal vesicle is a vessel formed of coiled, sacculated tubes; one lies on each side at the back of the bladder. The ejaculatory duct is a common duct for the vas deferens and the seminal vesicle. It runs through the prostate gland to open into the prostatic part of the urethra.

Prostate gland

This is about the size and shape of a horse chestnut. It lies behind the symphysis pubis, below the bladder and in front of the rectum. The prostate gland surrounds the first part of the urethra, the ejaculatory ducts passing through it.

This gland is made up of a number of tubular glands and fibromuscular tissue, and is enclosed in a capsule.

Penis

This is made up of three cylindrical bodies: the right and left corpora cavernosa and a central corpus spongiosum. It is attached posteriorly to the perineum and the sides of the pubic bone. The glans is the tissue into which the corpus spongiosum is enlarged at the end of the penis; it is enclosed in the prepuce (or foreskin). The urethra enters the corpus spongiosum posteriorly and opens anteriorly at the external urethral opening on the tip of the glans penis. The corpora

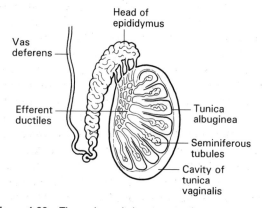

Figure 1.22   The male genital system: testis.

cavernosa and corpus spongiosum are made up of sponge-like tissue, formed by connective tissue and smooth muscle. This tissue encloses vascular spaces that engorge when stimulated by parasympathetic nerves.

PHYSIOLOGY

Menstruation

This begins at puberty around the age of 11–13 years and occurs at regular intervals of about 28 days until the menopause sets in at the age of 45–50 years. The menstrual cycle is controlled by FSH and LH (see p. 34). It is divided into three phases:

1. *Preovular (proliferative) phase.* This lasts for 14 days. Oestrogen is secreted by the ovarian follicle under the influence of FSH, and the endometrium grows thicker.
2. *Postovular (secretory) phase.* This phase lasts for 13 days. Progesterone, and to a certain extent oestrogen, is produced by the corpus luteum in the ovary. (If the ovum is not fertilized, the corpus luteum shrinks, and from the 22nd day the progesterone secretion starts to fall.) The endometrium becomes vascular and the glands are distended.
3. *Menstrual phase.* This lasts for 4–5 days. As the progesterone level falls, the endometrium degenerates and the unsupported capillaries break down, causing bleeding.

Penile erection and ejaculation

Spermatozoa are formed in the seminiferous tubules and pass along the vas deferens. During sexual excitement, impulses pass along the parasympathetic nerves to the arterioles of the penis. The arterioles dilate, and the vascular spaces of the penis become swollen with blood, leading to the stiffening and erection of the penis. During ejaculation, the semen produced by the seminal vesicles and prostate gland is discharged through the urethra.

Pregnancy

During the secretory phase in the female, fertilization takes place if the ovum (egg) combines with a sperm. After a short delay, the fertilized egg starts dividing until it forms a fluid-filled cavity called the blastocele. A single layer of cells, the trophoblast, forms around the blastocele. After implantation in the uterus, the trophoblast cells form the placenta and membranes. At one end of the blastocele, there is an accumulation of cells (the inner cell mass), which later forms the actual fetus.

The duration of pregnancy in humans averages 270 days from fertilization or 284 days from the first day of the menstrual period before conception.

The enlarged corpus luteum of pregnancy secretes oestrogen and progesterone, and after 8 weeks the placenta produces these hormones. At term, once labour begins, stimuli from the genital tract cause reflex secretion of the hormone oxytocin. This stimulates uterine contraction, which in turn dilates the cervix. The fetus descends and is expelled owing to a combination of factors such as muscular action and action pushing by the mother, the action of oxytocin and autonomic reflexes.

Lactation

Milk is formed by the cells of a glandular epithelium. Lactation occurs in two phases: milk secretion and milk expulsion. The secretion of milk is controlled by the hormones prolactin and ACTH. Milk expulsion is the transfer of milk from the alveoli to the nipple. Sensory receptors in the nipple, stimulated by the suckling infant, send impulses up the spinal cord to the hypothalamus, where they cause the release of oxytocin (see p. 34). This hormone, in addition to causing uterine contraction, contracts the smooth muscle cells of the ducts around the alveoli of the breast, which forces the milk from the alveoli to reach the nipple.

SKIN

ANATOMY

The skin is one of the largest components of the body and forms 15% of the total body weight. It is made up of epidermis and dermis.

The epidermis, the outer layer, is made up of stratified squamous epithelium, the upper layers of which contain keratin. Pigmentation of the skin is due to a black pigment, melanin, which is present in the deeper layers of the skin.

The dermis is made up of collagen and fibrous and elastic tissue. Its superficial layer projects into the epidermis as a number of small papillae. The deeper layers contain blood vessels, lymphatics and nerves.

Nerve supply. The skin is supplied with sensory and sympathetic nerves. Sensory nerve fibres in the skin that carry impulses to the brain include:

- free nerve endings;
- Meissner corpuscles around nerve endings in the papillae;
- Pacinian corpuscles found deep in the dermis.

Sympathetic nerve fibres supply the sweat glands and erector pili muscles.

Sebaceous glands are present everywhere in the skin except on palms and soles. A sebaceous gland is situated between a hair follicle and the erector pili muscle. It opens by a duct into the upper part of the follicle. Sebum is the name given to a collection of degenerated cells; it protects and lubricates the hair and skin.

Sweat glands. A sweat gland is a coiled tube found in the subcutaneous tissue with a long duct that opens on the surface of the skin. There are three types of sweat gland: (1) ordinary sweat glands, which are innervated by sympathetic nerves; (2) apocrine glands, which are present in the axillae, nipples and vulva; they have no nerve supply and a yellowish secretion is produced following stimulation by adrenaline; (3) ceruminous glands, which are present in the external auditory meatus and produce wax.

Hair. A hair is an outgrowth from a papilla at the bottom of a hair follicle (a narrow tube that runs from the surface of the skin to the dermis).

The erector pili muscle is a bundle of smooth muscle fibres attached at one end to the dermis and at the other end to a hair follicle. This muscle is supplied by sympathetic nerves. Contraction of erector pili muscles causes goose bumps.

Nails are specialized pieces of epidermis. A nail consists of nail bed and matrix.

PHYSIOLOGY
Functions of the skin

1. *Protection*. The skin protects the internal organs of the body against invasion by bacteria, trauma and water loss.
2. *Sensation*. Sensations such as pain, touch, pressure and temperature changes are picked up by the receptors in the skin and transmitted through the sensory nerves to the spinal cord and brain.
3. *Secretion*. This is of sweat (to aid temperature control) and in lactation, the breasts being modified sweat glands.
4. *Absorption*. The skin absorbs ultraviolet light and certain drugs.
5. *Storage*. The subcutaneous tissue acts as a store for fat and water.

Regulation of body temperature
(Fig. 1.23)

While discussing the body temperature, skin, subcutaneous tissue and muscles are described as the peripheral shell, and the content of skull, chest and abdomen as the inner core. The temperature of the inner core is maintained at a fairly constant level by heat loss and heat gain, whereas the peripheral temperature may vary.

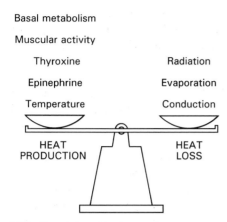

Basal metabolism

Muscular activity

Thyroxine   Radiation

Epinephrine   Evaporation

Temperature   Conduction

HEAT PRODUCTION   HEAT LOSS

Figure 1.23   Regulation of body temperature.

Heat loss occurs from the skin, expired air and faeces and urine. Heat loss occurs from the skin by conduction, convection, radiation and insensible loss. Water and heat loss by evaporation occurs through sweating. Sweat is secreted by sweat glands, which are present all over the skin. It contains sodium chloride, urea and lactic acid, and is secreted under the control of the hypothalamus and cerebral cortex. Sweating is increased by emotional state, exercise, a rise in body temperature and a fall in blood sugar. In hot weather, 1.5–2.0 L of sweat can be lost in one day.

Heat gain occurs by its production in the body and by uptake from the surrounding environment.

Heat production is due to metabolic activity in the body. The amount of heat produced by skeletal muscle varies from minimal at rest to maximal during exercise. The internal organs such as the heart and liver produce heat at a constant rate. The body absorbs heat from: (1) hot food, drinks and baths; (2) hot air in hot weather; and (3) direct radiation from the sun.

Normal body temperature. The body temperature is maintained between 36°C and 37°C (97°F and 99.5°F). In every individual, the temperature is low during the morning and high during the evening. In women, the temperature during the first half of the menstrual cycle is lower than that in the second half, rising by about 0.5°F during ovulation.

Temperature control. Body temperature is regulated by a combination of behavioural and physiological responses. In man, the behavioural responses are important. Thus if a person is hot, he moves to a cooler place and removes clothing. More blood circulates through the skin and he sweats. If a person is cold, he moves to a warmer place, puts on more clothes, blood circulation to the skin decreases and he shivers.

The hypothalamus in the brain senses the temperature of the blood perfusing the capillaries. It contains two centres for heat regulation. One responds to a fall in temperature by causing vasoconstriction and further production of heat, i.e. shivering. The other centre responds to a rise in temperature by causing vasodilatation, thus promoting heat loss. The physiological responses in man are controlled by the endocrine glands.

- Thyroid gland. Cold increases the production of thyroxine, which in turn increases heat production.
- Adrenal medulla. Cold increases the production of adrenaline, which increases heat production.

SKULL AND LOCOMOTOR SYSTEM

Skull

The skull is formed by the union of several bones, held together at the sutures. It protects the brain, eyes and ears, and provides attachment for the muscles acting on the head and teeth. The bones in the skull are listed in Box 1.12.

Some of the important sutures are the sagittal, which separates the two parietal bones; the coronal, which separates the frontal bone from the parietal bone; and the lambdoid, which separates the two parietal bones from the occipital bone.

Box 1.12 Bones of the skull	
Frontal	Zygoma (left and right)
Occipital	Mandible
Parietal (left and right)	Palatine (left and right)
Temporal (left and right)	Lacrimal (left and right)
Sphenoid	Nasal (left and right)
Ethmoid	Vomer
Maxilla	Conchae (left and right)

When the skull is viewed from within, it shows anterior, middle and posterior cranial fossae. The anterior cranial fossa is made up of the sphenoid and temporal bones. The middle cranial fossa is made up of the frontal, ethmoid and sphenoid bones, and the posterior cranial fossa is made up of the temporal and occipital bones.

Vertebral column and thoracic cage

The vertebral column is an important structure in the body since it carries the skull, thoracic cage and upper limbs. It protects the spinal cord and transmits the weight of the body to the lower limbs.

The vertebral column is made up of the following bones:

- cervical vertebrae (7)
- thoracic vertebrae (12)
- lumbar vertebrae (5)
- sacrum
- coccyx.

A typical vertebra shows a body, a vertebral arch, a vertebral foramen, an intervertebral foramen, a superior and inferior articular surface, a transverse process, a spine and an intervertebral disc.

A number of ligaments connect the vertebrae, both anteriorly and posteriorly.

The vertebral column in an adult shows a curve forwards in the cervical region; a curve backwards in the thoracic region; a curve forwards in the lumbar region; and a curve backwards above and forwards below in the sacral and coccygeal regions.

The vertebral column can be flexed, extended, moved laterally and rotated by movement between the adjacent vertebrae and alterations in the intervertebral discs.

Thoracic cage. The thoracic cage is made up of the sternum, ribs and costal cartilage, and the thoracic part of the vertebral column.

The sternum is a flat bone lying subcutaneously in the midline of the front of the chest. It is made up of the manubrium, the body and the xiphoid process.

There are 12 pairs of ribs that encircle the wall of the chest. They articulate behind with the vertebral column and in front with the sternum. Ribs 11 and 12 do not articulate with the sternum and are sometimes called floating ribs. Each rib has a head, neck, a tubercle and a shaft. The space between two ribs occupied by the external and internal intercostal muscles.

The thoracic cavity increases in size during inspiration and decreases during expiration. During inspiration, the muscles of the diaphragm contract along with the external intercostal muscles, thus increasing the length and width of the thoracic cavity. During expiration, the thoracic cavity returns to its normal size owing to elastic recoil.

Bones in the upper limb (Fig. 1.24)

The upper limb is made up of the scapula (shoulder blade), clavicle (collar bone), humerus, radius, ulna, carpal bones, metacarpals and phalanges.

The scapula is a triangular bone which forms part of the shoulder girdle. It is attached to the head, trunk and arm by a number of muscles. The scapula has an acromion, coracoid process and a glenoid fossa. The glenoid fossa lies at the upper

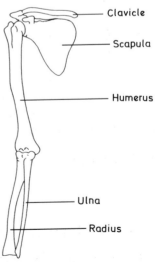

Clavicle

Scapula

Humerus

Ulna

Radius

Figure 1.24   Bones of the upper limb (excluding phalanges).

and outer border of the scapula and articulates with the head of the humerus to form the shoulder joint.

The clavicle is an S-shaped bone attached medially to the manubrium of the sternum and laterally to the acromion process of the scapula.

The humerus, a long bone, is made up of a head, a shaft and a lower end. The shaft has a number of muscles attached to it, including the deltoid muscle. The lower end has a lateral and medial epicondyle, along with the trochlea and capitulum.

Radius and ulna. The radius bone lies on the outer side of the forearm and has a head at the upper end which articulates with the capitulum of the humerus; a neck; a tuberosity to which the tendon of biceps muscle is attached; a shaft, to which various flexor and extensor muscles are attached; and a lower end with a styloid process and articular surface for the wrist bones.

The ulna is a long bone which lies on the inner side of the forearm and consists of an olecranon and coronoid process with an articular surface for the lower end of the humerus. At the lower end it has a styloid process and an articular surface for the lower end of the radius.

Carpal (wrist) bones. The wrist consists of eight bones arranged in two rows: proximal row – caphoid, lunate, triquetrium, pisiform; distal row – trapezium, trapezoid, capitate and hamate.

Metacarpals. There are five metacarpal bones in the hand and they have a base which articulates with the carpal bones, a shaft and a head. The head articulates with the phlanges.

Phalanges. The thumb has two phalanges and each finger three.

Bones in the lower limb (Fig. 1.25)

The lower limb is made up of the bones listed in Box 1.13.

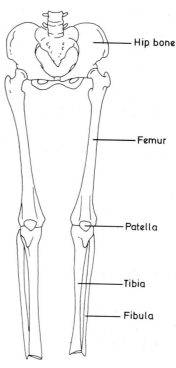

Figure 1.25   Bones of the lower limb (excluding metatarsals).

Box 1.13	Bones of the lower limb

Hip bone (innominate), which forms part of the pelvis
Femur
Patella
Tibia
Fibula
Tarsal bones
Metatarsal bones } form the foot
Phalanges

The pelvis is formed by the hip bone in front and at the sides, and by the sacrum and coccyx behind. It is divided into the false pelvis and the true pelvis by the line joining the two iliac bones.

The hip bone is an irregularly shaped, strong bone that articulates with a similar bone on the opposite side and the sacrum and coccyx behind. It consists of three bones: the ilium (plural ilia), ischium and pubis.

The femur consists of an upper end, a shaft and a lower end. The upper end has a head, which is connected to the acetabulum of the hip bone (forming the hip joint), a neck and a greater trochanter and lesser trochanter, to which the muscles are attached. The shaft is a long, smooth bone to which muscles connect. The lower end has large medial and lateral condyles to which the tibial bone and the patella are attached.

Patella. The patella, or knee cap, is a triangular sesamoid bone (a sesamoid bone being a bone formed in the tendon of a muscle) situated in the tendon of the quadriceps muscle of the thigh. It glides over the articular surface on the front of the lower end of the femur.

The tibia and fibula are the two bones of the leg below the knee. The tibia lies on the medial side and transmits the weight of the body. It has an upper end, a shaft and a lower end. The upper end is wide and consists of medial and lateral condyles. The upper end of the fibula is attached to the articular surface on the lateral condyle. The shaft is thick and its anterior border forms the prominent palpable shin. The lower end has a medial malleolus and an articular surface for the lower end of the fibula and the talus.

The fibula is a long, slim bone which lies on the lateral aspect of the leg. It has an upper end, a shaft and a lower end. The upper end articulates with the lateral condyles of the tibia, and the lower end articulates with the lower end of the tibia and talus.

Foot. The bones of the foot are: talus, calcaneum, navicular, cuboid and three cuneiform bones.

Metatarsals. There are five metatarsals, one for each toe. Each one has a base, a shaft and a head. The 1st, 2nd and 3rd metatarsals articulate with the cuneiform bones, while the 4th and 5th articulate with the cuboid bone.

Phalanges. The big toe has two phalanges while the rest have three. Each phalanx has a shaft and two ends.

JOINTS

There are three types of joints, based on their structure: fibrous, synovial, and cartilaginous.

1. *Fibrous joints.* In the lower tibiofibular joints, the bones are held together by a fibrous ligament.
2. *Synovial joints* (Fig. 1.26). Most joints are synovial, i.e. they are made up of cartilage, capsule, synovial fluid, synovial membrane and ligaments.
3. *Cartilaginous joints.* The bones are separated by cartilage; e.g. between the bodies of the vertebrae and in the manubriosternal joints.

Joints can also be classified according to their movements:

- Plane joint, e.g. acromioclavicular joint
- Hinge joint, e.g. elbow
- Saddle joint, e.g. 1st metacarpophalangeal joint at the wrist
- Condyloid joint, e.g. temporomandibular joint
- Pivot joint, e.g. radioulnar joint
- Ball and socket joint, e.g. hip joint.

Movements of joints can be:

- flexion, for example bending the elbow;
- abduction, for example lifting the arm away from the body;

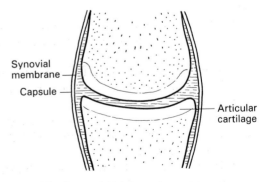

Figure 1.26   A synovial joint.

- adduction, as in bringing the arm to the side;
- rotation, for example moving the part round its own longitudinal axis;
- circumduction, a combination of abduction, adduction, extension and flexion.

IMPORTANT JOINTS IN THE BODY

1. *Temporomandibular joint*, formed by the articular surface of the temporal bone and the head of the mandible.

2. *Joints of the upper extremity*:
    - Acromioclavicular joint, formed by the acromion of the scapula and the lateral end of the clavicle;
    - Shoulder joint, formed by the glenoid cavity of the scapula and the head of the humerus;
    - Elbow joint, formed by the trochlea and capitulum at the lower end of the humerus, and the upper end of the ulna and the radius;
    - Wrist joint, formed by the lower end of the radius and ulna with the proximal row of carpal bones;
    - Carpal and phalangeal joints, formed by the distal row of carpal bones and the metacarpals. Phalangeal joints are formed by the metacarpals and the proximal phalanxes.

3. *Joints of the lower extremity*:
    - Pubic symphysis, formed by the symphyseal surfaces of the two pubic bones;
    - Sacroiliac joint, formed by the articulation of the sacrum on each side with iliac bone;
    - Hip joint, formed by the head of the femur and the acetabular fossa of innominate bone;
    - Knee joint, formed by the condyles of the femur, the upper end of the tibia and the patella;
    - Ankle joint, formed by the lower ends of the tibia and fibula articulating with the trochlea of the talus;
    - Joints of the foot: various tarsal bones are connected by joints.

MUSCLES

Some of the important muscles of the body are mentioned below.

1. *Muscles of the scalp and face*. The frontal and occipital muscles are attached to the front and back of the skull. The orbicularis oculi and orbicularis oris muscles are seen around the eye and the mouth.

2. *Muscles of chewing*. The masseter and temporalis muscles allow the opening and closing of the mouth.

3. *Muscles of the neck and shoulder*. Sternocleidomastoid and trapezium are the main muscles.

4. *Muscles of the upper extremity*. In the arm, the biceps, brachialis and triceps, and in the forearm, the superficial and deep flexors of the fingers and the flexor of the thumb, are the major muscles in the anterior aspect. On the posterior surface of the forearm, the extensor muscles of the wrist and fingers end as tendons into bones at the wrist or phalanges.

5. *Muscles of the lower extremity*. In the buttock, gluteus maximus medius and minimus; in the anterior aspect of the thigh, quadriceps femoris, rectus femoris and vastii muscles. In the medial aspect of the thigh, the adductor group of muscles and, posteriorly, the biceps femoris, semimembranosus and semitendinosus. Below the knee joint: anteriorly, tibialis anterior, extensor hallucis longus and extensor digitorum longus; posteriorly, gastrocnemius, soleus, tibialis posterior and flexor digitorum longus.

6. *Muscles of the abdomen*. Anteriorly and laterally, rectus abdominis, external and internal oblique muscles, transversus. Posteriorly, psoas and quadratus lumborum and iliacus.

7. *Diaphragm*. This muscular structure separates the thorax from the abdomen. Its fibres arise from xiphoid cartilage, the inner surface of the lower ribs at the sides and the bodies of the lumbar vertebrae behind. It is supplied by two phrenic nerves. The structures which pass through the diaphragm are: the aorta, inferior vena cava, oesophagus, and the thoracic duct.

FURTHER READING

Ackerman U 1992 Essentials of human physiology. Mosby, St Louis, MO

Gannong W F 1995 Review of medical physiology, 17th edn. Prentice Hall, New York

Hinchcliffe S, Montague S 1995 Physiology for nursing practice. Baillière Tindall, London

Ross J, Wilson K 1990 Anatomy and physiology, 7th edn. Churchill Livingstone, Edinburgh

Schmidt P, Adragna P J 1995 Human anatomy and physiology. Harcourt Brace, Orlando, FL

Snell R S 1995 Clinical anatomy for medical students, 5th edn. Little, Brown, Boston

Smith E, Paterson D, Scratcherd C 1988 Textbook of physiology, 11th edn. Churchill Livingstone, Edinburgh

2

Pharmacology

INTRODUCTION

Drugs are chemical substances which have an effect on the tissues of the human body; the study of drugs is called pharmacology. Pharmacology consists of two major divisions:

1. *Pharmacodynamics*, which is defined as how drugs, either by themselves or in combination, have an effect on the body.
2. *Pharmacokinetics*, which is defined as how the body affects drugs, in the form of absorption, distribution, metabolism and excretion.

In brief, pharmacodynamics is what drugs do to the body and pharmacokinetics is what the body does to drugs.

Pharmacodynamics

Drugs act on tissues in a number of ways, the most important being:

1. Action on *specific receptors*. Many drugs operate by acting on specific receptors, small parts of a cell that combine chemically with a drug.
2. Action on *metabolic processes*, as shown by antibiotics, sulphonamides and insulin. Some antibiotics act by stopping bacterial growth, such as cell wall formation (e.g. penicillins), and others by inhibition of protein synthesis (e.g. tetracyclines).

3. Action by *inhibiting enzymes*, for example anticholinesterases (e.g. neostigmine, which acts by preventing the destruction of acetylcholine; the effects in the central nervous system are due to its accumulation).
4. Action on *physicochemical properties* (e.g. volatile anaesthetics, see p. 54).

An important type of action is called competitive antagonism, which can be against (1) a specific receptor, for example β-adrenergic blockers, or (2) an enzyme, for example sulphonamides.

In the following sections, drugs will be described according to the system on which they act.

DRUGS ACTING ON THE CENTRAL NERVOUS SYSTEM

Terms commonly enountered are listed in Box 2.1.

Box 2.1 Drugs acting on the central nervous system

- A *hypnotic* is a drug that induces sleep
- A *sedative* is a drug that calms or soothes without inducing sleep
- A *tranquillizer* is a drug that quietens a person without him losing consciousness
- An *opioid* is a drug that produces sleep or drowsiness
- An *anticonvulsant* is a drug that prevents or controls convulsions
- An *anaesthetic* is a drug that induces reversible loss of consciousness
- An *analgesic* is a drug that relieves pain

HYPNOTICS

These drugs are used in small doses to reduce anxiety and/or as a premedication drug, and in high doses to produce sleep during the night.

Chloral hydrate is given orally as a solution and is rapidly absorbed from the intestine. It produces sleep within half an hour, lasting for 6–8 hours.
Dosage: 50–75 mg/kg orally.

Triclofos (Tricloryl) acts in a manner similar to that of chloral hydrate.

Chlormethiazole (Heminevrin) is a powerful sedative, antiemetic and hypnotic with an anticonvulsant action. It is used during treatment of the initial withdrawal phase of acute alcoholism, in the control of status epilepticus and as a sedative in intensive care or in pre-eclampsia.
Dosage: It is available as a 0.8% solution in 5% dextrose and is given intravenously (i.v.) at the rate of 8–20 ml/min.

Barbiturates

Barbitone, a derivative of barbituric acid (malonyl urea), was first introduced in 1903 as a hypnotic, following which a number of barbiturates were synthesized. Barbiturates are classified into long-, medium-, short- and ultra short-acting, based on the duration of action of a single dose. Examples are:

- Long-acting: barbitone, phenobarbitone (8–12 hours).
- Medium- and short-acting: amylobarbitone, pentobarbitone (2–8 hours).
- Ultra short-acting: thiopentone, methohexitone (act rapidly following i.v. injection).

They have an action on all levels of the central nervous system (especially on the cerebral cortex). In low dosage, they can antagonize analgesia; hence patients in pain when given barbiturates become restless. Most prevent convulsions in epileptics or following an overdose of local anaesthetic. They produce a fall in blood pressure in large doses. Barbiturates produce respiratory depression based on the amount of drug given.

The short-acting barbiturates are metabolized and excreted via the liver, whereas the long-acting ones are removed by renal excretion.
Mode of administration: Oral, intramuscular (i.m.) or i.v.
Contraindications: Patients suffering from porphyria (a congenital hereditary disorder). They should be used with great caution in patients with liver and kidney disease.

Barbiturate overdose and treatment: Signs of overdose include central depression (coma), respiratory and cardiac depression. Treatment consists of cardiac and respiratory support and forced alkaline diuresis using 10% mannitol, measuring the urine volume and pH, and replacement with intravenous fluids.

TRANQUILLIZERS

The benzodiazepines are a widely used group of tranquillizing drugs. They act on the reticular formation and limbic system in the brain. In small doses, they make the patient less anxious, but in high doses they cause drowsiness, amnesia and unconsciousness. They have the ability to decrease anaesthetic requirements by decreasing the minimum alveolar concentration (MAC) (see p. 54). There is little effect on blood pressure or cardiac output other than producing a rise in heart rate for a short period.

Diazepam may be given orally, i.v. or i.m.; injectable diazepam is available in doses of 10 mg (in 2 ml) dissolved in propylene glycol. This preparation is highly irritant to veins, so a newer preparation, Diazemuls, made up in lipid emulsion, has been made available.
Metabolism: Diazepam is metabolized in the liver and its breakdown product (desmethyldiazepam) is found to be active for up to 96 hours.
Indications: As a premedication drug, for induction of anaesthesia; in small doses in dental anaesthesia, for cardioversion and as a drug of choice to control convulsions.
Dosage: As a premedicant, diazepam 0.2 mg/kg orally 90 minutes before surgery.

Midazolam (Hypnovel) is a rapidly acting, water-soluble benzodiazepine. It is supplied as a colourless solution of 10 mg midazolam in 2 ml aqueous solution. This drug can be used as either an i.v. sedating or induction agent. For sedation, a total dosage of 2.5–10.0 mg i.v. is required, and for induction, a dosage of 0.1–0.5 mg/kg is needed. The recovery from midazolam is faster because of its short half-life. It has no active breakdown products.

Indications: As an i.v. sedation drug during endoscopy and dentistry.

Lorazepam (Ativan) is presented in doses of 4 mg in 2 ml dissolved in polyethylene glycol and propylene glycol. It has actions similar to those of diazepam. It produces anterograde amnesia (loss of memory for events occurring after its administration).
Indications: As a premedication drug and also to prevent an emergence reaction (i.e. hallucinations) following ketamine anaesthesia.
Dosage: On a weight-to-weight basis, lorazepam is five times more potent than diazepam. For premedication, 1–4 mg is given orally to be effective.

Temazepam is presented as 10 mg or 20 mg capsules. It is used as a night sedative or as a premedication drug.
Dosage: 20–40 mg 60 minutes before surgery.

Nitrazepam (Mogadon) is used as a hypnotic for night sedation.
Dosage: 5–10 mg.

Flumazenil (Anexate) is a benzodiazepine antagonist. It blocks the central effects, such as sedation and hypnosis, of benzodiazepines. Flumazenil is indicated for the reversal of sedation due to the use of midazolam (Hypnovel) in short diagnostic procedures such as endoscopy. It is also used in the intensive therapy unit in treating self-poisoning with benzodiazepines. It may induce an acute withdrawal syndrome and convulsions.
Dosage: In adults, it is injected as 200 µg of flumazenil i.v. over 15 s, with increments until the desired effect is achieved.

NEUROLEPTIC DRUGS

These are the drugs that cause quietening of emotional behaviour and psychomotor slowing. They are also called major tranquillizers or anti-psychotics. The major subgroups of neuroleptics are:

- phenothiazines, for example chlorpromazine, promazine, prochlorperazine and perphenazine;
- butyrophenones, for example droperidol and haloperidol.

Phenothiazines

Chlorpromazine (Largactil) produces lethargy, apathy and sleep by acting on the hypothalamus. It has a marked antiemetic action (preventing vomiting by its action on the vomiting centre and the chemoreceptor trigger zone). It causes tachycardia and a fall in blood pressure due to peripheral vasodilatation, and decreases bronchial, salivary and gastric secretion. It can also cause cholestatic jaundice in about 0.5–1.0% of patients. It has a mild antihistamine action. The drug is metabolized in the liver.

Indications: As a premedicant, and to treat intractable hiccup and vomiting.

Dosage: It can be given orally, i.m. or i.v. A very dilute solution of 1 mg/ml (10 mg in 10 ml normal saline) can be used for treating peripheral vasoconstriction in patients who have been adequately fluid resuscitated.

For premedication, 25–50 mg may be given i.m. 1 hour preoperatively, with an analgesic such as pethidine (50–100 mg).

Side-effects: Postural hypotension and agranulocytosis.

Promethazine hydrochloride (Phenergan). Many of its actions on the central nervous system are similar to those of chlorpromazine, although its sedative effects are more marked. There are no other marked effects on heart, skeleton, muscle, kidneys or liver. Promethazine causes bronchodilatation and has a marked antihistamine action. It is metabolized in the liver.

Indications: In premedication and to treat allergies such as hay fever, urticaria and motion sickness.

Dosage: For premedication, 25 mg i.m. 1 hour before surgery along with 75–100 mg pethidine.

Side-effects: An overdose can cause circulatory collapse and central depression.

Prochlorperazine (Stemetil) is an effective antiemetic agent that has few side-effects.

Indications: As an antiemetic during surgery, in psychiatry and in the treatment of migraine.

Dosage: As a deep i.m. injection (12.5 mg) repeated at 4–6 hourly intervals for the antiemetic effect.

Perphenazine (Fentazin) has a number of actions similar to chlorpromazine. The hypotension it causes is insignificant. It is an effective antiemetic.

Indications: As an antiemetic, as a premedicant and also in psychiatry.

Dosage: 4 mg orally or 5 mg i.m.

Side-effects: It can cause extrapyramidal signs (see below) if used frequently, as can all phenothiazines.

Trimeprazine (Vallergan) is used to relieve itching, as an antihistamine and as a premedication in children.

Dosage: 2–4 mg/kg body weight 1 hour before surgery.

Side-effects: It can cause restlessness postoperatively, associated with a flushed appearance.

Butyrophenones

These drugs, due to their specific action, induce a state in a patient whereby he looks tranquil but can be readily awakened. High doses can cause hallucinations, restlessness and extrapyramidal side-effects, including involuntary movements. These drugs have a powerful antiemetic effect.

Droperidol (Droleptan) resembles the phenothiazines in structure. It has a quick onset and shorter duration of action. Droperidol produces a picture of mental calm in a patient and is used along with fentanyl or phenoperidine as a neuroleptic agent in procedures (such as cardiac catheterization and angiograms) in which the patient's cooperation is needed, and in certain poor-risk patients. It is a powerful antiemetic, its action being mediated via the chemoreceptor trigger zone in the hypothalamus.

In high doses, droperidol produces extrapyramidal side-effects.

Indications: Intraoperatively as a neuroleptic agent or as an antiemetic.

Dosage: From 2.5 mg (between 15 and 20 kg body weight) to 5 mg (20–25 kg body weight) orally as a premedication for children; in adults, 2.5–5.0 mg i.v. as an antiemetic and up to 10 mg i.v. for neuroleptic analgesia.

ANTICONVULSANTS (ANTIEPILEPTICS)

Epilepsy is a sudden, excessive and rapid discharge of nervous activity in the grey matter of the brain. It has a number of causes, such as pathological (eclampsia during pregnancy or brain tumours), metabolic (hypoglycaemia and febrile convulsions in children), drugs, etc. Sometimes convulsions are seen in the operating theatre, either from an overdose of local anaesthetic drug or following the administration of a large dose of ether. The types of epilepsy usually seen are grand mal, petit mal, focal and temporal lobe.

The treatment of epilepsy consists of treating the cause, for example a brain tumour, avoiding factors that precipitate epilepsy, such as stress or alcohol, and the use of anticonvulsants. Anticonvulsants are drugs that inhibit the discharge of nervous activity or its spread from the grey matter in the brain, producing an overall depressing or hypnotic effect. The drugs of choice in epilepsy are as follows:

- *Grand mal, focal seizures, temporal lobe epilepsy:*
  - First choice: phenytoin
  - Second choice: carbamazepine, phenobarbitone, sodium valproate
- *Petit mal*
  - First choice: sodium valproate, ethosuximide
  - Second choice: clonazepam.

Phenytoin (Dilantin, Epanutin) is an effective antiepileptic in all types of epilepsy except petit mal. It is absorbed slowly from the intestine and is metabolized in the liver. It is painful on injection.

Indications: All types of epilepsy except petit mal and in the control of digitalis-induced arrhythmias.

Dosage: In adults, an initial dose of 100 mg twice a day orally, increasing to 600 mg over 24 hours. To control digitalis-induced arrhythmia, it is given 50–100 mg i.v. every 15 minutes until a sinus rhythm is seen on the ECG.

Side-effects: It can cause drug interactions, and enhances the metabolism of other drugs such as steroids, warfarin and tricyclic antidepressants, thus increasing their daily requirement. It causes insomnia and gastric disturbances. In young children, prolonged treatment causes hypertrophy of the gums.

Sodium valproate (Epilim) controls fits with minimal side-effects.

Indications: Petit mal epilepsy.

Dosage: 200 mg three times a day for adults initially, increasing to 1000–2000 mg per day.

Carbamazepine (Tegretol). In the past, carbamazepine was used in the treatment of temporal lobe epilepsy, but now it is more often employed in the treatment of trigeminal neuralgia.

Indications: Trigeminal neuralgia, temporal lobe epilepsy, intractable hiccups.

Dosage: 100–200 mg twice a day initially, increasing to 600–800 mg daily.

Side-effects: Jaundice and thrombocytopaenia.

Ethosuximide (Zarontin) is used in the treatment of petit mal epilepsy.

Dosage: 250 mg three times a day orally, increasing to up to 2 g per day.

Side-effects: Nausea, vomiting and drowsiness.

Clonazepam (Rivotril) is a benzodiazepine.

Indications: As a second choice drug in grand mal and petit mal epilepsy, and as a first choice in myoclonus and status epilepticus.

Dosage: 0.5 mg orally twice a day; in status epilepticus, 1 mg i.v. slowly.

Status epilepticus

Status epilepticus is a condition in which epileptic fits are continuous and not controlled by oral medication; they can be dangerous to life due to hypoxia and the inhalation of stomach contents. Treatment consists of diazepam 10 mg i.v. over a 2 minute period or repeated, or as an infusion at the rate of 20 mg per hour (40 mg in 500 ml of 5% dextrose). An alternative to diazepam is clonazepam 1 mg i.v. slowly over a 30 s period.

AGENTS USED FOR GENERAL ANAESTHESIA

Anaesthesia is defined as the absence of sensation, and general anaesthetics are those agents which produce loss of consciousness and sensation in a reversible manner.

Stages of anaesthesia

The depth of anaesthesia can be interpreted with the aid of stages, i.e. I to IV (see below). These stages were first described in relation to ether anaesthesia, and since then modifications have been made to these stages if anaesthesia is induced with intravenous induction agents. The following four stages were described by Guedel in relation to ether anaesthesia.

Stage I: analgesia. This lasts from the beginning of induction until loss of consciousness. During this stage, respiration is quiet but irregular, and all the reflexes are present.

Stage II: delirium or excitement. This begins at loss of consciousness and ends at the onset of surgical anaesthesia. During this stage, the patient is unconscious and respirations are irregular, with episodes of breath-holding. The reflexes are still active, and if the stomach is not empty, vomiting can occur.

Stage III: surgical anaesthesia. This stage lasts from the onset of regular respiration to the occurrence of respiratory failure due to toxic doses of the anaesthetic. It is divided into four planes.

1. Plane A. Respiration becomes regular and automatic. The eyelid reflex is lost, muscle tone and the laryngeal reflexes are still present, but the pharyngeal reflex disappears late in this plane.

2. Plane B. Muscle tone decreases, but the respiratory muscles are still active. The pupils are fixed and central, and the laryngeal reflexes are lost.

3. Plane C. Muscle relaxation is nearly complete and the intercostal muscles become paralysed. This is the plane most usually desired for surgical anaesthesia.

4. Plane D. Muscle relaxation is full, respirations are depressed and a tracheal tug is seen.

Stage IV: medullary paralysis. The respiration becomes gasping in nature and eventually stops. Blood pressure is low and the pulse weak. The skin becomes cold and the pupils widely dilated. Death is imminent from overdose of anaesthetic.

The above stages were seen only when chloroform or ether were used, but in the current situation the early stages seem to pass quickly. For example, if thiopentone is used as an induction agent, the patient rapidly passes into stage III, plane B or C, depending on the dose of thiopentone given, without showing signs of stage I or II.

Anaesthesia for surgical procedures

To allow the surgeon to perform a surgical procedure in a relaxed sleeping patient, the anaesthetist uses a technique called balanced anaesthesia. Balanced anaesthesia comprises anaesthesia, analgesia and muscle relaxation.

Anaesthesia is induced with an induction agent (p. 60); in children, a volatile anaesthetic agent can be used (see below). Surgical anaesthesia is then maintained using a volatile agent and oxygen, often in a carrier gas (nitrous oxide or air). Analgesia is provided with one of the agents suitable for the surgical procedure (see p. 58), and, if required, muscle relaxation is provided by a muscle relaxant (also called a neuromuscular blocker) (see p. 73) or a suitable local anaesthetic nerve block.

After the induction of anaesthesia, the patient either breathes spontaneously or is ventilated with a mixture of oxygen, nitrous oxide and a volatile agent. All the volatile anaesthetic agents diffuse readily into the central nervous system, having been carried from the lungs to the brain by the blood. During the induction of anaesthesia, volatile agents from the anaesthetic machine enter the body tissues (against a concentration gradient, i.e. from a high level outside to a zero level in the tissues). When the patient is adequately anaesthetized, he is maintained with the same or a slightly lower concentration of the agent, and there is no further uptake of the gases as the tissues become fully saturated. When the anaesthesia is completed, during the recovery period the anaesthetic gases are eliminated (against a concentration gradient, i.e. from a high level inside the body to outside where the concentration is zero).

The amount of time taken for the induction of an anaesthetic depends on the rate at which the tension of anaesthetic agents in the lung (called the alveolar anaesthetic tension) equals the tension in the anaesthetic machine delivering it (called the inspired anaesthetic tension). Some of the factors that play an important role in determining the alveolar anaesthetic tension are:

- inspired anaesthetic tension;
- solubility of the agent in blood;
- lung ventilation (also called alveolar ventilation);
- cardiac output of the patient.

The above-mentioned factors will be explored further to make the understanding of uptake and elimination of anaesthetic gases a little easier.

Inspired anaesthetic tension. A high inspired anaesthetic tension shortens the time required for the induction of anaesthesia (e.g. the anaesthetist normally sets up 4% enflurane or 3% halothane on the vapourizer during the induction to hasten the patient to sleep).

Solubility of the agent in blood is also known as the partition coefficient of the agent between blood and gas at body temperature. If the blood/gas partition coefficient of an agent is high, it is removed from the alveoli in the lungs by its blood supply (pulmonary capillary blood), thus decreasing its tension in the lungs and slowly increasing it in the blood and brain. This leads to

slower induction. As opposed to this, nitrous oxide, which has a low blood/gas partition coefficient, is taken up slowly by the pulmonary capillary blood. Thus the tension in the lung alveoli reaches the inspired tension comparatively fast, causing rapid equilibration.

Lung ventilation (alveolar ventilation). If the alveolar ventilation is increased (e.g. a hyperventilating patient when breathing spontaneously or manual hyperventilation in a paralysed patient), the uptake of the anaesthetic agent is considerably increased.

Cardiac output of the patient. If a patient has a high cardiac output (e.g. anxiety or thyrotoxicosis), a large amount of the anaesthetic agent is removed from the blood, thus increasing the time taken for the induction of anaesthesia. In patients with a low cardiac output (shocked, hypotensive patients), anaesthetic agents are slowly removed from the alveoli in the lungs. Thus the inspired concentration equals the alveolar concentration and the induction becomes rapid.

Another factor that contributes towards the uptake of anaesthetic gases is the rubber/gas partition coefficient (see below). Some of the anaesthetic agents (e.g. halothane) are soluble in rubber. This used to be of practical importance when anaesthetics were delivered to the patient via rubber circuits; nowadays, circuits tend to be made of PVC or polythene so this effect is much less pronounced. During the induction of anaesthesia, a large amount of anaesthetic agent was absorbed by the rubber until it was saturated; during this period, the patient would get an inadequate amount of gas. This circuit, which was saturated with the anaesthetic, would give up the agent during a subsequent anaesthetic. Box 2.2 gives an example of two rubber/gas partition coefficients.

Box 2.2 Rubber/gas partition coefficients	
Anaesthetic agent	Rubber/gas partition coefficient
Halothane	120
Nitrous oxide	1.2

Other factors that influence the uptake of anaesthetic gases include concentration and second gas effects. A description of these in simple terms is beyond the scope of this book.

Minimum alveolar concentration (MAC) is defined as the alveolar concentration of an agent that prevents a response to a stimulus in 50% of subjects.

Metabolism and excretion of volatile anaesthetic agents. A large portion of the volatile anaesthetic agent is excreted via the lungs, a small amount being excreted unchanged in urine and sweat. Some of it is biotransformed in the liver with the aid of liver enzymes such as cytochrome P450. By biotransformation, these agents, which are highly lipid (fat) soluble, are converted into water-soluble substances.

Biotransformation of agents, such as trichloro-ethylene to trichloroethanol, leads to a prolonged effect. Halothane, isoflurane and enflurane liberate inorganic fluoride during their metabolism. The inorganic fluoride liberated by methoxyflurane can cause nephrotoxicity (kidney failure), and the metabolite of halothane has been said to cause hepatitis.

Insoluble agents (such as nitrous oxide) will be released from the blood into the alveoli, from where they can be removed by ventilation. Soluble agents such as halothane will be removed slowly from the blood.

Volatile anaesthetic agents

These can be classified as either halogenated hydrocarbons or ethers.

Halogenated hydrocarbons

Fluorine, chlorine and bromine are called halogens, and the name for the chemical combination of hydrogen and carbon is hydrocarbon. When halogens are added to hydrocarbons, they develop anaesthetic properties. Many of the currently used anaesthetic agents are hydrocarbons with fluorine substitution. Inhalational (volatile) agents are usually administered via vapourizers. Most vapourizers in general use today are specifically

calibrated to deliver a known percentage concentration (dose) of agent. The different volatile agents have very different potencies and properties and are therefore administered via agent-specific vapourizers (e.g. a halothane vapourizer for halothane only). To prevent accidental filling of a vapourizer with the wrong agent, 'keyed' filling devices and colour coding have been introduced; each bottle of volatile will only thread onto its own filling tube, which in turn will only fit into its own vapourizer.

Halothane (Fluothane) is a colourless liquid with a sweet, pleasant odour. Because of its pleasant smell, halothane is the easiest agent to use for the purely inhalational induction of anaesthesia. It is made stable by the addition of thymol and by storing it in amber glass bottles. Thymol can accumulate in the halothane vapourizer, and the vapourizer therefore needs regular drainage following the manufacturer's instructions. Like all general anaesthetics, halothane depresses the central nervous system, and in addition causes an increase in cerebral blood flow and intracranial pressure. This agent is not used, or should be used with caution, in patients with head injury (with suspected raised intracranial pressure).

Halothane causes a fall in arterial blood pressure, depending on the depth of halothane anaesthesia, and bradycardia. Arrhythmias such as ventricular extrasystoles or nodal rhythm are seen in patients spontaneously breathing high concentrations of halothane. The cause is retention of carbon dioxide (due to underventilation), which releases catecholamines. Halothane sensitizes the heart to the effect of the catecholamines, thus causing dysrhythmias. The treatment consists of improving ventilation, decreasing the halothane concentration and, if necessary, changing the inhalational agent.

Halothane potentiates the effect of muscle relaxants (d-tubocurarine). It has no effect on the renal system but causes a fall in the tidal volume and increases respiratory rate (shallow rapid breathing). It inhibits the contractility of the uterus. The effect of halothane on the liver has gained considerable prominence in the last few years, and it has been shown that halothane can very rarely cause postoperative jaundice. The usual recommendation is not to use halothane within 6 months of the last exposure in adults. Although a few cases of halothane hepatitis have been reported in children, repeated halothane administration in children seems to be safe.

Metabolism: Halothane is metabolized in the liver by microsomal enzymes.

Indications: As it is a potent inhalational anaesthetic agent, halothane is used for many surgical procedures. As it causes hypotension, halothane is used along with d-tubocurarine to induce deliberate hypotension (see p. 194).

Dosage: A vapour concentration of 2–4% is required for the induction of anaesthesia, and one of 0.5–1.5% for the maintenance of anaesthesia.

Side-effects and precautions: Halothane has been known to cause hepatitis, hence the interval between exposures needs to be considered.

Other halogenated hydrocarbons

Chloroform is not available now. It was highly potent and able to cause death due to vagal arrest (acute episode of bradycardia) during induction, or to ventricular fibrillation during maintenance of the anaesthesia. It was notorious in causing liver damage (delayed chloroform poisoning).

Ethyl chloride is stored in liquid form in a glass container (which will explode if dropped) under slight pressure but is converted to gas at room temperature. It is highly volatile and causes rapid induction and recovery. In the past, it was used for the induction of anaesthesia by spraying on an open mask. Ethyl chloride was notorious in causing breath-holding when used in this way. When a child inhaled after breath-holding, the high concentration of ethyl chloride often caused ventricular fibrillation and cardiac arrest.

Its present use is as a topical anaesthetic for the drainage of localized abscesses, insertion of i.v. cannulae and testing for the level of sensory block following spinal or epidural anaesthesia. It should not be used unless there are full antistatic measures in place.

Anaesthetic ethers

After the discovery that diethyl ether had anaesthetic properties, a number of ethers were developed. All the new ones are fluorinated ethers. Some examples of these are given below.

Diethyl ether is a colourless, highly volatile liquid decomposed by air, light and heat. It produces loss of consciousness, as do all other volatile anaesthetic agents. During light planes of anaesthesia, there are no significant changes in heart rate and blood pressure, but with deeper levels there is a considerable fall in blood pressure. At lighter planes of anaesthesia, it causes an increase in respiratory rate and tidal volume, but at deeper ones it causes respiratory failure. It causes relaxation of the bronchial smooth muscle (hence it might be beneficial in status asthmaticus). Ether has a tendency to increase bronchial, salivary and gastric secretions. Patients receiving prolonged ether anaesthesia show a high incidence of postoperative nausea and vomiting. Ether causes relaxation of the uterus during deep anaesthesia. It can cause hyperglycaemia (due to mobilization of glycogen from the liver).

Metabolism: About 15% of the inhaled ether is metabolized to carbon dioxide and water.

Indications: Because it is explosive, its use in modern operating theatres has declined. It is still used frequently and successfully in the developing countries, by single operators with minimal equipment.

Dosage: Diethyl ether can be given through a vapourizer (Boyle's bottle) or an open mask. Up to 15–20% vapour concentrations are required for the induction of anaesthesia. To maintain deep anaesthesia, concentrations of 10% are required, compared with 5% for light anaesthesia. An EMO (Epstein, Mackintosh, Oxford) vapourizer delivers a concentration of between 0 and 25%, and if a patient is paralysed with a muscle relaxant, a 24% concentration of ether in air maintains unconsciousness. Recovery following 2–4% ether concentration is fairly quick, and the incidence of nausea and vomiting is insignificant.

Side-effects and precautions: Ether should not be used in children with fever in hot operating conditions as they will be prone to develop ether convulsions, the chances of which become higher if atropine is used as a premedication. If ether convulsions do occur, the treatment consists of stopping the ether, cooling the patient with a fan or sponging with cold water. Diazepam 1–2 mg or thiopentone 100 mg i.v. will stop the convulsions.

The use of ether is contraindicated in patients with diabetes mellitus and severe liver disease. As diethyl ether is flammable, it should not be used along with diathermy apparatus.

Enflurane (Ethrane). This volatile anaesthetic agent is non-explosive and non-inflammable in the presence of air or oxygen. Like any other anaesthetic agent, it produces loss of consciousness. In addition, enflurane is known to cause increased activity in the brain similar to an epileptic attack; hence enflurane is not recommended in patients with a history of epilepsy. At light planes of enflurane anaesthesia, the cardiovascular system is stable, but in deep planes there is a fall in blood pressure. It has minimal effect on other systems.

Indications: Because of the smooth induction and maintenance, enflurane is being used in a number of surgical procedures.

Dosage: Initially, 4–5% vapour concentration is required for the induction of anaesthesia followed by 2–5% for maintenance.

Precautions: It should be avoided in patients with a history of epilepsy.

Isoflurane (Forane) resembles enflurane in a number of ways, with a slight difference in its chemical composition. It produces a more rapid induction of anaesthesia than does halothane. It also produces a dose-dependent fall in blood pressure with less effect on cardiac output. Respiratory depression occurs in a dose-dependent manner similar to that of enflurane. A very small amount of isoflurane undergoes biotransformation, so the chances of toxicity are extremely low.

Sevoflurane and desflurane

These two inhalational agents, although synthesized in the 1960s (desflurane) and 1970s (sevoflurane), did not come into use until 1993, first being employed in Japan and North America.

Sevoflurane is a non-flammable volatile liquid, delivered via a vapourizer specifically calibrated for use with sevoflurane so that the concentration can be accurately controlled. The MAC of sevoflurane decreases with age and with the addition of nitrous oxide. Table 2.1 below indicates the effect of MAC on sevoflurane.

Anaesthesia is maintained with concentrations of 0.5–3.0% sevoflurane, with or without the use of nitrous oxide in elderly patients; lesser concentrations of sevoflurane are required to maintain surgical anaesthesia. Sevoflurane has minimal effect on intracranial pressure. It depresses the cardiovascular system in a dose-related fashion.

Metabolism: In humans, less than 5% of the absorbed sevoflurane is metabolized. It is defluorinated via the enzyme cytochrome P450, resulting in the production of hexafluoro-isopropanol, with a release of inorganic fluoride and carbon dioxide. It should be used with caution in patients with renal failure.

Table 2.1 Effect of MAC on sevoflurane

Age of patient (years)	Sevoflurane in 65% N_2O/35%O_2 (%)	Sevoflurane in O_2 (%)
1–3	2.0	3.3–2.6
5–12	Not available	2.4
25	1.4	2.5
35	1.2	2.2
50	0.98	1.8
60	0.87	1.6
80	0.7	1.4

Sevoflurane's low solubility in blood (blood:gas partition coefficient 0.65) results in a rapid increase in alveolar concentration (rapid induction), which rapidly decreases upon discontinuation of sevoflurane (hence the rapid recovery).

Sevoflurane is chemically stable, and its degradation by soda lime or baralyme at high temperatures produces a toxic olefin. Sevoflurane can nonetheless be used in circle systems with a carbon dioxide absorber, although the US (but not the UK) licence prohibits its use for longer anaesthetics with fresh gas flows of less than 2 L/min.

Contraindications: Sevoflurane should not be used in patients with known sensitivity to sevoflurane, and is contraindicated in patients with known or suspected genetic susceptibility to malignant hyperpyrexia. (*No* inhalational agent except nitrous oxide is safe in the latter condition.)

Desflurane is an ether with lower solubility in blood (blood/gas partition coefficient 0.45) and low tissue solubility. This produces a rapid rise in alveolar concentration during anaesthesia (rapid induction), a rapid fall in alveolar concentration during elimination (quick recovery), and a rapid equilibration between the tissues and blood.

Desflurane has a vapour pressure of 669 mmHg at 20°C compared with 240 for isoflurane (three times the level), and as the vapour pressure exceeds 1 atmosphere at 22.8°C (the boiling point), the same vapourizer type as used for the other inhalational agents cannot be used. A new vapourizer technology is used and is described on page 153.

The MAC for desflurane is 6.0 (five times that of isoflurane), decreasing with age and the use of nitrous oxide, midazolam or fentanyl. Desflurane decreases cerebral vascular resistance and can cause a rise in intracranial pressure in a dose-related manner. It decreases blood pressure in a dose-related manner, but maintains cardiac output and causes tachycardia. It does not decrease coronary blood flow.

Desflurane strongly resists biodegradation and degradation by soda lime.

Anaesthetic gases

Nitrous oxide (N_2O) is a colourless gas with a sweet smell. It is supplied in blue cylinders as liquid compressed to a pressure of 650 lb/in². It causes some increase in respiratory rate and has no effect on muscle, the liver or kidneys. It has a tendency to cause nausea and vomiting, and causes depression of bone marrow if given for longer than 24 hours.

Indications: As a supplement with oxygen (66% and 33%) in most surgical procedures; in a 50:50 mixture with oxygen (also called Entonox) for pain relief during labour and also during dental extraction in a dentist's chair. Nitrous oxide will only produce unconsciousness at greater than 100% inhaled (i.e. in a hyperbaric chamber); it is *not* an anaesthetic under clinical conditions.

Dosage: Nitrous oxide is a poor anaesthetic, but a good analgesic. It must always be administered with at least 21% oxygen to prevent the patient becoming hypoxic.

Side-effects and precautions: During recovery from nitrous oxide and oxygen anaesthesia, hypoxia (also called diffusion hypoxia) can occur. This is due to the reversal phase, in which large volumes of insoluble nitrous oxide are eliminated from the blood into the alveoli, thus decreasing the alveolar concentration of oxygen. This diffusion hypoxia can be prevented by giving oxygen in the period following extubation and in the recovery room. For the effects of nitrous oxide on closed gas-filled cavities in the body, such as the middle ear, gut and pneumothorax, readers are asked to seek an explanation from their anaesthetists.

Carbon dioxide (CO_2) is a colourless, odourless gas with a slightly acid taste. It is supplied in liquid form in grey cylinders at a pressure of 50 bar at 15°C. Carbon dioxide is non-inflammable and does not support combustion. Its uses during anaesthesia are:

- to induce hyperventilation to facilitate blind nasal intubation;
- to increase cerebral blood flow during carotid artery surgery;
- to bring the carbon dioxide levels to normal levels at the end of a period of hyperventilation.

Following several accidents involving carbon dioxide cylinders, the Royal College of Anaesthetists recommends that carbon dioxide is only attached to the machine at the specific request of the anaesthetist and that the cylinder is removed when no longer required.

Air. Compressed air is used extensively in medicine: to drive ventilators, as a source of power for pneumatic instruments or in oxygen–air anaesthetic techniques, when nitrous oxide is not used.

Air is supplied in the UK in cylinders of capacities 1280, 4800 and 6400 L (sizes F–J) compressed to 13 700 kPa. Medical air cylinders are painted grey with black and white shoulder quadrants and are fitted with bull-nose valves.

Cyclopropane is a colourless gas with a pungent taste and a strange smell. It depresses the central nervous system, as do all other anaesthetic agents. During light anaesthesia, blood pressure and cardiac output are increased, with a small fall in heart rate. At deeper planes of cyclopropane anaesthesia, blood pressure falls and heart rate rises. Cyclopropane is a marked respiratory depressant and has no significant effect on the liver, kidneys and muscular system, nor on the contractility of the uterus. Cyclopropane is highly explosive and should only be used with full antistatic measures.

Metabolism: Cyclopropane is excreted unchanged by the lungs.

Indications: Its use in the UK is non-existent. Anaesthetists who have used this gas in the past reserved it for 'bad-risk' patients and for inducing babies and small children. It is not suitable for major surgery without the use of muscle relaxants. As cyclopropane is a rapidly acting agent, the patient will be fully anaesthetized within 5 minutes without adequate muscle relaxation. Recovery from anaesthesia is fairly rapid (within a few minutes), but there is a high incidence of nausea and vomiting.

Dosage: A concentration of 5–10% produces light anaesthesia, 15–30% moderate-to-deep anaesthesia, and around 30–40% total respiratory paralysis. Because of its high cost, it should be used in a closed circuit with a carbon dioxide absorber.

Side-effects and precautions: Patients breathing spontaneously can develop ventricular arrhythmias (hypoventilation leading to a build-up of carbon dioxide). The treatment consists of decreasing the cyclopropane concentration and increasing the ventilation. To prevent hypotension or atelectasis of the alveoli at the end of cyclopropane anaesthesia, oxygen is given in the immediate postoperative period.

ANALGESICS

Analgesics are usually prescribed to relieve pain, which could be mild to severe (such as postoperative pain or pain due to trauma or cancer). They are either powerful narcotics or weak analgesics.

Opioid analgesics are either found naturally or prepared synthetically. One of the major problems with opioid analgesics is their addiction potential (i.e. people get hooked on them!). A few definitions should be introduced:

- *Agonists* are those opioids which exert actions such as analgesia, euphoria, stimulation of the chemoreceptor trigger zone (CTZ) (causing vomiting) and respiratory depression and addiction. Examples are morphine and diamorphine.
- *Antagonists* are those agents which oppose agonist actions, for example naloxone.
- *Partial agonists* are drugs that exhibit a few agonist and a few antagonist actions, for example pentazocine, nalorphine and buprenorphine.

Some of the common opioid analgesics used during and following surgery and those available in theatre will be described.

Postoperative analgesia

Morphine is obtained from opium, which is the dried juice from the unripe poppy heads of *Papaver somniferum*. It causes depression of the cerebral cortex and respiratory centre and miosis (pinpoint pupils). The use of large doses of morphine produces a slowing of the pulse rate and a fall in blood pressure. Morphine can produce a fall in the respiratory rate and tidal volume, and it also causes constipation. Morphine crosses the placental barrier and causes respiratory depression in neonates.

Its peak analgesic effect is 20 minutes after i.v. and 90 minutes after i.m. injection, the action lasting for 4 hours.

Morphine is metabolized in the liver and excreted via the kidneys. People receiving morphine on a regular basis are in danger of becoming addicted to it.

Indications: In the treatment of acute pain following surgery and myocardial infarction.

Dosage: 15–30 µg/kg body weight (approximately 8–20 mg) for acute pain and 8–10 µg/kg body weight (10–15 mg) as a premedication 1.5 hours before surgery (p. 146).

Side-effects and precautions: Side-effects include confusion, nausea, vomiting and respiratory depression. Morphine should be used with caution in elderly patients and is contraindicated in patients with liver failure and hypothyroidism.

Papaveretum (Omnopon) is less powerful than morphine in its sedative and analgesic properties. The papaveretum preparation consists of 50% anhydrous morphine, the other 50% being made up of papaverine, codeine, thebaine and narcotine.

Indications: In the treatment of acute pain following surgery and as a premedication.

Side-effects and precautions: Side-effects are the same as for morphine. Papaveretum should be avoided in patients over the age of 70 years.

Pethidine is less potent than morphine in its analgesic action. It causes cerebral depression, induces nausea and vomiting and may produce a fall in blood pressure. The respiratory depression caused by pethidine is dose dependent. Pethidine crosses the placental barrier, causing respiratory depression in the neonate. It is broken down in the liver and excreted via the kidneys.

Indications: As a premedication and pain reliever in the intraoperative and postoperative periods. It is also used in the early stages of labour.

Dosage: For premedication, 0.5–1.0 mg/kg body weight i.m. repeated 3–4 hourly.

Side-effects and precautions: Nausea, vomiting and depression are the common side-effects. Pethidine is contraindicated in patients with liver disease. It is also a drug that can cause addiction.

Pentazocine is a partial agonist. In small doses it causes sedation, and in larger doses restlessness and euphoria. Respiratory and cardiovascular depression are not as marked as with morphine.

Indications: In the relief of acute and chronic pain.

Side-effects: The same as for morphine except that pentazocine causes dysphoria.

Dosage: 15–60 mg can be given i.v. or i.m. for the relief of acute pain.

Buprenorphine is a 'partial agonist' with opioid actions. It is difficult to reverse with naloxone.

Indications: Relief of moderate-to-severe pain.

Dosage: 300–600 µg i.m., slow i.v. or sublingual, action lasting from 4 to 6 hours.

Side-effects and precautions: Nausea, vomiting and dizziness are very common.

Narcotic analgesics used in theatre

Alfentanil is a derivative of fentanyl. It has a faster onset of action and a much shorter duration of action (10–15 minutes). It is suitable as an i.v. infusion during anaesthesia.

Dosage: For spontaneous respiration in adults, 500 µg. Given i.m., 30–50 µg/kg. For i.v. infusion, 50–100 µg/kg over 10 minutes, then 1 µg/kg/min.

Side-effects: Respiratory depression and muscular rigidity.

Fentanyl is a highly potent analgesic with an onset of action in 1–2 minutes and an effect lasting for 20 minutes. In doses up to 200 µg, it may not cause respiratory depression.

Indications: As an analgesic in the intraoperative period.

Dosage: 3–5 µg/kg body weight i.v.

Side-effects and precautions: Nausea, vomiting and respiratory depression.

Phenoperidine is a powerful analgesic related to pethidine. When given i.v., it acts within 2–3 minutes, the effect lasting for up to 1 hour. It has little action on the cardiovascular system but causes respiratory depression.

Indications: As an analgesic during the intraoperative period.

Dosage: 20–50 µg/kg body weight when patients are being ventilated.

Side-effects and precautions: Nausea, vomiting and respiratory depression.

Non-steroidal anti-inflammatory drugs

Non-steroidal anti-inflammatory drugs (NSAIDs) inhibit prostaglandin synthesis, thus decreasing the inflammatory response to surgical trauma and hence reducing the feeling of peripheral pain. They have also been shown to have a central effect, decreasing the perception of pain. They can be given pre-emptively: preoperative administration of NSAIDs has been shown to inhibit the enzyne cyclo-oxygenase and decrease tissue prostaglandin synthesis, thus reducing pain after surgery.

The following drugs are commonly used NSAIDs in the UK.

Diclofenac inhibits cyclo-oxygenase, thus preventing the formation of prostaglandins and thromboxanes. It acts as an analgesic and anti-inflammatory agent.

Dose: 75–100 mg/day as tablets in divided doses.

Rectal administration is thought to reduce the gastrointestinal upset associated with diclofenac and is an especially convenient route of administration in theatre. It is advisable to ensure that patients are aware that a suppository will be given to them if this is the planned method of administration (as lawsuits have resulted in convictions for assault). The dose is 100 mg/day when given as a rectal suppository.

Diclofenac can also be given in a dose of 75 mg i.m. once or twice a day.

Side-effects: These include gastrointestinal upset, gastrointestinal bleeding, prolongation of the bleeding time, exacerbation of asthma and renal failure. (Bleeding time may be prolonged in any patient given an NSAID.)

Ketorolac is a potent analgesic with moderate anti-inflammatory activity. It can be used with or without opiates to treat postoperative pain (a morphine-sparing effect). Like all NSAIDs, it can cause gastrointestinal upset or bleeding, asthma, renal failure or blood clotting disturbances.

Dose: 10 mg i.m./i.v., up to a maximum of 30 mg/day.

Narcotic antagonists

Naloxone (Narcan) is the specific antagonist of all the narcotics (e.g. fentanyl, morphine and pethidine). The agonist actions (respiratory depression and analgesia) are completely reversed within 1 minute of i.v. injection, the action lasting 30 minutes.

Indications: It is used to antagonize respiratory depression caused by the narcotic agents. It has a definitive role in reversing the respiratory depression caused by intrathecal morphine (in this instance, analgesia is not reversed) and treating neonatal respiratory depression. However, the action of naloxone may not last as long as the opioid it is reversing, and there is a danger of 'renarcotization' at 30 minutes. Patients should therefore be closely monitored for a suitable period of time after naloxone treatment.

Dosage: In adults, 0.2–0.4 mg i.v. for an immediate effect and a further 0.4 mg i.m. for prolonging the effect.

Side-effects and precautions: Because naloxone has a short action, its administration may need to be repeated and patients must be observed closely for a suitable period of time.

INTRAVENOUS INDUCTION AGENTS

An ideal intravenous induction agent should satisfy the following criteria. The drug should:

- be stable in solution, be water soluble and have a long shelf-life;
- be non-irritant to the veins or tissues if accidentally injected outside the vein;
- produce sleep in one arm–brain circulation time, i.e. the amount of time the drug takes to travel from the arm to the brain; in a normal fit person this is 15 s, but the time is prolonged in the elderly and those with a low cardiac output;

- produce rapid recovery with little hangover effect;
- not produce excitatory effects such as tremor, involuntary muscle movements, hiccups and laryngospasm;
- not cause undue respiratory and cardiovascular depression;
- have a very low incidence of hypersensitivity reactions.

None of the currently available i.v. induction agents possesses all these characteristics. The important classes of i.v. induction agent are:

1. Barbiturates: thiopentone, methohexitone
2. Imidazoles: etomidate
3. Phenols: propofol
4. Phencyclidines: ketamine.

Thiopentone is a thiobarbiturate presented as a yellowish white powder. It is supplied mixed with sodium carbonate as thiopentone is soluble only in strong alkaline solutions (pH 10.5).

When given i.v., it produces loss of consciousness within 15–20 s (one arm–brain circulation time) in a fit adult patient, because thiopentone is taken up by brain tissue. When its plasma and brain concentration falls, the patient regains consciousness. Thiopentone is not completely metabolized but is redistributed to fat and other vascular tissues in the early stages.

On i.v. injection, there is a fall in blood pressure due to peripheral vasodilatation, which becomes marked in patients with hypovolaemia. Thiopentone can induce laryngospasm during induction, and respiratory depression (including apnoea) for a short duration. It is metabolized in the liver and excreted via the kidneys.

Indications: For the induction of anaesthesia and in the treatment of status epilepticus.

Dosage: 3–5 mg/kg body weight; it is available as a single dose vial of 500 mg in 20 ml.

Side-effects and precautions: Laryngospasm, bronchospasm and, if injected outside the vein, severe pain. If thiopentone is accidentally injected intra-arterially, it can cause acute pain; if not treated urgently, thrombosis and gangrene of the fingers occur. The use of thiopentone is

contraindicated in patients with a history of porphyria. It should be used with caution in patients with a known difficult airway or known fixed or low cardiac output (as in aortic stenosis or hypovolaemia).

Methohexitone (Brietal) is a methylated barbiturate that causes loss of consciousness in one arm–brain circulation time. The patient recovers his consciousness in 2–3 minutes, the drug being redistributed to fat and other tissues. The arterial blood pressure does not fall as markedly as thiopentone. Unlike thiopentone, methohexitone will not stop seizures (as in epilepsy or electroconvulsive therapy).

Indications: As patients recover more quickly and are more alert than when thiopentone is used, methohexitone is used in outpatient anaesthesia and electroconvulsive therapy.

Dosage: 1.5 mg/kg body weight. A 1% solution is made up by adding 10 ml of water to a vial containing 100 mg methohexitone.

Side-effects and precautions: Hiccups and involuntary movements are quite often seen.

Etomidate, an imidazoline derivative, causes loss of consciousness in one arm–brain circulation time. The patient recovers within 2 minutes. It does not cause a fall in blood pressure (cardiovascularly stable).

Indications: The induction of anaesthesia in frail, hypovolaemic patients, and also in outpatient anaesthesia.

Dosage: 0.3 mg/kg body weight.

Side-effects and precautions: Nausea, vomiting and involuntary movements.

Propofol is presented in a concentration of 10 mg/ml in a lipid emulsion and is a di-isopropyl phenol. Induction occurs within one arm–brain circulation time, and the recovery is rapid. Pain on injection can be prevented by mixing it with 1% plain lignocaine or injecting an analgesic before the propofol.

Dosage: 1–2 mg/kg for the induction of anaesthesia. For total i.v. anaesthesia, 6–10 mg/kg/h is given as an infusion.

Ketamine is an acidic solution that can be used to induce sleep when given either i.m. or i.v. If given i.v., it produces loss of consciousness in one arm–brain circulation time. It is also called a dissociative anaesthetic agent. Ketamine produces intense analgesia followed by loss of consciousness. If given to adults, ketamine induces hallucinations and bizarre dreams. If they are disturbed during recovery from ketamine, patients may react violently. For this reason, the patient is given 5–10 mg diazepam to prevent hallucinations and dreams and is not disturbed until he fully recovers.

Ketamine causes a rise in blood pressure, heart rate, intraocular pressure and intracranial pressure.

Indications: In patients with difficult airways (burns or trauma of face and upper airway) and in poor-risk patients. Ketamine is used for the induction of anaesthesia in children below 10 years of age for neuroradiological procedures, radiotherapy and cardiac catheterization. It is also used to treat bronchospasm in status asthmaticus.

Dosage: When given i.v. (2 mg/kg), it produces anaesthesia within 30 s, lasting for 5–10 minutes. If given i.m. (10 mg/kg), it produces a loss of consciousness in 4 minutes that lasts for 15–30 minutes. It can also be given as a continuous infusion, and the anaesthetic effects can be reversed using 0.5–1.0 mg physostigmine without affecting the analgesia.

Side-effects: Hallucinations, dreams, hypertension, vomiting and increased secretions. Ketamine is contraindicated in patients with hypertension, angina and raised intracranial pressure.

DRUGS ACTING ON THE RESPIRATORY SYSTEM

Prophylaxis and treatment of bronchial asthma

Sodium cromoglycate (Intal) does not prevent bronchoconstriction, nor does it cause bronchodilatation. It acts by preventing the release of the histamine which is produced as a result of an antigen–antibody reaction. (The antigen is the allergic source coming from outside, such as dust or feathers; the antibody is the immunoglobulin produced in response to the antigen.)

Indications: As prophylaxis against an attack of bronchial asthma.

Dosage: It is inhaled 4–8 times a day from a single-dose, 20 mg cartridge (Spincap) inhaler.

Salbutamol (Ventolin) has a highly selective action on bronchial musculature when given by an aerosol (inhaler or nebulizer). The action is immediate and longlasting; the maximum effect is seen in 5 minutes, and its action lasts for 4–6 hours.

Indications: Bronchospasm from any cause, including bronchial asthma.

Dosage: It is given as a metered aerosol inhaler (giving 100 µg during each inhalation). In the wards and recovery room, a mixture of 1 ml (2.5 mg) salbutamol plus 1 ml normal saline is given to the patient, nebulized with oxygen.

In an operating theatre emergency, an i.v. injection of salbutamol (2–4 µg/kg) can be given. Salbutamol is also prescribed orally 2–4 mg four times a day.

Terbutaline is similar to salbutamol in action, reaching its peak effect 30 minutes after subcutaneous injection.

Aminophylline is related to caffeine. It stimulates the respiratory centre, causes a small rise in blood pressure and induces dilatation of the smooth muscles of the bronchioles.

Indications: In the treatment of bronchial asthma and bronchospasm of any cause.

Dosage: It can be given orally 100–300 mg 3–4 times a day or as a rectal suppository (360 mg). In an emergency, a 10 ml ampoule (containing 250 mg) of aminophylline can be injected slowly i.v. to relieve bronchospasm.

Respiratory stimulants

Doxapram (Dopram) stimulates respiration by acting directly on the medullary respiratory centres. In low doses, it increases the tidal volume, and in high doses also increases the respiratory rate.

The injection of doxapram causes a small rise in blood pressure and heart rate.

Indications: To reverse the respiratory depression caused by narcotics (fentanyl, papaveretum and morphine). An advantage of doxapram is that (unlike naloxone) it does not reverse the analgesia caused by these drugs.

Dosage: 1–5 mg/kg body weight i.v. in the postoperative period to reverse respiratory depression, repeated at 2-hourly intervals. It can also be used in the ward in the treatment of respiratory failure as an infusion, the recommended rate being 1–3 mg/min of a 0.2% solution.

DRUGS ACTING ON THE CARDIOVASCULAR SYSTEM

DRUGS ACTING ON THE HEART
Inotropic and chronotropic drugs

These terms need to be defined before discussion of the various drugs included in this category.

- *Inotropic drugs* are those which alter the force or the contraction of the heart beat, for example digoxin, dopamine and dobutamine.
- *Chronotropic drugs* are those which influence the heart rate by increasing or decreasing it. A good example is isoprenaline.

Digoxin (Lanoxin) is prepared from the leaf of Digitalis lanata. It is chemically related to steroids and the sex hormones. Digitalis has no effect on the normal heart, but in patients with congestive cardiac failure, it increases the force of contraction, decreases the size of the dilated heart and increases the cardiac output. It also slows the conduction of impulses from the atrium to the ventricle, thus slowing the ventricular rate in atrial fibrillation. It increases the urinary output (diuretic effect) indirectly by increasing the cardiac output.

Metabolism: Digitalis can be given orally or i.v.; the absorption of the drug depends very much on its formulation. Digoxin acts in 1–4 hours and the effect lasts for 1–2 days. It is broken down and excreted by the kidneys.

Indications: In the treatment of congestive cardiac failure and atrial fibrillation.

Dosage: Orally 0.5 mg initially, followed by 0.25 mg 6 hourly. In an emergency (theatre), 0.5 mg (diluted) slowly i.v. initially, followed by 0.5–0.25 mg every 6 hours.

Precautions and side-effects: Digoxin is not given after a myocardial infarction and should be given with caution in patients with renal impairment. Nausea, vomiting and bradycardia are early signs of overdose.

Isoprenaline (Saventrine) is an inotrope related to other catecholamines (such as adrenaline). Isoprenaline has a powerful stimulating action on the heart and increases the heart rate. It produces a fall in blood pressure by peripheral vasodilatation. Isoprenaline causes dilatation of the bronchial smooth muscle and also inhibits the release of histamine.

Indications: To treat bradycardia following heart block.

Dosage: In the treatment of heart block, 1 mg isoprenaline is added to 500 ml of 5% dextrose and given at the rate of 2–4 µg/min.

Side-effects: Tachycardia, chest pain, palpitations, headache, nausea and vomiting. It should be used with great caution in patients with thyrotoxicosis.

Dopamine (Intropin) is a naturally occurring transmitter found in the brain and kidneys, being the precursor of noradrenaline and adrenaline. It exerts an inotropic effect by increasing the cardiac output, with a slight rise in systolic pressure, and has a specific vasodilatory effect on the renal artery, thus increasing renal blood flow.

Indications: In the treatment of hypotension, following open heart surgery and in the early stages of renal failure.

Dosage: Dopamine is available as 200 µg in a 5 ml ampoule that is added to 500 ml of 5% dextrose, giving a dilution of 400 µg/ml. To improve renal blood flow, dopamine is started at the rate of 2–5 µg/kg/min. At doses greater than 5 µg/kg/min, its cardiac effects predominate.

Side-effects and precautions: Tachycardia and peripheral vasoconstriction as the dosage is increased. It is not advisable to use it in patients with phaeochromocytoma or cardiac arrhythmia. It should always be administered via a central vein as extravasation can cause skin necrosis.

Dobutamine (Dobutrex) has no effect on renal blood flow but does have a specific action in increasing the contractility of the heart. In higher doses, it is less likely than dopamine to cause tachycardia, and it can be given through a peripheral vein if necessary.

Indications: Cardiogenic shock following myocardial infarction; after cardiac surgery.

Dosage: It is available as 250 mg in a 10 ml ampoule, which is diluted in 500 ml of 5% dextrose. It is given at the rate of 2–10 μg/kg/min.

Sometimes a combination of dopamine and dobutamine is used, the former to improve renal perfusion and the latter to improve cardiac function in patients with cardiogenic shock.

Chronotropic drugs are those which increase the heart rate, examples being adrenaline and noradrenaline. As these agents also increase blood pressure, they will be discussed below under vasopressors.

Antidysrhythmics

Antidysrhythmics are those agents which are used to treat cardiac arrhythmias. They are classified according to their site of action on the action potential of a cardiac nerve fibre. It is not necessary for readers to have a detailed explanation of their mode of action. A few antidysrhythmics that are used in the operating theatre are described below.

Quinidine (Delanide) is used in the treatment of ventricular extrasystoles and ventricular paroxysmal tachycardia.

Dosage: 300 mg three times a day orally.

Lignocaine (Xylocaine) is used to treat ventricular dysrhythmias following myocardial infarction. It is one of the drugs seen in the cardiac arrest drug box.

Dosage: a loading dose of 1–2 mg/kg body weight followed by an infusion of 1–4 mg/min for 48 hours. Overdose can lead to seizures.

Mexiletine (Mexitil) is used in the treatment of ventricular arrhythmias following myocardial infarction.

Dosage: 100–250 mg i.v. as a bolus, followed by an infusion, the oral dose being 400–600 mg initially, followed by 200 mg four times a day.

Propranolol (Inderal) is used to treat a range of supraventricular and ventricular arrhythmias.

Dosage: 1 mg i.v. repeated up to a maximum of 10 mg. Alternatively, practolol (Eraldin) 5 mg is given slowly i.v. during an emergency in the operating theatre. (See also beta-blockers, p. 68.)

Amiodarone (Cordarone) is used to treat resistant supraventricular tachycardias.

Verapamil (Cordilox) is used in the treatment of supraventricular tachycardias. It is given i.v. (during an emergency), the dose being 5–10 mg over 30 s. Incorrect usage can be associated with severe complications, including death.

Cardiac arrhythmias in the operating theatre

Cardiac arrhythmias can be seen in patients who are spontaneously breathing a mixture of gases, especially halothane. If the patient hypoventilates due to increased anaesthetic depth, carbon dioxide retention occurs, which stimulates the release of catecholamines (adrenaline and noradrenaline) in the body. These in turn make the cardiac muscle irritable and, especially in the presence of halothane, dysrhythmias such as ventricular extrasystole and heart block are seen. The treatment consists of reducing the concentration of halothane and improving the patient's ventilation (manually or by intermittent positive-pressure ventilation). By getting rid of the excess of carbon dioxide, most of the dysrhythmias disappear. If some irregularity still persists, a change of inhalational agent, optimization of oxygenation or specific antidysrhythmic drug treatment is required.

VASOPRESSORS

Vasopressors are those drugs which increase the blood pressure. In anaesthetic practice, sympathomimetic agents that stimulate the heart or vasoconstrictors are used. In patients with hypotension caused by vasodilatation (spinal and epidural analgesia), or following the removal of a phaeochromocytoma, vasopressors such as ephedrine and noradrenaline are used. In all these cases, it is essential to treat any hypovolaemia (blood loss) before giving vasopressors.

Some of the vasopressors used in the operating theatre are described below.

Adrenaline is a naturally occurring hormone that can be synthesized commercially. In therapeutic doses, it induces a rise in systolic blood pressure with a fall in diastolic pressure; in large doses, it causes a rise in both systolic and diastolic pressure. Adrenaline induces relaxation of the bronchial smooth muscles.

Indications: To prolong the effect of local anaesthetics by causing vasoconstriction at the site of injection (see local anaesthetics on p. 73); it is also used in the treatment of bronchial asthma, anaphylactic shock and cardiac arrest.

Dosage: When adrenaline is used to increase the duration of local anaesthetics, a solution (lignocaine with adrenaline) with a concentration of 1:200 000 is used. For directions on how to make up the dilutions, see the Appendix.

Use of adrenaline during anaesthesia: Adrenaline is used by surgeons to decrease bleeding from the skin incision during surgery on the thyroid gland or mastoid region and during plastic surgery. Adrenaline solutions should have a maximum concentration of 1:100 000 or 1:200 000, and the total dose should not exceed 10 ml of 1:100 000 solution in 10 minutes of surgery.

Ephedrine is a sympathomimetic amine produced synthetically; it has both alpha and beta effects (see beta-blockers on p. 68 for an explanation). It causes an increase in blood pressure and cardiac output. Ephedrine stimulates respiration and dilates the bronchial smooth muscles.

Indications: To treat the hypotension caused by sympathetic blockade during spinal and epidural anaesthesia. It is especially useful in pregnant women because it does not cause constriction of the blood vessels supplying the placenta.

Dosage: To correct hypotension during spinal and epidural anaesthesia, 30 mg is diluted in 10 ml of normal saline and bolus doses of 1–5 mg are given as required. Intramuscular injections of 15 mg can be given to produce a longer-lasting effect.

Side-effects and precautions: Anxiety, restlessness, tachycardia and hypertension. It is contraindicated in patients with coronary artery disease.

Mephentermine sulphate is a sympathomimetic amine with both alpha and beta effects. It increases the arterial blood pressure, heart rate and cardiac output.

Indications: It has been used to treat and maintain blood pressure following the withdrawal of a noradrenaline drip in patients who have undergone removal of a phaeochromocytoma.

Dosage: 15 mg mephentermine is given i.m. or i.v. to treat hypotension. When given i.m., it acts within 5–10 minutes and lasts for up to 2 hours; when given i.v., it acts within 2 minutes, the action lasting for less than 1 hour.

Methoxamine hydrochloride (Vasoxine) is a sympathomimetic agent with an alpha effect. Methoxamine increases the blood pressure by causing marked peripheral vasoconstriction (alpha effect). The cardiac output and heart rate are decreased.

Indications: To prevent and treat hypotension during spinal and epidural anaesthesia, except in pregnant women where the alpha vasoconstriction will reduce the placental blood supply.

Dosage: 5–10 mg given slowly i.v. improves the blood pressure within 2 minutes, the action lasting for an hour.

Metaraminol tartrate (Aramine) is a sympathomimetic agent with both alpha and beta effects. It increases the cardiac output and arterial blood pressure.

Indications: In the treatment of hypotension following spinal and epidural anaesthesia.

Dosage: 1–5 mg given slowly i.v. restores the blood pressure within 3 minutes, the action lasting for 25 minutes. A dose of 2–10 mg given i.m. acts within 10 minutes and lasts for an hour.

Noradrenaline (Levophed) is a naturally occurring hormone that can also be manufactured synthetically. Noradrenaline has powerful alpha and weak beta effects. It produces an increase in systolic and diastolic blood pressure due to a marked peripheral vasoconstriction. The cardiac output remains unchanged, with a slower heart rate.

Indications: To treat hypotension following the removal of a phaeochromocytoma.

Dosage: It is given as an i.v. infusion; 2 mg when added to 500 ml of 5% dextrose gives a dilution of 4 µg/ml. The drip is started at 2 ml/min and the rate adjusted according to the blood pressure.

Precautions: Noradrenaline must always be given through a central vein because it will cause gangrene of the skin if it leaks subcutaneously.

Phenylephrine hydrochloride (Neophryn) is a sympathomimetic with strong alpha and weak beta effects. The blood pressure is increased due to peripheral vasoconstriction without any changes in heart rate.

Indications: In the treatment of hypotension (following hypotensive anaesthesia) and for the relief of nasal congestion (nasal surgery). During halothane anaesthesia, phenylephrine is less likely to cause dysrhythmias than is the alternative, adrenaline.

Dosage: To correct hypotension, 0.5 mg is given i.v. or i.m. or as an infusion. To relieve nasal congestion, 1–4 drops of 0.5–1.0% phenylephrine are instilled into the nose.

VASODILATORS AND ANTIHYPERTENSIVE AGENTS

A variety of drugs lower blood pressure. In this section, a few drugs prescribed to lower blood pressure in daily practice (antihypertensives) and deliberately lower blood pressure in the operating theatre (hypotensive agents and vasodilators; see p. 69) will be described.

'Deliberate hypotension' is used by the anaesthetist (see p. 194) to:

- make the operative surgical field bloodless;
- decrease the blood pressure in the immediate postoperative period following coronary artery surgery.

Drugs acting on the central nervous system (hypothalamus)

Most general anaesthetics and barbiturates depress the hypothalamus and cause a fall in blood pressure.

Methyldopa (Aldomet) probably acts on the brainstem vasomotor centre where it causes a stimulation of alpha receptors, which inhibits the outflow from the vasomotor centre and therefore leads to vasodilatation and a fall in blood pressure.

Indications: In the treatment of hypertension, with or without a diuretic.

Dosage: Methyldopa is started at 250 mg three times a day orally and gradually increased to 2 g per day after 48 hours.

Side-effects and precautions: Sedation, mental depression, postural hypotension and occasionally haemolytic anaemia. It is contraindicated in patients with liver disease or phaeochromocytoma.

Clonidine (Catapres) acts by stimulating alpha receptors in the hypothalamus, causing a fall in blood pressure, heart rate and cardiac output.

Indication: Hypertension.

Dosage: 200–300 µg/day orally.

Precautions: If clonidine is abruptly withdrawn, marked hypertension develops. Hence patients receiving clonidine treatment should have alternative antihypertensive therapy started if they cannot take their clonidine orally postoperatively. (All patients should continue to take their antihypertensives until operation.)

Hydralazine hydrochloride (Apresoline) produces a fall in blood pressure by acting on the alpha receptors in the hypothalamus and directly acting on the arterioles peripherally.

Indications: In present practice, it is used in hypertensive crises and pre-eclamptic toxaemia.

Dosage: 10–40 mg i.v., followed by an infusion.

Drugs acting on preganglionic sympathetic fibres

Local anaesthetic drugs such as lignocaine or bupivacaine, when used for spinal and epidural analgesia, paralyse the preganglionic sympathetic fibres, thus causing a fall in blood pressure and peripheral vasodilatation.

Drugs acting on the autonomic ganglion (ganglion blockers)

Autonomic ganglia carry both parasympathetic and sympathetic fibres, and the drugs that interfere at this site are called ganglion blockers. These blockers have been used to produce deliberate hypotension. Although a number of ganglion-blocking agents have been described, the only drug still used in the operating theatre is trimetaphan (Arfonad).

Trimetaphan (Arfonad) is a rapidly acting ganglion blocker with an onset of action of 1–3 minutes and lasting for 10–15 minutes after one dose. The hypotensive action of trimetaphan is potentiated by the patient adopting a slight head-up position.

Indications: To produce induced or controlled hypotension.

Dosage: It can be given in a bolus dose of 50 mg and repeated at 10–15-minute intervals (10–20 mg). For a continuous infusion, a 0.1% solution (500 mg trimetaphan in 500 ml of 5% dextrose) is used with an initial rate of 2–4 ml/min. The infusion is adjusted according to the blood pressure.

Side-effects: Tachycardia and tachyphylaxis. Tachyphylaxis is the state in which repeated doses have less and less effect; this develops within minutes.

Drugs acting on postganglionic sympathetic neurons

These drugs act by decreasing the sympathetic activity, thus causing a fall in heart rate, blood pressure and cardiac output. Examples in this group are guanethidine, reserpine and debrisoquine.

Guanethidine (Ismelin) is used as an anti-hypertensive agent. In pain relief clinics, guanethidine is used to improve local blood flow in the extremities.

Dosage: For the treatment of blood pressure, 10 mg orally increasing each week. To improve blood flow to a limb, 10–20 mg guanethidine, 100 IU heparin and 1% lignocaine made up to 10 ml with normal saline is injected into the periphery of the affected limb after it has been isolated from the rest of the circulation by an occlusive tourniquet. The tourniquet is then left inflated for at least 20 minutes.

Drugs acting on adrenergic receptors

The activity of the sympathetic nervous system is mediated by two different receptors called alpha (α) and beta (β). Adrenergic receptor-blocking drugs act by competing with adrenaline and noradrenaline for the α- and β-receptors on the effector organs such as heart, blood vessels and bronchi. The α-receptors are present in the peripheral blood vessels and the β-receptors in the heart and bronchi.

When the α-receptors are stimulated, the peripheral vessels are constricted, thus maintaining the blood pressure or increasing it. Beta-receptors are divided into two groups: β_1-receptors are present on the heart muscle, and β_2-receptors are present on bronchi, arteries, the uterus and skeletal muscle.

Alpha-adrenergic receptor blockers

These drugs block the alpha responses of adrenaline, producing hypotension (due to vaso-dilatation), compensatory tachycardia, congestion of mucous membranes and pupillary constriction.

Tolazoline (Priscol) has powerful but brief action on the peripheral vessels. It is used as a trial drug in vascular diseases.

Phentolamine (Rogitine) is a short-acting agent, with an onset of action in 2 minutes and lasting up to 15 minutes following an i.v. injection. After i.v. injection, it causes a fall in blood pressure and an increase in cardiac output and heart rate secondary to a fall in peripheral resistance (vasodilatation).

Indications: In the control of blood pressure fluctuations following open heart surgery and to control hypertension during surgery for the removal of a phaeochromocytoma.

Dosage: To control blood pressure, 5 mg should be given slowly i.v.

Phenoxybenzamine (Dibenamine) is a powerful α-adrenergic blocking agent. It has a slow onset of action (1 hour), the drug lasting for a very long time. Its action cannot be easily reversed. Phenoxybenzamine causes a fall in blood pressure by decreasing the peripheral resistance (vasodilatation).

Indications: In the treatment of peripheral vascular disease and in the control of hypertension in phaeochromocytoma.

Dosage: It is given orally 20 mg three times a day, increasing up to 120 mg a day.

Side-effects and precautions: Nausea, vomiting, sedation and postural hypotension.

Prazosin is a powerful α-adrenergic blocker that lowers the blood pressure without associated tachycardia.

Beta-adrenergic receptor blockers

These drugs block only the beta effects of adrenaline – the cardiac effects – resulting in a decreased heart rate and cardiac output (due to reduced myocardial contractility). Some of the beta-blockers (β_1) are cardioselective and some non-selective (i.e. they also act on β-receptor sites in the lungs).

The main uses of beta-blockers, with their mode of action and adverse side-effects, are given in Box 2.3. This is followed by a description of important beta-blockers.

Box 2.3 Uses of beta-blockers	
Disease	*Mode of action of beta-blockers*
Angina pectoris	Reduce cardiac work
Cardiac arrhythmias	Decrease the drive to the cardiac pacemaker
Hyperthyroidism	Reduce cardiac output and heart rate
Phaeochromocytoma	Block beta effects of circulating adrenaline and noradrenaline
Glaucoma	Decrease the production and outflow of aqueous humour

Side-effects: The beta-blockers produce heart failure, vasoconstriction, bronchoconstriction and hypoglycaemia.

Cardioselective (β_1) beta-blockers

Practolol (Eraldin) is 2.5 times less active than propranolol.

Indications: To control cardiac arrhythmias occurring during anaesthesia.

Dosage: Practolol is given as 4–10 mg i.v. repeated at 5-minute intervals.

Atenolol is used in the treatment of hypertension.

Dosage: 100 mg once a day, increasing to 200 mg after 2 weeks.

Non-cardioselective ($\beta_1 + \beta_2$) blockers

Oxprenolol (Trasicor) slows the heart rate, associated with a fall in cardiac output.

Indications: In the control of angina pectoris and cardiac arrhythmias.

Dosage: It is given as 20 mg two or three times a day orally for arrhythmias and 40 mg three times a day for angina.

Side-effects: It can precipitate bronchoconstriction in patients with bronchial asthma.

Propranolol (Inderal) decreases the heart rate and cardiac output and, in the hypertensive patient, causes a fall in blood pressure after prolonged treatment.

Indications: To control tachyarrhythmias during anaesthesia and manage tachycardia in patients with phaeochromocytoma. Propranolol is effective in the treatment of angina. In the operating theatre, 0.5–5.0 mg is given slowly i.v. to correct arrhythmias. In the treatment of angina pectoris, it is given as 80 mg four times a day.

Side-effects and precautions: Sleepiness during the day, impotence and bad dreams are the common side-effects. Propranolol precipitates bronchospasm in patients with bronchial asthma.

The other non-selective beta-blockers available are sotalol, timolol eye drops and pindolol.

Labetalol (Trandate) has both α- and β-adrenoreceptor blocking actions. It is used when rapid control of blood pressure is essential.

Indications: In hypertensive crises and phaeochromocytoma.

Dosage: It is given initially 5–10 mg i.v. repeated after 5 minutes if necessary.

Side-effects and precautions: Postural hypotension and bradycardia. It can precipitate bronchospasm in patients with bronchial asthma.

Esmolol is a newer, ultra short-acting beta-blocker useful for the minute-to-minute control of high blood pressure. It is most commonly given as an infusion.

Dosage: For supraventricular tachycardia 50–200 µg/kg/min; for perioperative tachycardia and hypertension 80 mg loading dose over 15s followed by a 150 µg/kg/min infusion.

Drugs acting on vascular smooth muscle

Some drugs act directly on the smooth muscle of arterioles and veins (without influencing the nerve supply), thus causing vasodilatation. Examples are given below.

Glyceryl trinitrate (GTN) (Nitroglycerin, Trinitrin) is available as a tablet, spray, patch or i.v. solution. It produces relaxation of the smooth muscles of large veins and postarteriolar blood vessels.

Its main use has been in the relief of the acute pain of angina pectoris. The action begins within 2 minutes and lasts for up to 30 minutes if the tablet is dissolved under the tongue. Glyceryl trinitrate is also used to decrease blood pressure by causing venous dilatation.

Dosage: 0.3–1.0 mg orally as required, the i.v. dose being 100–200 µg/min.

Side-effects and precautions: Light-headedness; in overdose, it causes methaemoglobinaemia.

Sodium nitroprusside (Nipride) has a direct vasodilator action on the smooth muscle of the vessel wall. It causes a fall in blood pressure and tachycardia without altering cardiac output.

Indications: To induce hypotension during surgery. It has also been used in the control of hypertension during the removal of a phaeochromocytoma.

Dosage: Sodium nitroprusside is given as an i.v. infusion; 50 mg is dissolved in either 500 ml or 100 ml of 5% dextrose and the infusion titrated according to the blood pressure. The maximum recommended dose is 3.5 mg/kg body weight.

Side-effects and precautions: Tachycardia. When the lethal dose (71.5 mg/kg body weight) is exceeded, toxicity occurs. The signs of toxicity are acidosis and the blood pressure not returning to normal in spite of the infusion being stopped. The toxicity is treated by using vitamin B_{12}, sodium nitrite and thiosulphate.

Sodium nitroprusside solution degenerates in light and should be wrapped in aluminium foil during administration to avoid deterioration.

Drugs acting on blood volume

Diuretics are those drugs which cause an increase in urine output. They are used in the treatment of oedema and ascites in congestive heart failure and renal failure. Diuretics act by affecting renal and extrarenal mechanisms.

Extrarenal diuretics, for example digoxin and aminophylline, act by increasing the cardiac output.

Renal mechanisms vary:

1. Some diuretics, such as osmotic diuretics (e.g. mannitol), act on the proximal convoluted tubule, increasing the osmolality of the tubular fluid and preventing water resorption.

2. Drugs such as frusemide (Lasix) and bumetanide (Burinex) act on the ascending limb of the loop of Henle and actively prevent sodium resorption. This leads to the formation of a large volume of urine.

3. Drugs such as triamterene, amiloride and spironolactone act by preventing the resorption of sodium and chloride in the distal tubule.

Some of the common diuretics used in the operating theatre are given below.

Acetazolamide (Diamox) acts as an inhibitor of the enzyme carbonic anhydrase, which is present in the distal tubules.
Indications: In the treatment of glaucoma and the oedema of heart failure.
Dosage: 250–500 mg once a day orally, the action lasting for 12 hours.

Frusemide (Lasix) (see above for its mechanism of action).
Indications: i.v. in the treatment of acute pulmonary oedema and congestive heart failure.
Dosage: In an emergency, 20–40 mg i.v. brings about a rapid response. In the treatment of heart failure, 40–80 mg is given orally.
Side-effects and precautions: Electrolyte imbalance (low potassium). Large i.v. doses can cause deafness.

Bumetanide (Burinex) acts as a loop diuretic (see above).
Indications: As for frusemide.
Dosage: 1 mg Burinex equals 40 mg frusemide in potency. In an emergency, 1–2 mg may be given i.v.

Mannitol is used to reduce the brain volume in cerebral oedema and in the prevention of renal failure (during hepatobiliary and aortic surgery).
Dosage: Mannitol is available as a 10 or 20% solution; the recommended dose is 0.5–1.0 g/kg body weight.

DRUGS ACTING ON THE UTERUS

Uterine stimulants

Uterine stimulants are those drugs used to encourage labour and delivery of the fetus.

Oxytocin (Syntocinon) acts mainly on the pregnant uterus, causing it to contract rhythmically.
Indications: To induce labour at term and contract the uterus after the birth of the fetus to prevent postpartum bleeding.
Dosage: 10–50 units are added to 5% dextrose and the rate adjusted to between 0.1 and 0.8 units per hour. Five units can be given i.v. during caesarean section. It is less likely than ergometrine to cause either vomiting or uncontrolled hypertension (see below).

Ergometrine maleate is a rapidly acting uterine stimulant that contracts the uterus in 30 seconds following an i.v. injection and 2–4 minutes after an i.m. injection. Its action lasts for 3–6 hours.
Indications: To contract the uterus following the delivery of placenta or during caesarean section.
Dosage: 0.25–0.5 mg i.v. or 0.2–1.0 mg i.m.
Side-effects and precautions: Headache, vomiting and hypertension. It should be used with caution in patients with pre-eclampsia and hypertension.

Prostaglandins are a group of polyunsaturated fatty acids. Prostaglandins E_2 (PGE_2) and prostaglandins $F_{2\alpha}$ ($PGF_{2\alpha}$) are used to stimulate the uterus.
Dosage: Labour can be induced with an infusion at the rate of 0.5–2.0 µg/min. Prostaglandins can be given orally as 0.5 mg of PGE_2 or 5 mg of $PGE_{2\alpha}$ to induce labour.
Side-effects: Nausea and vomiting.

Uterine inhibitors

Beta-adrenergic stimulant drugs such as salbutamol and ritodrine relax the uterus. Hence they are used to prevent premature labour in the first trimester.

Papaverine and **amyl nitrate** inhibit the muscles of the cervix, and **halothane** relaxes the uterus.

DRUGS ACTING ON THE ENDOCRINE SYSTEM

Hormones and drugs commonly seen in the operating theatre are briefly described here. Readers are asked to refer to a standard pharmacology textbook for details.

Pancreas

Insulin is a polypeptide that is synthesized and stored in the β-islet cells of the pancreas. It causes a fall in blood sugar level by increasing the glucose uptake in peripheral tissues.

Indications: The main indication for a synthetic insulin is diabetes mellitus.

Dosage and preparation: There are three types of insulin preparation:

1. short-acting (with rapid onset): neutral insulin injections such as Actrapid, soluble or regular insulin;
2. intermediate duration of action (with slower onset): insulin zinc suspension (e.g. Semilente and Semitard);
3. long duration of action: insulin zinc suspension (crystalline, ultralente or ultratard).

The choice of insulin(s) and the dose are adjusted to the individual patient and there is no fixed dose regimen.

Insulin and surgery: If a patient receiving a long-acting insulin is scheduled for minor surgery in the morning, her morning dose of insulin is omitted. If a patient who is on a long-acting insulin is scheduled for major surgery, she is admitted to the ward and the insulin preparation changed to a rapid-acting one such as Actrapid. When the blood sugar is adequately controlled, surgery is carried out.

Some diabetics are treated with **oral hypoglycaemics** such as chlorpropamide (Diabinese), tolbutamide (Rastinon) and glibenclamide (Daonil). If these patients are scheduled for minor surgery, the tablets are omitted on the day of surgery. If they are to undergo major surgery, some centres change the treatment from oral hypoglycaemics to Actrapid during the surgical period.

Adrenal gland

The synthetic corticosteroids that are available have an anti-inflammatory effect. The steroids available and used in theatre will be described.

Hydrocortisone (Efcortesol) has an immediate effect, which is short lived after an i.v. or i.m. injection.

Indications: Anaphylaxis, shock, status asthmaticus and as an anti-inflammatory agent. It is sometimes used to prevent laryngeal oedema after repeated attempts at intubation.

Dosage: 100 mg i.v.

Dexamethasone (Decadron) is used as an anti-inflammatory agent in the operating theatre, for example following maxillofacial surgery.

Dosage: 8 mg i.v. followed by 4–8 mg i.m. 8 hourly for 24 hours.

Methylprednisolone (Solu-medrone) is used by transplant surgeons as an immunosuppressant.

Patients who are on steroid therapy when they are scheduled for surgery are managed as follows:

• Patients who are receiving oral prednisolone should receive a slightly higher dose until after surgery, the dose then being tapered back to preoperative levels.

• If the patient was receiving regular steroids until about 3 months before surgery, hydrocortisone is given 100 mg i.m. before surgery and at 8-hourly intervals for 24 hours.

• If the patient was receiving a high dose of steroids for several years until up to 6 months before surgery, a regimen similar to that described above is followed.

DRUGS ACTING ON BLOOD

Histamine and H₁ and H₂ receptor antagonists

Histamine is a naturally occurring amine that is released in response to injury or an antigen–antibody reaction. Some drugs such as d-tubocurarine and morphine also release histamine. The actions of histamine are:

- increasing the acid and pepsin content of gastric juice;
- stimulation of any smooth muscle (e.g. bronchial muscle causing bronchospasm);
- dilating the arterioles and causing hypotension;
- dilatation and increased permeability of capillaries, leading to extravasation of plasma into the extracellular fluid and causing hypotension (from fluid loss) and oedema (from tissue swelling).

The action of histamine can be antagonized either by adrenaline or by preventing histamine from reaching its site of action (receptors), as by H_1 and H_2 receptor antagonists. H_1 receptors cause the latter three effects mentioned in the list above. H_2 receptors have an effect on gastric acid secretion.

H₁ receptor antagonists

H_1 receptor antagonists are also known as anti-histamines. These are effective against histamine-induced bronchoconstriction (except in asthma), histamine-induced capillary permeability and itching. Some antihistamines are effective in motion sickness. These are effective orally, i.m. or i.v.

Side-effects: Sedation, fatigue, tremors and dry mouth.

Some of the important antihistamines available in theatre are given below.

Chlorpheniramine maleate (Piriton) is used in an emergency (allergy to blood transfusion or penicillin) in a dose of 10–20 mg i.v. or i.m.

Dimenhydrinate (Dramamine) has a powerful antiemetic effect. It is effective against vomiting due to irradiation and the toxaemia of pregnancy.

Dosage: 50 mg diluted given slowly i.v. in an emergency, or 50–100 mg tablets 4 hourly.

The other common antihistamine, promethazine, is described on page 50.

H₂ receptor antagonists

H_2 receptors are present on the gastric parietal cells. As discussed above, H_2 receptor antagonists inhibit gastric acid secretion.

Cimetidine (Tagamet) is given orally or i.v. It effectively decreases the volume and pH of gastric acid secretion. It is used in the treatment of peptic ulcer and reflex oesophagitis, and as a prophylactic anaesthetic premedication (see premedication on p. 146).

Ranitidine (Zantac) is given either orally as 150 mg twice a day, or i.v. or i.m. in a dose of 50 mg. It is used in the treatment of benign gastric and duodenal ulceration and reflex oesophagitis. During emergency anaesthesia, ranitidine 50 mg i.v. can be used to inhibit any further gastric acid secretion. H_2 antagonists will have no effect on any acid already in the stomach.

Anticoagulants

Anticoagulants are those drugs which stop the formation of a further thrombus, i.e. a new thrombus (prophylactically) or the extension of a pre-existing thrombus (therapy). There are two types of anticoagulant: (1) directly acting and (2) indirectly acting.

Directly acting

These include heparin, which is rapidly effective and only acts for a few hours; it should be given i.v. or i.m.

Heparin is a highly acidic polysaccharide and is also found widely in the granules of mast cells in the connective tissue surrounding blood vessels. Heparin has a strong electronegative charge, and by its action on prothrombin and thrombin, prolongs the clotting time.

Indications: In theatre, it is used as an anticoagulant during open heart surgery and vascular (aortic) surgery. Pre- and postoperatively, it is also given in a low dose s.c. to prevent deep vein thrombosis.

Dosage: Heparin is available as biologically active units; the dose for open heart surgery is 300 IU/kg body weight. For prophylaxis, s.c. heparin is given in a dose of 5000 IU 8 hourly.

Side-effects: Occasional allergic reactions. It is incompatible with dextrose and hydrocortisone.

Protamine sulphate is used as an antidote to heparin. Protamine has a highly positive charge and can neutralize the negatively charged heparin molecule.

Indication: To reverse the effects of heparin.

Dosage: 1 mg protamine is given i.v. for each 100 IU heparin injected. At the end of open heart surgery, residual heparin activity is checked using the prothrombin time, and protamine is injected accordingly.

Indirectly acting

These include the coumarin and inandione groups (**Warfarin**) and **phenindione** (Dindevan). These drugs take 72 hours to become effective, and their action lasts for several days. Indirectly acting drugs are given orally.

These oral anticoagulants are stopped 72 hours prior to surgery, and the prothrombin time tested. If necessary, vitamin K is given to antagonize the effects, and the patient is allowed to proceed to surgery.

DRUGS ACTING ON THE NEUROMUSCULAR SYSTEM

LOCAL ANAESTHETIC AGENTS

Local anaesthetic agents are those agents which can produce a reversible depression of conduction of the nerve impulse. They can be injected into the subcutaneous tissue (infiltration), near to nerves (brachial plexus or individual nerve block), into the epidural or subarachnoid space, or as an i.v. local analgesic (Bier's block).

General pharmacological actions and side-effects of local anaesthetics

They can penetrate the blood–brain barrier and stabilize excitable cells (e.g. neurons); thus some agents can control status epilepticus if given i.v. in adequate doses. If given in large doses, they can cause convulsions and coma. Local anaesthetics such as lignocaine and procaine also have general analgesic properties. Some of the local anaesthetics, for example procainamide and lignocaine, have been used in the control of ventricular arrhythmias. All local anaesthetics except lignocaine and cocaine cause peripheral vasodilatation; cocaine causes vasoconstriction.

In a mild toxic reaction (or overdose), the patient becomes pale and restless and the symptoms pass off without treatment. In a severe reaction, convulsions followed by cardiorespiratory arrest can occur. Management of a toxic dose of local anaesthetic consists of 100% oxygen, artificial ventilation and cardiac massage as required.

Use of adrenaline to prolong the action

The effect of a local anaesthetic wears off when it is removed from the site of administration by absorption into the bloodstream. Thus anything which delays its absorption into the circulation will prolong its local action and reduce its toxicity. Adrenaline, when used in a concentration of 1:200 000, will double the duration of action (e.g. to 1–2 hours). Adrenaline should not be used with a local anaesthetic when performing blocks on the finger, toe or penis, as adrenaline-induced vasoconstriction may lead to gangrene at these sites.

Some of the common local anaesthetic agents used are given below.

Lignocaine (Xylocaine) is a rapidly acting agent whose action is intense and longlasting.

Indications: Lignocaine is widely used for a number of procedures by local infiltration, topical application (4% Xylocaine for endotracheal tubes and spray) and nerve, epidural and caudal blocks. It is also used to control dysrhythmias following myocardial infarction.

Dosage: Lignocaine is used as follows, with or without the use of adrenaline:

- For a nerve block: 1% solution with adrenaline (10 ml for single nerves).
- For infiltration analgesia: 0.5% solution 100 ml (500 mg) with adrenaline and 40 ml (200 mg) without adrenaline.
- For spinal analgesia: 1.0–1.5 ml of 5% heavy Xylocaine (plain).
- For epidural and caudal blocks: 15–50 ml of a 1.5% solution with adrenaline.
- For a topical spray of pharynx and larynx: 4 ml of 4% solution.

For the treatment of arrhythmias, see page 64.

Bupivacaine (Marcain) has a longer duration of action (3–6 hours) and a slower onset than lignocaine.

Indications: For nerve blocks and epidural analgesia in labour and for surgery. Nowadays, heavy bupivacaine (0.5%) is used for spinal analgesia.

Dosage: Bupivacaine is available as 0.25%, 0.5% and 0.75% solutions, the first two being available either plain or with adrenaline. Heavy bupivacaine (0.5% with dextrose) is available for spinal analgesia.

The maximum dose is 2–3 mg/kg with or without adrenaline in a 4-hour period. For spinal analgesia, 3–4 ml heavy or plain Marcain is used. 'Heavy' Marcain is so called because it is denser than spinal fluid and therefore sinks to whichever part of the body is lowermost – the position of the patient will influence the distribution of the anaesthetic and thus the level of the block. Local anaesthetic with adrenaline is never used at sites where the adrenaline-induced constriction of blood vessels could be damaging, for example in finger, toe, penile or spinal blocks (although its use in epidural blocks is safe).

Ropivacaine is an amide type of local anaesthetic with properties similar to those of bupivacaine.

Prilocaine (Citanest) has a longer duration of action than lignocaine and is less toxic.

Indications: Nowadays, it is used regularly for i.v. regional analgesia (Bier's block) and for epidural and nerve blocks.

Dosage: For i.v. regional analgesia, 30–40 ml of 0.5% plain solution is used. The maximum recommended dose is 400 mg with plain solution and 600 mg with adrenaline.

Side-effects: It can cause methaemoglobinaemia.

Cocaine is the only local anaesthetic drug to cause vasoconstriction. In addition to its local anaesthetic effects, it causes cerebral excitement, tachycardia, hypertension and a rise in respiratory rate due to sympathetic stimulation.

Indications: It is used only as a surface analgesic and a vasoconstrictor in nose (submucosal resection and polypectomy) and eye (dacryocystorhinostomy) surgery to produce analgesia and to decrease bleeding during the operation.

Dosage: Because cocaine causes vasoconstriction, adrenaline is not necessary and can be dangerous. A dose of 1.5 g/kg should not be exceeded. In eye surgery, a 4% solution is used, and for operations on the nose 10% and 20% solutions are employed.

Side-effects: It is a drug of addiction. An overdose causes headache, nausea and convulsions. The treatment of overdose consists of sedation and use of alpha- and beta-blockers to decrease the sympathetic overactivity caused by the cocaine.

MUSCLE RELAXANTS

As described in the section on physiology, there is at the junction between nerve and muscle a specialized portion of muscle membrane called a neuromuscular junction (NMJ). At rest, the sodium ion level is high extracellularly and the potassium ion level high intracellularly, thus maintaining an electrical potential across the membrane of the cell; the potential inside is usually about –90 mV. At the NMJ, acetylcholine (ACh), a neurotransmitter, is stored in synaptic vessels. On arrival of a nerve impulse, ACh is released and reacts with the receptors at the NMJ, which facilitates the movement of sodium inside and potassium outside the membrane. The NMJ loses its polarization and is called depolarized when the membrane potential is reduced from –90 mV to –45 mV. This potential is moved (propagated) along the muscle fibre, causing it to contract. After a few milliseconds, the acetylcholine that was released earlier now becomes completely hydrolysed to inactive choline and acetic acid in the presence of the enzyme cholinesterase. The cell membrane once again becomes impermeable to sodium ions (being extruded) and potassium ions (being pushed back into the cell). Thus the muscle fibre becomes repolarized and ready to respond to any further action potential.

If the mechanism described above is blocked, the nerve impulses reaching the muscle will be blocked (leading to muscle relaxation). There are two main types of blockers, which are described below:

1. *Depolarizing blockers*. Drugs in this category imitate the action of ACh at the NMJ (see above), but their action persists for up to 3–4 minutes. The initial depolarization which these drugs (e.g. suxamethonium) cause produces a short period of muscle contraction (seen as fasciculation). After fasciculating, the muscle relaxes because, as long as the drug is present at the muscle receptor, it cannot repolarize and thus cannot contract again. When the drug breaks down (see suxamethonium), the muscle recovers contractability.

2. *Non-depolarizing or competitive blockers*. These drugs compete with Ach for receptors at the NMJ. They do not cause depolarization themselves but block the NMJ receptor from depolarization by ACh. This results in paralysis of the muscles. The action of these drugs can be reversed with anticholinesterase drugs (see p. 77), which will prevent the destruction of ACh by cholinesterases, thus allowing the concentration of ACh to build up relative to the concentration of the blocking agent.

Dual block is seen when depolarizing relaxants are used in high doses or over a long period of time. This type of block may or may not be reversed by anticholinesterase drugs.

The depth or level of the neuromuscular block can be monitored using a peripheral nerve stimulator. The peripheral nerve stimulator is also used to help test the effectiveness of the reversal of the neuromuscular block by anticholinesterase (see p. 77).

Depolarizing muscle relaxants

Suxamethonium (Scoline, Anectine) is a short-acting relaxant. When it is injected i.v., it acts within 30 s, the action lasting up to 5 minutes. On i.v. injection, suxamethonium causes profound paralysis preceded by muscle fasciculations. When large and repeated doses of suxamethonium are used, it causes bradycardia and sometimes cardiac arrest.

Suxamethonium causes a dangerous rise in serum potassium in patients with burns, major injuries or abnormal muscles (e.g. muscular dystrophy). Suxamethonium causes an abrupt rise in intraocular pressure; hence it is contraindicated in patients with perforating eye injury (to avoid prolapse of the eye contents during this rise).

Suxamethonium is broken down by the enzyme plasma cholinesterase. If the plasma cholinesterase level is low, as in liver disease or malnutrition, or as a result of genetic factors, suxamethonium will not be broken down and hence will be long acting.

Suxamethonium does not cross the placenta. Neonates are resistant to its action.

Indications: It is used to facilitate rapid and easy intubation; suxamethonium is a useful short-acting muscle relaxant for endoscopies and electroconvulsive therapy. It can also be used for longer operations, in which it is given as a continuous infusion.

Dosage: 1.0–1.5 mg/kg body weight. For a continuous infusion, 500 mg suxamethonium is added to 500 ml of 5% dextrose and 600 μg atropine. The drip rate is adjusted according to the requirement of the patient. Special care must be taken to ensure that the drip is taken down once the operation is over; in no circumstances should a patient be returned to the recovery room with it still connected. Some hospitals add dye to the suxamethonium drip as well as the standard labelling, so that the drip is identifiable even from a distance.

Side-effects and precautions: Following the use of suxamethonium, young fit patients experience muscle pains for several days. It is not given to patients with congenital muscle disorders, a history of malignant hyperpyrexia, liver disease or known plasma cholinesterase deficiency. If suxamethonium is unknowingly given to the latter (pseudocholinesterase deficient) patients, a prolonged apnoea occurs. This is treated with intermittent positive-pressure ventilation and fresh frozen plasma.

Competitive or non-depolarizing muscle relaxants

These muscle relaxants are further divided into those with a short-to-medium duration of activity and those of long duration. Examples of those of short-to-medium duration are given below.

Atracurium (Tracrium) is a potent non-depolarizing relaxant of medium duration, a single dose lasting for 20–25 minutes. It has no cumulative effects (i.e. repeated doses last the same length of time). It undergoes spontaneous non-enzymatic degradation under normal body pH (7.4) and temperature (37°C) by the Hofmann elimination reaction. The drug is broken down irrespective of liver or renal damage.

Dosage: 0.6 mg/kg for intubation and maintenance of relaxation; 25% of the initial dose as 'top-ups'. For continuous infusion, the rate is 0.4 mg/kg body weight per hour. In large doses, atracurium can cause histamine release. It is presented as 25 mg in 2.5 ml, 50 mg in 5 ml, or 250 mg in 25 ml ampoules.

Vecuronium (Norcuron) is one of the cleaner muscle relaxants with no effect on the heart (the opposite of pancuronium, which causes tachycardia due to a vagolytic effect). Its action lasts for 20–30 minutes. The drug is excreted in bile;

hence it should be used with caution in patients with liver failure.

Dosage: 0.1–0.15 mg/kg body weight.

Mivacurium is a non-depolarizing muscle relaxant that produces good intubating conditions in 2–3 minutes and lasts 12–20 minutes. It is broken down by plasma cholinesterase.

Dosage: For intubation, 0.15–0.25 mg/kg; as a continuous infusion, 5–6 µg/kg/min.

Rocuronium is a steroidal neuromuscular blocking drug structurally similar to vecuronium. It is not metabolized but is excreted unchanged in the bile and urine. It has a duration of action similar to that of vecuronium.

Dosage: For intubation, 0.6 mg/kg; as a continuous infusion, 0.3–0.6 mg/kg/hour duration.

Examples of muscle relaxants of long duration are as follows.

d-Tubocurarine (Tubarine) takes 180 s to begin to act, the effect lasting for 30–40 minutes. Curare produces a fall in blood pressure with a rise in heart rate due to blocking of the sympathetic ganglia. It does not cross the placenta from mother to child. It is metabolized in the liver, so patients with liver disease require large amounts of this drug.

Indications: It is useful for long abdominal and thoracic operations.

Dosage: 0.45 mg/kg body weight. It is safely reversed with neostigmine in normal conditions.

Side-effects and contraindications: Its action is potentiated by hypercarbia and metabolic acidosis. It has a tendency to release histamine and can thus aggravate bronchospasm in patients with bronchial asthma.

Pancuronium (Pavulon). On i.v. injection, the patient is adequately paralysed within 90–120 s, the action lasting for 35–40 minutes. Pancuronium causes a rise in heart rate, blood pressure and cardiac output (a vagolytic effect). It is broken down in the liver and excreted in bile.

Indications: The same as for curare.

Dosage: 0.1 mg/kg body weight.

Side-effects and precautions: Its action is potentiated by respiratory acidosis.

Doxacurium is a non-depolarizing muscle relaxant that resembles pancuronium. It has its onset of action in 4–6 minutes, lasting for 40–70 minutes.
Dosage: 0.05–0.08 mg/kg.

Pipecuronium is a non-depolarizing muscle relaxant with an onset of action of 3–5 minutes and a duration of action of 40–70 minutes.
Dosage: 0.14 mg/kg.

Doxacurium and pipecuronium, because of their long duration of action, may not find a place in anaesthetic practice in the UK in preference to the continuous infusion of atracurium and vecuronium.

ANTICHOLINESTERASES

Anticholinesterases are those agents which inhibit or inactivate cholinesterases (which normally break down acetylcholine; see p. 74), thus raising the concentration of acetylcholine at all sites at which it is being released. High concentrations of acetylcholine at sites other than the NMJ (muscarinic receptors) will produce salivation, bradycardia, bronchospasm and abdominal colic (muscarinic effects). To counteract these unwanted effects, atropine is given.

Neostigmine is a synthetic anticholinesterase and has a prominent action on the NMJ and gastrointestinal tract. Its other actions are as mentioned above.
Indications: To antagonize the effects of competitive muscle relaxants and in the treatment of paralytic ileus (of the gastrointestinal tract) and myasthenia gravis.
Dosage: It is given orally for paralytic ileus and myasthenia gravis in a dose of 15–30 mg 3–4 times a day. To antagonize the muscle relaxant, neostigmine is given in a dose of 0.05–0.08 mg/kg body weight with atropine 0.02 mg/kg body weight (the ratio of neostigmine to atropine being nearly 2:1).

Side-effects and precautions: It is used with caution in patients with heart disease and asthma. Atropine should always be given with neostigmine to avoid bradycardia, salivation, etc.

Physostigmine (Eserine) is more potent than neostigmine and has the ability to penetrate the blood–brain barrier (which neostigmine cannot).
Indications: In myasthenia gravis, to reverse the central nervous depressant effects of atropine, hyoscine and benzodiazepines. Physostigmine drops are also used in the treatment of glaucoma.
Dosage: 0.5–1.0 mg i.v.

Pyridostigmine (Mestinon) is 50% less potent than neostigmine.
Indications: As for neostigmine.

PARASYMPATHETIC ANTAGONISTS AND ANTICHOLINERGIC AGENTS

The neurotransmitter at all preganglionic and postganglionic nerve endings is acetylcholine (except for sympathetic postganglionic nerve endings, which are adrenergic).

The receptors at the ganglion are described as nicotinic. All effector cell receptors (except those of the NMJ) are muscarinic. Antagonists of nicotinic receptors may be pure ganglion-blocking drugs (e.g. trimetaphan), muscle relaxants (e.g. vecuronium) or have a combined effect (e.g. d-tubocurarine). Antagonists of muscarinic receptors include the drugs atropine and glyco-pyrrolate.

Atropine is an alkaloid from the plant *Atropa belladona*. It initially stimulates the cerebral and medullary centres; this is followed by depression at high dosage. By blocking the muscarinic actions of acetylcholine, atropine prevents sweating, increases body temperature and causes the blood vessels in the skin to dilate (the atropine flush). Atropine increases the heart rate by blocking the heart's muscarinic receptors (called a vagolytic action because the effect on the heart is similar to that of cutting the vagus nerve). It causes a decrease in bronchial secretions, and the bronchial musculature is relaxed.

Indications: To antagonize the muscarinic actions of neostigmine. It is also used as a premedicant to decrease salivary and bronchial secretions (i.e. as an antisialogogue). Atropine is used to correct bradycardia. It is also used as drops to dilate the pupils in the eye (a mydriatic effect).

Dosage: It is given as 0.02 mg/kg body weight i.v. along with neostigmine (0.05–0.08 mg/kg) during the reversal of residual muscular paralysis.

For premedication, 0.2 mg/kg is given i.m. 1 hour before surgery. It is given 0.02 mg/kg i.v. for the treatment or prevention of bradycardia.

Side-effects and precautions: Atropine overdose causes dilatation of the pupils, blurred vision, dry mouth, delusions and sometimes convulsions. The treatment consists of physostigmine 0.5–1.0 mg i.v. Atropine should be avoided in patients with marked tachycardia (e.g. thyrotoxicosis and cardiac disease) or high fevers.

Hyoscine is similar to atropine in a number of actions. In small doses it causes bradycardia and in large doses tachycardia. It causes amnesia, and in elderly patients induces excitement and restlessness. Hyoscine dries up salivary and bronchial secretions effectively (antisialagogue effect) and is a powerful antiemetic agent.

Indications: As an antisialagogue, antiemetic and amnesic (during caesarean section) during general anaesthesia.

Dosage: 5–6 µg/kg body weight (approximately 0.2–0.4 mg) i.v.

Side-effects and precautions: It can cause drowsiness and all the side-effects of atropine. It should be avoided in patients above the age of 65 years.

Glycopyrrolate (Robinul) is an anticholinergic with no sedative properties because it cannot cross into the brain. It is a good antisialagogue and causes a slight change in heart rate with no effect on pupil size. It is used in combination with neostigmine (Robinul–neostigmine) in the reversal of neuromuscular block.

Dosage: 0.001 mg/kg.

DRUGS ACTING ON THE GASTROINTESTINAL SYSTEM

Antiemetics

The vomiting centre is situated in the hypothalamus and the chemoreceptor trigger zone near the fourth ventricle of the brain. Vomiting occurs due to stimulation of the emetic centre by various causes. The emetic substances could be opioid analgesics, such as morphine and pethidine, which act on the chemoreceptor trigger zone. Certain drugs, such as digitalis, may cause nausea by acting on the gastrointestinal tract as well as on the chemoreceptor trigger zone.

Postanaesthetic vomiting is due to a combination of factors, such as the type of surgery (especially ear surgery, tonsillectomy and cervical dilatation), the use of nitrous oxide and narcotics, and early mobilization in the postoperative period.

Vomiting can also occur during pregnancy, when flying and following exposure to radiation.

The antiemetic effect of drugs on the vomiting centre is due to anticholinergic action, and that on the chemoreceptor trigger zone is due to dopaminergic action. The important antiemetic agents available in the operating theatre are promethazine (see tranquillizers), dimenhydrinate (see antihistamines), prochlorperazine (see tranquillizers), hyoscine (see anticholinergics and parasympatholytics) and droperidol (see major tranquillizers).

Metoclopramide (Maxolon, Primperan) has a central action on the chemoreceptor trigger zone and a peripheral action on the upper gastrointestinal tract. It increases peristalsis and emptying of the stomach. This action on the gastrointestinal tract is blocked by opiate analgesics.

Indications: To help to empty the gastric contents during labour and emergency anaesthesia, and also to act as an antiemetic.

Dosage: 10 mg i.v. or i.m. every 8 hours.

Side-effects: It causes extrapyramidal dystonia (see phenothiazines) and should be used cautiously in children.

Domperidone (Motilium) is used in the treatment of nausea and vomiting, the dose being 10–20 mg every 4–8 hours.

Ondansetron (Zofran) is structurally related to serotonin and produces selective 5-hydroxy-tryptamine receptor antagonism. It is used as an antiemetic in oncology patients and in the management of postoperative nausea vomiting.
Dosage: 4–8 mg i.v. or orally.

Granisetron is a 5-HT3 receptor antagonist that produces an antiemetic effect for 24 hours following a single dose.
Dosage: 40 µg/kg i.v.

OTHER DRUGS USED IN ANAESTHESIA

Famotidine is a potent highly selective H_2 receptor antagonist. It inhibits the secretion of gastric acid for 12 hours. This drug has no adverse effects on the haemodynamic system.

Omeprazole blocks gastric acid secretion by selective inhibition of the H+-K+-ATPase proton pump in the parietal cell membrane. It is superior to H_2 receptor antagonists for the treatment of reflux oesophagitis and Zollinger–Ellison syndrome.

FURTHER READING

Dundee J W, Clarke R S J, McCaughey W 1991 Clinical anaesthetic pharmacology. Churchill Livingstone, Edinburgh

Dahl J B, Kehlet H 1993 The value of pre-emptive analgesia in the treatment of post operative pain. British Journal of Anaesthetics 70: 434–439

Orme M L 1986 NSAIDS and the kidneys. British Medical Journal 292: 1621–1622

Rang H P, Dale M M 1995 Pharmacology, 2nd edn. Churchill Livingstone, Edinburgh

Stoetling R K 1991 Pharmacology and physiology in anesthetic practice. J B Lippincott, Philadelphia

Sasada M P, Smith S P 1991 Drugs in anaesthesia and intensive care. Castle House Publications, Tunbridge Wells

Souter A J et al 1994 Controversies in the perioperative use of NSAID'S. Anesthesia and Analgesia 79: 1178–1190

Wood M, Wood A J 1990 Drugs and anesthesia. Williams & Wilkins, Baltimore

3

Microbiology

HISTORY

Since antiquity, it has been known that diseases such as leprosy and gonorrhoea are contagious. In 1665 a haberdasher from Holland, Antony van Leeuwenhoek (1632–1723), known as the 'father of microbiology', examined water from a tub using his home-made lenses and found little animals, which were in fact protozoa (tiny organisms).

The French chemist Louis Pasteur (1822–1895) proved that the conversion of sugar to alcohol in the production of wine was caused by the activity of living microorganisms. He also pointed out that specific microorganisms cause specific diseases in man and animals.

Robert Koch (1843–1910) from Germany proved in 1876 that *Bacillus anthracis* causes anthrax. In 1882 he also isolated *Mycobacterium tuberculosis*, the causative organism of human tuberculosis.

Alexander Ogston, a Scottish surgeon, showed in 1880 that cocci (round bacteria) produced inflammation and were the main cause of acute abscesses. He isolated Staphylococci and Streptococci.

Ivanowsky (1892) and Beijernick (1898) became aware that there were some organisms even smaller than bacteria; they showed that mosaic disease of the tobacco plant could be transmitted to healthy plants by means of tissue juices freed from bacteria by filtration. Thus a new group of minute organisms called viruses came to be recognized.

In 1940 Chain and Florey opened the antibiotic era by showing that penicillin was an effective chemotherapeutic agent.

Immunology, the subject that deals with the defence mechanisms of the body against bacteria and viruses, has grown along with the knowledge of microorganisms and of effective vaccines for preventing infectious diseases.

CLASSIFICATION OF BACTERIA

Bacteria are classified on the basis of their morphology, staining reactions and metabolism, and have been divided and subdivided into orders, families, genera and species (Table 3.1).

Table 3.1 Principal diseases and their causative pathogens

Genus	Species	Mode of transmission	Disease
Gram-positive bacteria			
Actinomyces	A. israelii	Endogenous	Actinomycosis: abscess in facial region, abdomen
Mycobacterium	M. tuberculosis	Airborne	Pulmonary tuberculosis
Corynebacterium	C. diphtheriae	Airborne and close contact	Diphtheria
Bacillus	B. anthracis	Skin contact with contaminated hides, bone meal	Anthrax
Clostridium	C. welchii	Wounds contaminated with soil	Gas gangrene
	C. tetani	Wounds contaminated with soil	Tetanus
Streptococcus	Strep. viridans	Endogenous bacteraemia	Dental abscess; endocarditis
	Strep. pyogenes	Airborne, contact with a carrier	Acute tonsillitis
	Strep. faecalis	Endogenous	Urinary tract, wound infection, cholecystitis
	Strep. pneumoniae	Endogenous or airborne	Lobar pneumonia
Staphylococcus	Strep. aureus	Endogenous or carrier by direct or indirect routes	Boils, styes, osteomyelitis, septicaemia
Gram-negative bacteria			
Neisseria	N. meningitidis	Endogenous or airborne spread from carrier	Meningococcal meningitis
	N. gonorrhoeae	Acquired during sexual intercourse or birth	Gonorrhoea, ophthalmia neonatorum
Haemophilus	H. influenzae	Endogenous or from carriers	Bronchopneumonia, meningitis, epiglottitis
Bordetella	B. pertussis	Airborne, close contact	Whooping cough
Vibrio	V. cholerae	Water and food borne. Close contact with carriers	Cholera
Pseudomonas	P. aeruginosa	Endogenous or contact with contaminated areas or instruments	Infected wounds, chronic otitis media, septicaemia
Escherichia	E. coli	Endogenous or exogenous	Wound infections, peritonitis, septicaemia, gastroenteritis
Klebsiella	K. aerogenes	Endogenous or exogenous	Urinary tract infections
Proteus	P. mirabilis	Endogenous, sometimes exogenous	Urinary tract and wound infections
Salmonella	S. typhi	Water or food borne by ingestion	Typhoid fever
	S. paratyphi a,b,c	Water or food borne	Paratyphoid
Shigella	Sh. dysenteriae	Ingestion or by hand-to-mouth routes involving faecal contamination	Bacillary dysentery
Bacteroides	Bact. fragilis	Endogenous	Appendicitis and peritonitis, brain abscess
Mycoplasma	M. pneumoniae	Airborne	Mycoplasma pneumonia

Higher bacteria are thin filamentous organisms that are sheathed and show simple branching, for example the Actinomycetacea family comprising Actinomyces and Nocardia.

Lower bacteria are simple unicellular structures. The following terms will be used:

- Gram-positive, Gram-negative; as well as by using their physical shape, bacteria can be divided into groups by their reaction to stains such as the Gram stain.
- Coccus cells are spherical, for example Staphylococci, Streptococci, Diplococci and Sarcinae.
- Bacillus cells are straight and cylindrical (rod shaped).
- Vibrios are curved and comma shaped.
- Spirilla are spiral, non-flexible rods.
- Spirochaetes can be differentiated from Spirilla as they show active cell flexion. They do not possess flagella (tails) but are still mobile. There are three genera of pathogenic Spirochaetes:
  - Borreliae are larger and more refractile; they can be identified by ordinary staining methods. They have large coils with a wavelength of 2–3 μm.
  - Treponemata are slimmer with a coil wavelength of 1–15 μm. Silver impregnation techniques and dark-ground microscopy can identify them.
  - Leptospirae are very fine, with a coil wavelength of 0.5 μm or less. One or both poles of the organism are hooked. They are identified under dark-ground illumination.
- Mycoplasmata. These are very small organisms (50–300 nm in diameter), behave like bacteria but have no rigid cell wall. Thus they assume various shapes and are very delicate. They were originally known as 'pleuropneumonia-like organisms' (PPLOs).
- Chlamydiae are spherical bodies of about 300 nm in diameter and are intracellular parasites.
- Rickettsiae and coxiellae are intermediate between bacteria and viruses. They range from being spherical (300–500 nm in diameter) to being thin rods (up to 2 μm in length). They can be seen by the light microscope but do not pass through filters.

METHODS OF IDENTIFICATION
Gram's method

This is the most important staining procedure used in medical bacteriology. Based on their staining properties, bacteria can be divided into two classes:

- *Gram-positive organisms* retain the violet stain following treatment with acetone or ethanol.
- *Gram-negative organisms* lose the violet stain in the decolourization process, but take up a counterstain and appear pink.

All cocci are Gram-positive except for the genus Neisseria. All rod-shaped bacteria are Gram-negative except for the genera Bacillus, Clostridium, Corynebacterium and Mycobacterium.

GROWTH OF BACTERIA

A standard method of obtaining organisms in pure culture is by plating out on a solid medium.

A small quantity of material (for example pus or sputum) is streaked onto the surface of the medium in a culture plate (petri dish) using a sterile wire loop. Periodically, the initially inoculated material is streaked with a sterile wire loop and reinoculated into different areas of the medium. When the plate is incubated, a crop of colonies appears. Isolated colonies can be picked off, and the characteristics of the pure cultures can be studied in fresh medium.

The commonly used media are:

- For general purposes: nutrient agar, blood agar, heated blood agar (chocolate agar), cooked meat medium and MacConkey's agar.
- For intestinal organisms: MacConkey's agar, deoxycholate citrate agar (DCA) and selenite F broth.
- For mycobacteria: Dorset's egg medium, Lowenstein–Jensen medium and Dubos medium.
- For *Corynebacterium diphtheriae*: Loeffler's medium and tellurite medium.

The important pathogens and commensals seen in clinical practice are summarized below.

Rods

Non-spore forming

1. Gram-negative
- Enteric bacteria, e.g. *Escherichia coli, Klebsiella pneumoniae, Pseudomonas aeruginosa* and *Vibrio cholerae.*
- Respiratory pathogens, e.g. *Haemophilus influenzae* and *Bordetella pertussis.*
- Genitourinary pathogens, e.g. *Haemophilus ducreyi.*
- Blood and tissue pathogens, e.g. Brucella and Bacteroides.

2. Gram-positive
- Gastrointestinal pathogens, e.g. bovine tuberculosis.
- Respiratory pathogens, e.g. *Corynebacterium diphtheriae.*
- Blood and tissue pathogens, e.g. *Listeria monocytogenes.*

Endospore forming

1. Gram-negative
The bacteria included in this class are of no medical importance.

2. Gram-positive
- Aerobic or facultative (produce spores only in contact with free oxygen), e.g. *Bacillus anthracis.*
- Anaerobic or microaerophilic (produce spores and germinate only in an atmosphere without oxygen), e.g. Clostridium species such as *Clostridium tetani, Clostridium perfringens* and *Clostridium botulinum.*

Cocci

Diplococci

1. Gram-negative
- Neisseria species, e.g. *Neisseria gonorrhoeae* and *Neisseria meningitidis.*

2. Gram-positive
- Streptococcal species, e.g. *Streptococcus pneumoniae, Streptococcus pyogenes* and the Enterococcus group (*Streptococcus faecalis*).

- Staphylococcal species, e.g. *Staphylococcus aureus.*

Helical, flexible bacteria

- Treponema species, e.g. *Treponema pallidum.*

Bacteria without cell walls

- Mycoplasma.

Minute bacteria

Two orders:
- Order I: Rickettsiales: genus Rickettsia.
- Order II: Chlamydiales, e.g. *Chlamydia trachomatis.*

IMPLICATIONS OF THE CARRIER STATE

In a number of infectious diseases, the causative organisms are not eliminated completely at the time of recovery of the patient. Following diphtheria or streptococcal sore throat, the organisms may still persist in the throat; similarly, following typhoid fever, dysentery or poliomyelitis, patients continue to excrete the organisms in their faeces. These types of patient are convalescent excreters or carriers. The number of people who continue to harbour and excrete these organisms after 2 months can be up to 5–10%; sometimes the carrier state remains indefinitely. Temporary carriers or excreters excrete the organisms for more than a year. Chronic carriers, for example patients with typhoid fever, excrete the organisms for a long period.

As long as a patient continues to excrete bacteria he or she is an infective risk to others.

Contact carriers

Some people who come into contact with a patient suffering from an infectious disease may acquire the organisms and harbour them without suffering from the disease. Such persons are called contact carriers or symptomless excreters. This state may be temporary or chronic. Over half the population, and an even higher proportion of hospital workers, carry *Staphylococcus aureus* in their nose and on their skin; they are an important source of disease.

The diseases often found in contact carriers are diphtheria, streptococcal sore throat, meningococcal meningitis and hepatitis B. As these contact carriers go unrecognized, they constitute a special hazard for the rest of the uninfected population.

INFECTION

Sources of infection

The organisms causing disease in man are derived from three sources: human beings, animals and other sources.

Humans

Some organisms, such as Bacteroides and *Escherichia coli*, live harmlessly in the bowel, but acting together they can cause peritonitis if the bowel wall is mechanically damaged. Escherichia coli is also the most common cause of urinary tract infection.

Haemophilus influenzae, Streptococcus pneumoniae and *Streptococcus viridans* live harmlessly in the upper respiratory tract but can cause bronchitis, sinusitis, bronchopneumonia and otitis media. Sometimes *Streptococcus viridans* may enter the bloodstream and settle on a damaged heart valve, causing subacute bacterial endocarditis.

Animals

Diseases primarily affecting animals which are transmitted to man are called zoonoses. Cows may excrete *Mycobacterium bovis* (causing tuberculosis) or *Brucella abortus* (giving rise to brucellosis) in their milk.

Other sources

Pseudomonas aeruginosa, Proteus and clostridial species live freely in the soil and as commensals in the intestines of man and animals. They may infect burns, wounds and the urinary tract. *Clostridium tetani* and *Clostridium perfringens* can gain access to deep wounds contaminated with soil, causing tetanus and gas gangrene.

Legionella pneumophila, which grows in soil and water, may contaminate the water in air conditioners and humidifiers.

Sepsis, asepsis and antisepsis

Sepsis means the presence of pathogenic organisms growing in tissues or blood.

An antiseptic is a substance that combats sepsis. It can be applied to exposed living tissues without damage to the tissues; examples are dilute alcohol and tincture of iodine.

Asepsis means the absence of any living organisms. Aseptic technique is a procedure aimed at eliminating live organisms; modern surgical and microbiological procedures are based on aseptic technique.

Local infection control policies

In any hospital, infection control policies are based on:

- eradicating the source of infection;
- interrupting the mode of transmission;
- increasing the individual's resistance.

Surveillance of infection

A microbiologist (infection control officer), assisted by an infection control nurse, is usually responsible for maintaining up-to-date records of all hospital infections. The main sources of these records are:

- laboratory records of pathogenic organisms isolated;
- data collected from:
  - doctors, nurses and occupational health departments;
  - routine visits to all wards and departments;
  - general practitioners.

Infection control policies relating to specific infections

Infection caused by Gram-negative bacilli

Gram-negative bacilli contribute to 40–50% of all cases of sepsis in surgical wounds. Isolation of some types of coliform bacteria from the wound indicates contamination rather than true infection. Infection is usually due to *Pseudomonas aeruginosa*, Klebsiella, Proteus and *Escherichia coli*. Burns become infected with Pseudomonas, resulting in delayed healing and failure of grafts. If septicaemia (the condition in which bacteria actually grow and reproduce in the blood) occurs, death can follow.

Sources of infection. Most of the Gram-negative bacilli are usually normal intestinal flora and sometimes free-living organisms.

Mode of infection. Coliform infections are common following operations on the gastrointestinal tract, for example appendicectomy. Sometimes they infect non-abdominal wounds by cross-infection (i.e. contamination from some other patient, often by way of the medical or nursing staffs' hands).

Some patients acquire new, more aggressive strains of coliform on admission to hospital, which then go on to cause urinary tract and wound infections. Some outbreaks of coliform infections have been traced to contaminated suction apparatus, endotracheal tubes, anaesthetic machines and handcreams.

Control of infection. This depends on appropriate ward and theatre hygiene. It usually involves using sterilizing methods rather than disinfecting and regular checks on the sterility of moist equipment such as humidifiers, in which coliforms can multiply. Good handwashing technique between patient contacts is also essential.

Infections caused by Staphylococci

Staphylococcus aureus is responsible for 30–40% of all cases of sepsis occurring in surgical wounds. It is widely distributed among patients and hospital staff and is a major source of cross-infection.

Source of infection. Deep-seated infection within a few days of an operation and before the wound has been dressed indicates a theatre infection. Ward infections are superficial and follow the dressing of wounds and burns in the ward.

Control of infection

1. *Isolation.* All patients with *Staphylococcus aureus* infection should be isolated and barrier-nursed. Infected members of staff and carriers should not be allowed into operating theatres and wards until they are cured.

2. *Search for carriers.* Swabs are taken from the nose, throat, skin, minor septic spots and pimples of individuals who are suspected of being a possible source of infection.

3. *Treatment of carriers.* If they are patients, carriers should be isolated; if working personnel, they should be taken off work and prescribed local treatment with an antibacterial preparation such as a cream containing chlorhexidine and neomycin (for nose) and hexachlorophane soap (for skin).

Infections caused by Streptococci

Group A haemolytic Streptococci are the source of infection in burns, plastic surgery operations and wound sepsis. The sources of infection are nasal and throat carriers.

Oral penicillin is used to treat carriers.

Viral hepatitis

Source of infection. Viral hepatitis is caused by the hepatitis A, hepatitis B and hepatitis C viruses.*

Hepatitis A causes small outbreaks of infection; the virus is excreted in the faeces, and the infection is acquired by mouth.

Hepatitis B virus reaches people through contaminated blood. Sharing needles (e.g. i.v. drug abusers) and multiple blood or blood product transfusions are common causes. Babies can

---

*Viruses are small infective agents that grow and reproduce only in living cells. They have the power to enter specific living cells, within which they multiply, giving rise to signs of disease.

become infected from their mothers during birth, and this method of transmission is relatively common in the Far East.

Control of infection. Control of the hepatitis A virus depends upon preventing the contamination of food or water by faeces, and hygienic measures to prevent faecal spread of the disease.

Serum hepatitis (hepatitis B virus) can be prevented by: (1) screening blood for the virus, (2) the use of separate needles for each patient, (3) vaccination of hospital staff against the disease, and (4) universal body fluid precautions (e.g. gloves and eye protection when handling body fluids) to avoid exposure to infected blood.

PHYSIOLOGY OF BODY DEFENCE MECHANISMS

The body's defence mechanisms against infection can be divided into two types: non-acquired and acquired.

Non-acquired mechanisms

Outer defences

Mechanical barriers. An intact skin is a highly effective barrier against bacteria, compared with mucous membranes, which are permeable.

Mechanical removal. Mucous membranes of the respiratory tract trap bacteria in a layer of mucus and carry them towards the oesophagus by ciliary action. Coughing, sneezing, blinking, tears, sweat, saliva and gastrointestinal secretions remove many bacteria.

Bactericidal activity (cidal = destroying). Skin has bactericidal properties against *Streptococcus pyogenes*, *Escherichia coli*, Salmonella and Pseudomonas.

Gastric juice, because of its acidity, kills all bacteria except *Mycobacterium tuberculosis*. Prostatic secretions that enter the bladder at the end of micturition contain an antibacterial agent. Breast milk contains various antibacterial substances

and an antiviral agent. The enzyme lysozyme is present in high concentration in tears and has the ability to destroy bacteria.

Normal flora or commensals act as defensive organisms but may also cause disease. The mechanism by which they fight disease-causing organisms is competition for space and food.

Inner defences

Body fluids. Serum from a normal person, if incubated for a few hours with certain species of bacteria, will kill them (bactericidal action) and may dissolve some Gram-negative non-pathogenic organisms such as *Escherichia coli*, *Haemophilus influenzae* and Salmonellae (bacteriolytic action).

Body fluids also have the property of neutralizing bacterial endotoxins, enzymes and viruses. The substances responsible for these actions are lysozymes, complement and natural antibodies.

Phagocytosis. Phagocytes are body cells (polymorphs and macrophages) that are specialized in the capture, ingestion and destruction of invading bacteria.

Acquired defences

These defence mechanisms depend on the previous contact of the body with microorganisms or their products. They are divided into two types:

1. antibody-relayed immunity (humoral immunity), which depends on the production of specific antibodies;*
2. cell-relayed immunity (cellular immunity), which depends on the development of specifically sensitized cells (T-lymphocytes).[†]

---

*An antibody is an immunoglobulin produced as a result of the introduction of an antigen into the tissues of an animal. An antigen is a substance which, when introduced into the tissues of an animal, can provoke an immune response.

[†]T-lymphocytes are derived from lymphoid tissues such as the spleen and lymph nodes. They circulate in the blood and extravascular fluids and encounter antigens anywhere in the body.

The acquired defence mechanisms differ from the non-acquired in the following respects:

- They take time to develop because of the late arrival of antibodies and sensitized lymphocytes.
- They are more powerful because of the specific and amplified action of antibodies and lymphocytes against bacteria and their products.
- Once immunity to an organism is acquired, the body retains this response to the specific organism as a cellular memory, often for life. Reinfection with the same organism is vanishingly rare.

CHEMOTHERAPEUTIC AGENTS AND ANTIBIOTICS

Chemotherapeutic agents are drugs that are either lethal or inhibitory to the organisms that cause infectious diseases. An antibiotic is an antimicrobial substance produced synthetically or from micro-organisms genetically altered to produce it.

Alexander Fleming in 1929 found that the products of the mould *Penicillium notatum* were strongly active against a wide range of bacteria, but attempts to concentrate the active agent (penicillin) were unsuccessful until Chain and Florey at Oxford, in 1940, isolated penicillin preparations of high antibacterial activity.

Type of action

Antibacterial agents are divided into two types, based on their action:

1. *Bactericidal* drugs destroy bacteria; examples are penicillins, cephalosporins, aminoglycosides and polymyxin.
2. *Bacteriostatic* drugs are those which merely inhibit the growth of organisms, such as sulphonamides, tetracyclines and chloramphenicol.

Mode of action

Sulphonamides act by competitive inhibition of a bacterial enzyme that has as its substrate the structurally similar substance para-aminobenzoic acid, an essential nutrient for many bacteria.

Trimethoprim inhibits the bacterial enzyme dihydrofolate reductase.

Penicillins, cephalosporins, bacitracin, vancomycin and cycloserine interfere with cell wall synthesis and secondarily cause cell fragility and thus bacteriolysis.

Tetracyclines and chloramphenicol act as specific inhibitors of protein synthesis.

Streptomycin and other aminoglycosides inhibit protein synthesis.

Polymyxin becomes firmly bound to the cytoplasmic membrane and acts by damaging it.

Range of action

1. Antibiotics active against Gram-positive organisms include penicillins and erythromycin.
2. Antibiotics active against Gram-negative organisms include polymyxin and nalidixic acid.
3. Antibiotics active against both Gram-positive and Gram-negative organisms (broad-spectrum antibiotics) include tetracyclines, chloramphenicol, ampicillin and sulphonamides.

ANTIBIOTICS IN REGULAR USE

Penicillins and related compounds, such as the cephalosporins, contain a β-lactam ring in their chemical structure and hence are called β-lactam antibiotics. They are divided into four groups:

- Group 1: benzylpenicillin (penicillin G) and penicillins with similar activity, e.g. phenoxymethylpenicillin (penicillin V).
- Group 2: penicillins with broad-spectrum activity, e.g. ampicillin, amoxycillin and carbenicillin.
- Group 3: penicillins resistant to staphylococcal penicillinase (β-lactamase), e.g. cloxacillin and flucloxacillin.
- Group 4: Penicillins more active against Gram-negative bacilli than Gram-positive organisms, e.g. mecillinam.

Group 1 penicillins. Benzylpenicillin (Crystapen) is the antibiotic of choice in infections caused by *Staphylococcus aureus*, *Streptococcus pyogenes*, *Streptococcus pneumoniae*, Clostridium and other gas gangrene organisms, and in syphilis. Similarly, *Corynebacterium diphtheria*, *Neisseria meningitidis* and *Neisseria gonorrhoea* are sensitive to penicillins.

Benzylpenicillin is destroyed by gastric hydrochloric acid, so it is given by intramuscular (i.m.) injection. Penicillin V (Crystapen) and phenethicillin (Broxil), which are acid resistant, can be given by mouth.

Dosage: Benzylpenicillin (Crystapen) 300–600 mg is given four times daily by the i.m. route or in a dose of up to 24 g by intravenous (i.v.) injection. Penicillin V (Crystapen) 250–500 mg is given every 6 hours.

Group 2 penicillins. Ampicillin (Penbritin) is less active than benzylpenicillin against all Gram-positive organisms except *Streptococcus faecalis*. It is active against many Gram-negative bacilli, such as Salmonellae, Shigellae, *Escherichia coli*, *Proteus vulgaris* and *Haemophilus influenzae*. It is inactivated by β-lactamase and is normally given by mouth.

Amoxycillin (Amoxil) resembles ampicillin in its activity.

Group 3 penicillins. Cloxacillin (Orbenin) and flucloxacillin (Floxapen) are unaffected by the β-lactamase enzyme produced by penicillin-resistant *Staphylococcus aureus*. Both of these are absorbed when administered orally.

Dosage

Drug (Trade name)	Dose	Route	Interval (hours)
Ampicillin (Penbritin)	250 mg to 1 g 500 mg	Oral i.m. or i.v.	6 6
Amoxycillin (Amoxil)	250 mg 500 mg	Oral i.m. or i.v.	8 6
Carbenicillin	5 g	i.v. slowly	6
Ticarcillin (Ticar)	15–20 g	i.v.	Divided doses
Mezlocillin (Baypen)	2 g 500 mg to 2 g	i.v. i.m.	6–8 6
Piperacillin (Pipril)	100–300 mg/kg body weight	i.m. or i.v.	8–12

Dosage

Drug (Trade name)	Dose	Route	Interval (hours)
Flucloxacillin (Floxapen)	250 mg 500 mg	Oral i.v.	6 6
Cloxacillin (Orbenin)	500 mg 250 mg/500 mg	Oral i.m. or i.v.	6 6

Group 4 penicillins. Mecillinam (Selexidin) is highly active against Escherichia coli and other Gram-negative intestinal bacteria.

Dosage: 5–15 mg/kg body weight is given 6-hourly i.m. or i.v.

Side-effects: Hypersensitivity and urticarial rash. Penicillin allergy is one of the most common drug allergies in the Western world.

Cephalosporins resemble penicillins in being bactericidal and of low toxicity. They have a broad spectrum of activity and can be used against Streptococci, Staphylococci (including penicillin-resistant strains) and a wide range of Gram-negative bacteria.

Cephalexin (Keflex, Ceporex), cephradine (Velosef) and cefaclor (Distaclor) are active when given by mouth. Cefuroxime (Zinacef), cefoxitin (Mefoxin), cefotaxime (Claforan) and ceftazidime (Fortum) are often effective against strains of Gram-negative bacilli resistant to other cephalosporins. They are given either i.m. or i.v.

Dosage

Drug (Trade name)	Dose	Route	Interval (hours)
Cephalexin (Keflex)	250 mg	Oral	6
Cephradine (Velosef)	250 mg 500 mg	Oral i.m. or i.v.	6 6
Cefaclor (Distaclor)	250 mg	Oral	8
Cefuroxime (Zinacef)	750 mg 1.5 g	i.m. i.v.	8 8
Cefoxitin (Mefoxin)	1–2 g	i.m. or i.v.	6–8
Cefotaxime (Claforan)	1 g	i.m. or i.v.	12
Ceftazidime (Fortum)	1–6 g	i.m. or i.v.	Divided doses

Side-effects: The principal side-effect of the cephalosporins is hypersensitivity. Haemorrhage due to interference with blood clotting factors has been reported.

Aminoglycosides. This group of antibiotics includes neomycin, kanamycin (Kantrex), gentamicin (Genticin, Cidomycin), amikacin (Amikin) and framycetin (Soframycin). They are similar in chemical structure, antibacterial activity, pharmacological properties and toxicity.

They are bactericidal and active against some Gram-positive and many Gram-negative organisms. Streptomycin and kanamycin are also active against *Mycobacterium tuberculosis*, while amikacin and gentamicin have activity against *Streptococci faecalis* and Pseudomonas.

Side-effects: Ototoxicity (impaired hearing) and nephrotoxicity (damage to the kidneys), which commonly occur in adults and patients with renal failure.

Plasma concentrations are measured approximately 1 hour after an i.m. dose or 20 minutes after an i.v. dose. Post-dose concentrations of gentamicin should not exceed $10\,\mu g/ml$ and the predose concentration should be less than $2\,\mu g/ml$ in order to minimize the risk of hearing or kidney damage.

Tetracyclines. This group includes tetracycline (Achromycin), oxytetracycline (Terramycin), chlortetracycline (Aureomycin), demeclocycline (Ledermycin), doxycycline (Vibramycin) and minocycline (Minocin).

Dosage

Drug (Trade name)	Dose	Route	Interval (hours)
Neomycin	1 g	Oral	4
Kanamycin (Kantrex)	250 mg	i.m.	6
Gentamicin (Genticin)	2–5 mg/kg body weight	i.m. or i.v.	8
Amikacin (Amikin)	15 mg/kg body weight	i.m. or i.v.	12
Framycetin (Soframycin)	2–4 g	Oral	Divided doses

Dosage

Drug (Trade name)	Dose	Route	Interval (hours)
Tetracycline (Achromycin)	250–500 mg 100 mg	Oral i.m.	6 12
Oxytetracycline (Terramycin)	250–500 mg	Oral	6
Chlortetracycline (Aureomycin)	250–500 mg	Oral	6
Demeclocycline (Ledermycin)	300 mg	Oral	12
Clomocycline (Megaclor)	170–340 mg	Oral	6–8
Doxycycline (Vibramycin)	200 mg initially, then 100 mg	Oral	Daily

They are normally given by mouth and are broad-spectrum antibiotics active against Gram-positive and Gram-negative bacteria as well as Rickettsiae, Chlamydiae and Mycoplasmas. They are also effective against many Gram-negative bacilli resistant to penicillin, including *Escherichia coli*, Salmonellae, Shigellae, coliform organisms and the Haemophilus and Brucella groups.

Side-effects: Large i.v. doses can cause severe liver damage. Tetracyclines should not be given to patients with renal failure as they aggravate biochemical abnormalities. They inhibit growth and the development of bones and teeth in the developing fetus and infant. Children up to the age of 8 years who receive tetracycline develop permanent unsightly staining of teeth.

Chloramphenicol (Chloromycetin) has a range of activity similar to that of the tetracyclines; it is normally given by mouth. It is the drug of choice in typhoid fever, meningitis and acute epiglottitis caused by *Haemophilus influenzae*.

Dosage: 500 mg is given orally 6 hourly, or 50 mg/kg daily in divided doses i.m. or i.v.

Side-effects: Depression of bone marrow function is a rare but potentially fatal complication. It also causes severe shock and death in premature infants (grey baby syndrome). The use of chloramphenicol should be restricted to short courses of treatment.

Erythromycin (Erythrocin) is a member of the macrolide group of antibiotics. It is effective against *Mycoplasma pneumoniae*, Legionella and Campylobacter. It is reserved for patients who are hypersensitive to penicillin or infected with penicillin-resistant organisms.

Dosage: 250–500 mg is given orally 6 hourly, or 2 g daily in divided doses i.v.

Side-effects: Gastrointestinal upsets; erythromycin estolate may cause jaundice and impaired liver function if treatment is prolonged.

Sulphonamides. As bacterial resistance has increased against sulphonamides, they are being replaced by other antibiotics. The folic acid antagonist cotrimoxazole (Bactrim) is indicated in urinary tract infections, prostatitis, exacerbations of chronic bronchitis, Salmonella infections, brucellosis and *Pneumocystis carinii* infections. Sulphonamides are of value in the prophylaxis of meningococcal infections caused by sensitive strains.

Antituberculous drugs. The drugs used in the treatment of tuberculosis are listed below.

Side-effects:

- Rifampicin causes severe hypersensitivity reactions and thrombocytopenic purpura. It also turns the urine a rose or orange colour.
- Isoniazid can cause peripheral neuropathy when a high dosage is used. Pyridoxine (vitamin B_6) 10 mg daily should be given prophylactically to prevent this.

Dosage

Drug (Trade name)	Dose	Route	Interval (hours)
Co-trimoxazole (Bactrim)	960 mg 960 mg	Oral i.m. or i.v.	12 12
Sulphadiazine (Sulphatriad)	1.0–1.5 g	i.m. or i.v.	4
Sulphafurazole (Gantrisin)	1 g	Oral	4–6
Sulphamethizole (Urolucosil)	200 mg	Oral	6
Trimethoprim (Monotrim)	200 mg	Oral	12

Dosage

Drug (Trade name)	Dose	Route	Interval (hours)
Isoniazid (Rimifon)	300 mg 1 g	Oral Oral	Daily Twice a week
Ethambutol (Myambutol)	15 mg/kg body weight	Oral	Daily
Streptomycin	1 g	i.m.	Daily
Pyrazinaruide (Zinamide)	20–30 mg/kg body weight	Oral	Daily

- Ethambutol causes visual disturbances, such as colour blindness and restriction of visual fields.

Other antibiotics

Polymyxin B (Aerosporin) is reserved for severe infections caused by *Pseudomonas aeruginosa*.

Spectinomycin (Trobicin) is active against a wide range of organisms including *Neisseria gonorrhoea*.

Metronidazole (Flagyl) is active against strict anaerobes, trichomonal urethritis, vaginitis, amoebic dysentery and giardiasis, and in the prevention and treatment of anaerobic infections associated with bowel surgery.

Dosage: 400 mg is given 8 hourly by mouth, or 500 mg 8 hourly for 7 days by i.v. infusion. Patients taking Flagyl should not drink alcohol, as the combination of the two causes flushing and nausea.

Amphotericin B (Fungilin, Fungizone) is used for the systemic treatment of severe generalized infections caused by yeasts and fungi, for example cyptococcosis and blastomycosis.

Dosage: 200 mg is given every 6 hours by mouth; it can also be given as an i.v. infusion.

ANTIVIRAL CHEMOTHERAPEUTIC AGENTS

Acyclovir (Zovirax) is highly active against herpes virus. It is valuable in the treatment of life-threatening infections with herpes simplex and the varicella zoster (chicken pox), particularly in patients undergoing immunosuppressive therapy.

Dosage: 200 mg is given five times daily orally, or 5 mg/kg body weight as an 8-hourly i.v. infusion.

Idoxuridine (Iododeoxyuridine) inhibits DNA viruses. It is highly toxic for systemic use but can be used in the form of eye drops for the treatment of herpetic keratitis.

Amantadine (Symmetrel) inhibits certain myxoviruses. When given orally, it is effective in preventing infection with type A influenza virus.

Dosage: 100 mg is given 12 hourly orally.

METHODS OF STERILIZATION AND DISINFECTION

Sterilization is defined as the destruction or removal of all living microorganisms in or on an object. *Disinfection* is defined as the destruction or removal of pathogenic microorganisms in order to make the object non-infective.

A summary of the various methods of sterilization and disinfection is given below:

1. Physical methods
   (a) Heat
      (i) Dry heat
      (ii) Autoclaving
      (iii) Steam/formaldehyde
      (iv) Pasteurization
      (v) Boiling
   (b) Cold
      (i) Gamma irradiation
      (ii) Ethylene oxide
      (iii) Ultraviolet light
2. Chemical methods
   (a) Salts
   (b) Halogens
   (c) Oxidizing agents
   (d) Alcohols
   (e) Soaps and detergents
   (f) Phenols
   (g) Diguanide compounds.

PHYSICAL METHODS

Heat

Dry heat

Contaminated swabs, dressings and human tissue are collected in disposable bags and burnt.

Autoclaving (steam under pressure)

This is the usual method of sterilizing surgical instruments, dressings, gowns, towels and culture media.

An autoclave is a closed chamber in which objects are subjected to steam at high pressures and temperatures above 100°C. Steam is a more efficient method of sterilization than is air at the same temperature. If air is present in the sterilizing chamber, a satisfactory temperature will not be achieved, and pockets of air may prevent penetration of the load of articles by the steam. The air must therefore be removed.

Types of autoclave. There are two types in frequent use:

1. *Downward-displacement autoclaves.* Air is removed in two stages and sterilization is effected by an atmosphere of pure steam. The minimum exposure time required for sterilizing instruments is 15 minutes at 121°C or 10 minutes at 126°C. Bulky dressings and surgical packs require exposures two or three times longer.

2. *High-vacuum/high-pressure autoclaves.* Air is removed by a powerful pump. Steam penetrates the load instantaneously, and very rapid sterilization of dressings and packs is possible in 3 minutes at 134°C.

The causes of failure to produce a sterile load are:

- faults in the autoclave and the way it is operated, for example poor-quality steam, failure to remove air and condensate, faulty gauges and timings, and leaking door seals;
- errors in loading, such as large packs, excessive layers of wrapping material and overpacking;
- recontamination after sterilization owing to an inadequate air filter, leakage into the chamber, wet or torn packs, or incorrect storage.

Methods of testing the effectiveness of autoclaves are:

- Automatic dial recording of temperatures and times of each sterilizing cycle.
- Heat-sensitive tape fixed to the outside of each pack.
- A chemical indicator placed in the most accessible part of each load, for example the routine use of Browne's TST strips or Browne's tubes.
- For high-vacuum/high-pressure autoclaves, daily tests in an empty chamber using a heat-sensitive tape fixed as a cross in the middle of 24–36 towels. If all the air has been removed, there will be a uniform colour change; if air remains, the colour change is incomplete at the centre (Bowie-Dick test).
- Daily checks for leaks by evacuating the chamber and confirming that the leak rate does not exceed 1.3 kPa over a 10-minute period.

Steam/formaldehyde

Autoclaving and dry heat are not practical for heat-sensitive articles such as plastics and optical devices. In a modified autoclave, steam under subatmospheric pressure will rapidly kill non-sporing organisms after the air in the chamber has been removed by a high-vacuum pump. All but a few resistant spores are killed; if formaldehyde vapour is added to the steam, it can destroy all spores and effect sterilization.

Pasteurization

This involves the immersion of instruments, such as endoscopes, for 10 minutes in water at a temperature of between 75 and 85°C. It is effective in destroying vegetative bacteria.

Boiling

At 100°C for 5 minutes, boiling kills all vegetative organisms, but a few spores may survive. Boiling is satisfactory for disinfecting contaminated cups, plates and cutlery but is not safe for instruments used in surgery.

Cold

Gamma irradiation

This method involves the use of gamma radiation from a cobalt 60 source and is used commercially.

Ethylene oxide

This is a well-established technique for sterilizing heat-labile articles. The essential part of this process consists of using a 15% ethylene oxide/85% carbon dioxide mixture and controlled humidity. It can be used for sterilizing artery and bone grafts, heart–lung machines, plastic articles such as disposable syringes, surgical instruments such as cystoscopes, catheters, bacteriological media and vaccines.

Ethylene oxide is toxic to man; when it contaminates the skin, it can cause vesicles and is also known to produce cancer.

Ultraviolet light

This is a form of surface radiation. As its penetrating capacity is poor, it is used for sterilizing surfaces, bone chips, grafts and blades.

CHEMICAL METHODS

Salts

Simple salts in high concentration inhibit bacteria, although they may not kill them.

Halogens

Chlorine is used to disinfect water. A very strong solution of hypochlorite (which liberates chlorine) is used to disinfect articles and surfaces contaminated with blood. It is effective against hepatitis B virus.

Iodine, as a 2–5% aqueous or ethanolic solution in potassium, is used to effectively disinfect intact skin before surgical operations. Povidone-iodine (Betadine) is a non-staining, non-irritant, water-soluble iodine complex. It is a topical disinfectant, killing all spores with a prolonged action. Betadine is used undiluted for skin preparation preoperatively and as a surgical scrub. Iodine allergy is common, and patients should be specifically asked for it prior to anaesthesia.

Oxidizing agents

These are effective against bacteria and viruses. Hydrogen peroxide is used for cleaning and disinfecting wounds. Potassium permanganate is used for disinfecting drinking water, fruit and vegetables.

Alcohols

Pure alcohol has no antibacterial activity. Seventy per cent alcohol kills vegetative bacteria and some viruses rapidly, and is also active against *Mycobacterium tuberculosis*. It is used for preparing the skin prior to injections and for disinfecting trolley tops and other clean surfaces in high-risk areas.

Soaps and detergents

Soaps have minimal germicidal activity, killing Streptococci, *Haemophilus influenzae* and the influenza virus. Anionic detergents, such as sulphated long-chain fatty alcohols, are excellent cleansing agents for floors, walls, ledges, furniture and trolleys.

Cationic detergents include the quarternary ammonium compound cetrimide (Cetavlon). Their surface-active properties make them excellent cleansing agents for intact skin, wounds and burns. They are active against most Gram-positive bacteria. Non-ionic detergents, such as ethylene oxide condensates, are excellent cleansing agents but have no germicidal activity.

Phenols

Clearsol contains 40% of phenols and is used as a general disinfectant in a dilution of 1%. It is used effectively against Gram-positive and Gram-negative organisms, including *Pseudomonas aeruginosa*.

Chloroxylenol (Dettol) is used at a dilution of 5% for general disinfection purposes and is used

effectively against most organisms, excluding certain Gram-negative ones.

Diguanide compounds

Chlorhexidine (Hibitane) is an established antibacterial agent. Hibitane hospital concentrate 5% is a solution of 5% chlorhexidine gluconate; an aqueous dilution of 0.5% of this concentrate is used for the surface disinfection of towels, tables, etc. Box 3.1 shows the various uses and required dilutions of hibitane. Hibitane concentrate is effective against a wide range of Gram-positive and Gram-negative organisms.

Box 3.1 Uses of Hibitane	
Hibitane concentration	*Use*
1% Hibitane in water (0.05%)	Prophylactic treatment of wounds
10% Hibitane in 70% methylated spirit (0.5%)	Presurgical skin disinfection
10% Hibitane in 70% industrial methylated spirit (0.5%)	For emergency presurgical disinfection of heat-labile instruments
1% Hibitane in 70% industrial methylated spirit (0.5%)	Presurgical rinsing of the hands
(Dilutions in brackets are the effective concentration of the antibacterial agent.)	

Hexacholorophane is an antibacterial agent and can be combined with soap in a 2% proportion. It is more effective against Gram-positive than Gram-negative bacteria.

Box 3.2 contains a summary of the methods of sterilization of various pieces of equipment.

Box 3.2 Methods of sterilization	
Anaesthetic apparatus	*Methods*
Rubber face masks, rebreathing bags, corrugated tubes, airways, endotracheal tubes	Immerse in 0.5% aqueous Hibitane or Savlon or Cidex for 10 minutes
Corrugated tubes, Y-pieces, Heidbrink valves, rubber airways, endotracheal tubes	Autoclave

Box 3.2 *(Cont'd)*	
Anaesthetic apparatus	*Methods*
Electrical apparatus: electrical leads and illuminators, diathermy cautery electrodes, electric bone saws, drills, electrical lamps	Read manufacturer's instructions. Autoclave or immerse in 10% Hibitane for 30 minutes. Ethylene oxide
Metalware	Autoclave at 134°C for 6 minutes
Linen (gowns, caps, operation drapes packed into packets)	Sterilize at 126°C for 30 minutes
Endoscopes such as cystoscopes, bronchoscopes, oesophagoscopes	Subatmospheric steam formaldehyde
Glassware	Autoclave after careful packing
Metal instruments:	
• Scissors, dissecting and artery forceps, metal bougies and catheters	Autoclave in open trays for 6 minutes
• Carbon steel instruments such as solid scalpels, twist drills and osteotomes	Dry heat or ethylene oxide
Nailbrushes	Autoclave at 130°C for 6 minutes
Rubber goods such as non-disposable tubing, drainage, sheeting, catheters	Autoclave
Plastics, polyvinyl chloride, polythene tubing, nylon tubing	Wet heat. Ethylene oxide or subatmospheric steam/formaldehyde steam sterilization
Suture material: unopened inner sachets	Immersion in a fluid recommended by the manufacturer for 30 minutes before use
Monafilament nylon and silkworm gut	Autoclave
Metal wire, mesh, suture clips	Autoclave
Braided, twisted, plated and floss silk	Autoclave

ACQUIRED IMMUNE DEFICIENCY SYNDROME

The acquired immune deficiency syndrome (AIDS) is the final stage of infection with a virus earlier known as HTLV III and now known as human immunodeficiency virus (HIV). It must be remembered, however, that not all patients infected with HIV go on to develop AIDS.

AIDS was reported for the first time in the USA in 1979; the first UK case was reported in 1981. Since then, AIDS has been reported from various parts of the world.

In the Western world, the disease is found in high-risk groups such as:

- homosexual men;
- intravenous drug abusers;
- children born to HIV-infected women;
- the heterosexual partners of HIV carriers;
- people who have required multiple blood or blood product transfusions.

Before donor blood was screened for the HIV virus, some patients became infected after receiving a contaminated blood transfusion.

The vast majority of cases in the USA and UK are homosexual and bisexual males, with a fair number of drug abusers as positive carriers.

In central Africa, AIDS is present in both sexes, the predominant spread being in heterosexuals.

Aetiology

The causative agent – HIV – is a member of the retrovirus group of viruses. It acts to destroy the defences that protect humans against infection by other agents.

Human beings can normally resist infection owing to the activities of a variety of specialized cells (e.g. phagocytes and lymphocytes), which are present in the lymph nodes and spleen. The phagocytes destroy invading bacteria; the lymphocytes, which are of two types, produce antibodies (B-lymphocytes) and attack virus-infected cells (T-lymphocytes). Some lymphocytes control the activity of other cells of the immune system. One subpopulation of these promotes the immune response to infection and are called T-helper (T_h) cells. Another subpopulation regulates the response, thus exerting control; these are known as T-suppressor (T_s) cells.

Before the HIV can infect cells, it attaches onto the surface of the T_h lymphocytes. As a result of infection, the T_h cells may be irreversibly damaged and lost from the blood; this can be detected as a reduced cell count or a change in the ratio of T_h to T_s cells. It is this decrease in the number of cells responsible for activating the immune response that reduces the individual's ability to resist infection. Despite this immuno-deficiency, an infected person can remain healthy. However, some patients develop a secondary 'opportunistic' infection, particularly with organisms against which T-lymphocytes normally afford protection.

Acquired immune deficiency can be suspected when a previously healthy individual develops pneumonia caused by the normally harmless parasite *Pneumocystis carinii*, or the uncommon tumour known as Kaposi's sarcoma.

Clinical features

Patients can be asymptomatic with a detectable level of anti-HIV antibody in their serum.

They may also present with symptoms such as fever, malaise, pharyngitis and arthralgia (acute glandular fever-like syndrome) within 1–8 weeks of exposure.

Patients may develop a chronic illness called AIDS-related complex (ARC) or 'pre-AIDS'. The symptoms range from generalized lympha-denopathy to fever, weight loss, diarrhoea and thrombocytopenia, but without opportunistic infections.

AIDS is characterized by 'opportunistic infections' such as *Pneumocystis carinii* pneumonia, candidiasis, toxoplasmosis, herpes simplex stomatitis, gingivitis and Kaposi's sarcoma.

The incubation period for AIDS is variable, ranging from 6 months to 5 years or longer. In a majority of infected individuals, HIV infection is unaccompanied by signs or symptoms and can be identified only by the presence of antiviral antibodies in the serum.

Mode of transmission

Sexual contact. HIV is present in semen and can be transmitted by vaginal or rectal intercourse. The incidence of heterosexual transmission in Africa is much higher, females and males being equally infected by HIV infection.

Blood-borne. HIV is present in the blood of infected individuals; hence transfusion of blood and blood products can cause transmission of the virus to the person receiving them.

The individuals who are at risk are haemo-philiacs receiving factor VIII and intravenous drug abusers who share needles and syringes contaminated with HIV-infected blood.

From mother to fetus. Infected mothers can transmit HIV infection to the fetus via the placenta during pregnancy, by infected blood during delivery, and to the neonate via breast milk.

Needlestick injuries. Accidental 'needlestick' injury while handling the blood of an AIDS patient can result in the transmission of HIV infection.

Preventative measures

These include:

- prevention of puncture wounds, abrasions and cuts in the presence of body fluids and blood, and the protection of existing wounds;
- control of surface contamination with blood and body fluids by the use of disinfectants and by taking proper care;
- application of simple protective measures to prevent contamination of personnel or clothing, and the practice of good basic hygiene such as regular handwashing;
- the safe disposal of contaminated waste.

It is essential to realize that operating theatre personnel will be handling patients or specimens that have not been identified as presenting a risk of infection. Hence extra care should be taken in handling of all patients.

Testing of health staff

Staff exposed to specimens or patients infected with HIV should be aware that laboratory tests are available to detect antibodies to the virus. The occupational health department in each hospital should make local arrangements for these tests. Staff who have an accident handling infected material should be offered the chance of having their serum tested or stored for future testing. In such circumstances, an 'immediate' specimen should be tested followed by further specimens at regular intervals.

Care of the patient

The infected patient should be looked after by staff trained in the precautions appropriate for HIV infection. Staff looking after patients who require isolation should be properly trained in isolation techniques and the use of gloves, gowns, aprons and eye protection.

Blood, body fluids and tissue specimens for diagnosis must be taken by experienced staff who must wear gloves, gowns, aprons and eye and face protection. Resheathing of the needle must not occur: all disposable sharps must be placed in a puncture-proof bin suitable for incineration. Non-disposable items should be placed in a suitably secure enclosure for sterilization or disinfection. After secure closure of the receptacle, the specimens must be labelled by whatever system is recognized locally to indicate a danger of infection. Labelled specimens should be sealed in plastic bags without using staples, metal clips or pins. The request form accompanying them should clearly mention the suspicion or knowledge of HIV infection and must be kept separate from the specimen container to avoid contamination.

The physician or surgeon is responsible for making the laboratory staff aware of the risk, and specimens should not be sent to the laboratory without an agreement between the doctor and senior laboratory staff.

Precautions for body handling and disposal

If a person known or suspected to be infected with HIV dies, either in hospital or elsewhere, it is essential that funeral personnel involved in handling the body are informed that there is a risk of infection. Sometimes powered devices implanted in the body during life (for example cardiac pacemakers) may present a risk of injury to staff if the body is cremated. These should be removed before cremation in a hospital using a 'no-touch' technique through a tiny incision. The skin should be stitched and the wound sealed with waterproof adhesive tape. The body should be replaced in a plastic body bag after local skin disinfection.

Waste disposal

Material that comes in contact with HIV-infected patients should be either autoclaved or incinerated as necessary.

Disinfection and sterilization

As the HIV retrovirus is stable at room temperature in both the wet and the dry state, it is essential to establish thorough disinfection and sterilization practices whenever contamination occurs.

Chemical disinfectants. The retrovirus is inactivated by alcohols, hydrogen peroxide, hypochlorite, formalin, Lysol and glutaraldehyde. Of these, hypochlorite, glutaraldehyde and isopropyl or ethyl alcohol are the most useful.

If HIV-positive blood, body fluids or excreta are spilled onto surfaces, either 2% glutaraldehyde or hypochlorite solution containing 10 000 p.p.m. (parts per million) chlorine should be used.

For general good hygiene or treatment of minor surface contamination, 1% phenolic disinfectant or a lower concentration of hypochlorite (1000 p.p.m. available chlorine) should be used.

Physical treatment. Ultraviolet light and gamma rays do not eliminate the HIV retrovirus.

Sterilization. HIV is destroyed by conventional sterilizing regimens using moist or dry heat treatment.

Maintenance and cleaning

It is the responsibility of the head of the department or a designated deputy to implement written codes of practice that should specify the procedures to be adopted for the protection of maintenance and service staff working in patient facilities and laboratories.

4

Physics and electronics

UNITS OF MEASUREMENT

Initially, measurements were made using commonly available objects. During Anglo-Saxon times, standards were adopted; for example, there was a standard yard in the form of an iron bar kept at Winchester. At the end of the 18th century, metric standards were developed in France, measuring length in metres and weight in kilograms.

Until 1960 there were two main systems of measurement in the UK: the imperial system, which was used for general purposes, and the metric system, used in certain branches of science. In 1960 the organization responsible for maintaining standards of measurements formally approved and introduced the Système International d'Unites (SI units).

SI units

This system is a refinement of the traditional metric system: there are six basic SI units (Table 4.1). There are 15 supplementary units

Table 4.1   Basic SI units

Physical quantity	Name of unit	Symbol
Length	Metre	m
Mass	Kilogram	kg
Time	Second	s
Electric current	Ampere	A
Thermodynamic temperature	°Kelvin	°K
Luminous intensity	Candela	cd

and derived units, which are mentioned in the Appendix.

Physical state of matter

Matter is made up of gases, liquids and solids, and these are all composed of molecules. A molecule is the smallest part of an element or compound which can exist by itself. It is made up of individual parts called atoms, the smallest components of a molecule that can take part in a chemical change.

Atoms and molecules have a weight. These weights are not 'real' but are factors by which they are heavier than hydrogen. The original reference of hydrogen with an atomic weight of 1 was replaced by carbon with an atomic weight of 12.

An atom contains a large nucleus surrounded by a cloud of electrons. The nucleus contains protons, which are positively charged, and neutrons, which have no charge. The electrons are negatively charged. Where an atom is electrically neutral, the total number of electrons is equal to the total number of protons. Most atoms are not electrically neutral and will react with other atoms to try to achieve neutrality; for example, two hydrogen atoms will combine with one oxygen atom to make electrically neutral water. Atoms carrying a positive or negative charge are therefore reactive. Charged atoms are called ions.

Speed is the rate of change of distance, for example 70 kilometers per hour (km/h).

Velocity is the distance travelled in a unit time in a given direction.

Force is that which changes or tends to change the state of rest or uniform motion of a body.

$$\text{Force} = \text{Mass} \times \text{Acceleration}$$

The unit of force is the newton (N), which produces an acceleration of 1 metre per second (m/s) in a mass of 1 kilogram (kg).

Friction is the resistance that must be overcome when one surface moves over another. The friction between two surfaces depends on how tightly they are pressed together. Friction is useful because if, for example, none existed between our feet and the ground, we would not be able to walk.

Work in science has a definite meaning. Mechanical work is done whenever anything is moved against a force or resistance. The unit of work energy is the joule (J). One joule of work is done when a force of 1 N moves through a distance of 1 m measured in the direction of force.

Energy is the capacity for doing work. There are two kinds of energy (Fig. 4.1):

1. The kinetic energy of a body is the energy it possesses by virtue of its velocity or movement (the swinging pendulum of Fig. 4.1A).
2. The potential energy of a body is the energy it possesses because of its position or state (the poised weight of Fig. 4.1B).

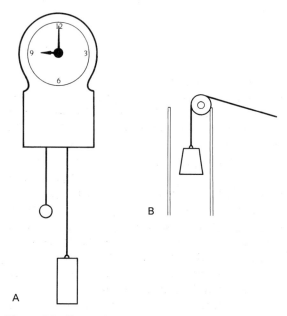

Figure 4.1 Types of energy: (A) kinetic, and (B) potential.

Power is the rate of doing work. When we speak of power, we mean how quickly work is done. The unit of power is the watt (W). One watt is used when 1 J of work is done in 1 s.

The mass of a body is the amount of material it contains.

Weight. The pull of the earth or the force of gravity on a body is called the weight of that body.

Density is the mass per unit volume of a substance.

$$Density = \frac{Mass\ of\ object}{Volume\ of\ object}$$

It is measured in kilograms per cubic metre (kg/m^3)

Pressure

Pressure is the distribution of force over an area:

$$Pressure = \frac{Force}{Area}$$

The unit of pressure is the newton per square metre (N/m^2), also called the pascal (Pa).

A gas will always flow from a high-pressure region to one of lower pressure if it is free to do so. An instrument called a manometer can measure these pressures; it consists of U-tubes made of glass or plastic and half-filled with a liquid (oil, water or mercury depending on the pressure to be measured) (Fig. 4.2). One side of the tube is connected to the pressure source to be tested. With both sides at the same pressure, both liquid columns are at the same level. A difference in pressure is shown by a difference in the levels of the columns of fluid.

The manometer measures pressure in terms of a head of liquid, but it is useful in medical

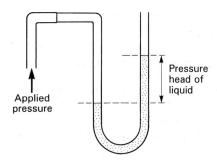

Figure 4.2   A manometer.

practice to have a direct-reading pointer instrument to measure pressure. A bourdon gauge is an instrument made up of a curved metal tube of oval cross-section, which tends to straighten out when the pressure inside it is increased. As the tube straightens out the toothed quadrant rotates and turns the pointer round the seal. The scale is calibrated in the first place using a series of known pressures measured by a manometer (Fig. 4.3).

Atmospheric pressure is the pressure exerted by the atmosphere on all objects. At sea level, this pressure is 101 kPa; this decreases at high altitudes. Air is made of three main components: oxygen, nitrogen and water vapour. In air, the percentage of oxygen is 21%, nitrogen 78% and water vapour 0.8%. The remainder is made up of other gases. These three components contribute to the total atmospheric pressure of 101 kPa, each constituent being said to exert a partial pressure. The composition of air at sea level is shown in Table 4.2.

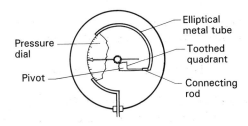

Figure 4.3   A bourdon pressure gauge.

Table 4.2   Composition of air at sea level

	Pressure (mmHg)	Percentage
Oxygen	149	20.9
Carbon dioxide	0.3	0.04
Nitrogen	564	74
Water vapour	47	6

Table 4.3   Composition of air at 4267 m

	Pressure (mmHg)	Percentage
Oxygen	95	21
Nitrogen	351	78
Water vapour	3.6	0.8

If we climb a mountain to 14 000 feet and measure the atmospheric pressure, it will be found to be around 60 kPa. At this height, the percentage of gases remains the same as at the sea level, i.e. the percentage of oxygen is 20–21%, but the partial pressure of oxygen will decrease, as shown in Table 4.3.

At this point, a few definitions which will later be related to anaesthetic gases (see Ch. 6) are introduced.

Vapour pressure (Fig. 4.4)

In a closed space, when evaporation takes place from a liquid, the volume above the liquid contains air molecules and vapour molecules. All the molecules will be bombarding the walls of the container and exerting a pressure. This pressure exerted by the vapour molecules is called the vapour pressure.

Saturated vapour pressure. If a liquid is heated, the number of molecules of vapour re-entering the liquid will at some stage be exactly the same as the number of molecules leaving it. The pressure exerted at this point is called the saturated vapour pressure. This principle is used in anaesthetic vapourizers.

Boiling point. The words 'boiling' and 'evaporation' are used to describe the change from liquid to vapour. Evaporation is a slow process that occurs at all temperatures; it occurs from

EVAPORATION

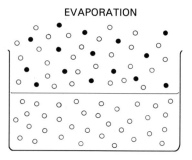

VAPOUR PRESSURE

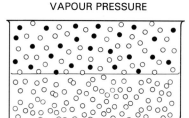

● = Air molecules
○ = Liquid vapour pressure

Figure 4.4   Saturated vapour pressure.

the surface of the liquid. Boiling takes place when bubbles of vapour are formed inside the bulk of the liquid. The constant temperature at which boiling takes place is the boiling point; the boiling point of water is 100°C.

The specific latent heat of vaporization is the heat required to change 1 kg of liquid into vapour at boiling point without a change of temperature. The unit of specific latent heat is the joule per kilogram (J/kg).

GAS LAWS

Dalton's law of partial pressures

In a mixture of gases, each gas exerts the same pressure as it would if it alone occupied the container. For example, if two gases, carbon dioxide and oxygen, are placed inside a cylinder, carbon dioxide exerting a pressure of 3 and oxygen exerting a pressure of 5, the total pressure in the

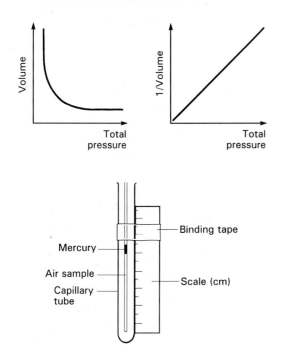

Figure 4.5   The gas laws: Boyle's and Charles'.

cylinder is 8. If oxygen is removed from the cylinder, the molecules of carbon dioxide spread out and the pressure in the cylinder remains at 3.

There are three other gas laws that show an interrelationship between the pressure (P), volume (V) and temperature (T) of a gas.

Boyle's law (Fig. 4.5)

Boyle's law states that at constant temperature, the pressure of a gas is inversely proportional to its volume:

$$P \alpha \frac{1}{V} \text{ (at constant temperature)}$$

Boyle's law holds accurately for real gases such as oxygen and nitrogen over a wide range of pressures.

Charles' law

Charles' law states that, at a constant pressure, a given quantity of a gas expands by a constant proportion of its volume for each degree rise in temperature:

$$T \alpha V \text{ (at constant pressure)}$$

Gay-Lussac's law

At constant volume, the pressure of a gas is directly proportional to its temperature:

$$P \alpha T \text{ (at constant volume)}$$

A general equation for the three laws is:

$$P \alpha \frac{T}{V}$$

Ideal or perfect gas

An 'ideal' or 'perfect' gas is one in which the attraction between molecules can be regarded as negligible and the volume of molecules small compared with the space in which they are enclosed. A 'perfect gas' obeys the laws of Boyle and Charles in all circumstances. These laws can then be combined to give the equation of state of a perfect gas, so PV/T is a constant.

Adiabatic changes in a gas

The gas laws mentioned above are a description of the behaviour of a gas when one of the three variables – pressure, temperature or volume – is maintained at a constant value. For these conditions to apply, heat energy must be added to or taken from a gas as the change occurs.

The state of a gas can, however, be altered without allowing the gas to exchange heat energy with its surroundings. This change of state is called an adiabatic change. A typical example of adiabatic change is when a gas cylinder connected to an anaesthetic machine or regulator is turned on quickly: the pressure of the gas in the connecting pipes and gauges rises rapidly. As the gas is compressed adiabatically, there is a considerable risk of fire, because of large temperature rises. Alternatively, if a compressed gas is made to expand adiabatically, cooling occurs. This is made use of in the working of a cryo

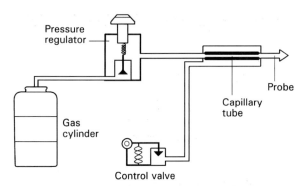

Figure 4.6   A cryoprobe.

Cryoprobe (Fig. 4.6)

Principle. The cooling effect of a cryoprobe is due to an adiabatic process.

A gas such as nitrous oxide or carbon dioxide flows from a cylinder through an adjustable pressure regulator, which is used to set the cooling rate. The gas flows through a capillary tube in the cryoprobe and expands in the probe tip, where a temperature as low as $-7°C$ can be produced. The cooling effect is controlled by a hand- or foot-operated valve that turns off the flow of gas through the probe. The gas is allowed to expand rapidly out of a capillary tube and the temperature falls as a result of this expansion.

Uses. The cryoprobe is used in eye surgery to weld detached retinas and in neurosurgery to remove single lesions (such as cysts in the brain or isolated cerebral tumours). It is also used in the management of chronic pain. Its application to nerves causes local destruction, resulting in long-term (3–6 months) analgesia.

Critical temperature

The critical temperature of a gas is that temperature above which a gas cannot exist as a liquid no matter how much pressure is applied. Oxygen has a critical temperature of $-118°C$, and in all practical situations it is a gas within the cylinder. As it is used, the pressure drop in the cylinder over a period is constant.

Nitrous oxide has a critical temperature of $36.5°C$. In the UK and countries with a cold climate, it always exists as a liquid in the cylinder, whereas in very hot countries it exists in gaseous form. When nitrous oxide is used, the liquid vapourizes to produce nitrous oxide gas at the top of the liquid. The gas at the top of the cylinder always exerts the same pressure because it is continually supplemented from the liquid reservoir. Once all the liquid is used, the nitrous oxide gas pressure will fall as the gas is used up.

In anaesthetic practice, it is not possible to find out how much nitrous oxide is left in the cylinder by measuring the pressure: the amount of nitrous oxide left in the cylinder can only be found by weighing it. *Tare weight* is the weight of an empty nitrous oxide cylinder, and when subtracted from the total weight of the cylinder gives the weight of nitrous oxide in the cylinder.

Filling ratio is the weight of a substance (e.g. nitrous oxide) in a cylinder divided by the weight of the same cylinder filled with water:

$$\frac{\text{Weight of substance (liquid + gas) in a cylinder}}{\text{Weight of water required to fill the cylinder completely}}$$

Cylinders of nitrous oxide have a filling ratio of 0.75; thus a 'full' cylinder contains about nine-tenths liquid, the rest being gas. As mentioned above, the means of keeping a check on the contents of nitrous oxide (and carbon dioxide) cylinders is by weighing them.

HEAT

Heat is another form of energy; it can be transferred from a hotter substance to a colder one. Temperature is the thermal state of a substance which determines whether it will give heat to another substance or receive heat from it.

TRANSMISSION OF HEAT

Heat is transmitted from a higher to a lower temperature by different mechanisms.

1. *Conduction* is the transfer of heat through a material that is not at uniform temperature, from points of high to points of low temperature.

Conduction is the method of heat transfer in solids. Heat can be transferred in this manner by a heating mattress for temperature control during surgery.

2. *Convection* is the transfer of heat energy by circulation of the material due to differences in temperature. Convection, by its very nature, can occur in fluids and gases. During anaesthesia, the process of breathing causes heat loss as the inspired gases will be at room temperature and the temperature of the expired gases will be from 34°C to 36°C.

3. *Radiation* is the transfer of heat by means of electromagnetic waves. Radiant heat travels through empty space and is the method by which heat energy reaches the earth from the sun. In intensive care units, infra-red heaters are employed to maintain the temperature of infants by radiant heating.

TEMPERATURE SCALES

A thermometer is an instrument for measuring temperature. It is calibrated by choosing two temperatures (called fixed points) and dividing the interval between them into a number of equal spaces called degrees. In this way temperature scales are derived. The lower fixed point, the ice point, is the temperature of pure melting ice at standard atmospheric pressure. The upper fixed point, the steam point, is the temperature of steam from pure boiling water at standard atmospheric pressure.

On the Celsius (or centigrade) temperature scale, the interval between the fixed points of 0°C and 100°C is divided into 100 degrees.

On the Fahrenheit scale, the ice point is 32°F and the steam point 212°F.

The relationship between the two scales is as follows:

$$°F = 9/5°C + 32$$

TECHNIQUES OF TEMPERATURE MEASUREMENT

Temperature is measured by either a non-electrical or an electrical technique.

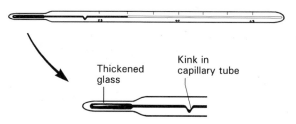

Figure 4.7   A clinical thermometer.

Non-electrical techniques

Any property that changes with temperature can be used in a thermometer to measure a temperature change. The most commonly used property is that of the expansion of a liquid, commonly mercury or alcohol, in a glass tube. Mercury is used because of its low freezing point (–39°C) and high boiling point (357°C), and because the thread can be seen easily; it expands regularly and gives readings consistent with other methods of measuring temperature.

Clinical thermometer (Fig. 4.7)

The normal body temperature for human beings is 36–37°C (97–99°F). When someone is ill, his body temperature often rises, and a clinical thermometer is used to take the temperature. The thermometer is placed in the mouth under the tongue. As the mercury rises, it forces its way past the kink in the tube. When the thermometer is removed from the patient and the mercury begins to contract, the thread breaks at the kink and the reading can be taken. In order to read the correct temperature, the thermometer must be left for a certain time (usually 1 or 2 minutes) in the patient's mouth, the time being marked on each thermometer. To set the thermometer ready for a second reading, it is given a sharp shake.

The two main disadvantages of a mercury thermometer are: (1) a period of 1–2 minutes is required to achieve a uniformity between the mercury and its surroundings; and (2) it may be difficult to introduce the thermometer into some orifices because of its rigidity and the risk of breaking the thermometer, with consequent injury to the patient.

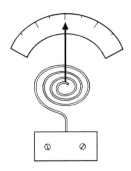

Figure 4.8 A bimetallic thermometer.

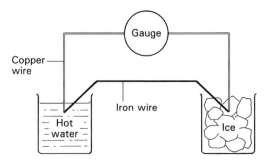

Figure 4.9 A thermocouple.

Alcohol is sometimes used instead of mercury in thermometers. It is suitable for measuring low temperatures because mercury solidifies at –39°C, but alcohol thermometers are unsuitable for high temperatures because alcohol boils at 78°C.

The other non-electrical method of temperature measurement is the Dial thermometer. Dial thermometers use either a bimetallic strip or a bourdon gauge principle.

Bimetallic thermometer (Fig. 4.8)

The sensing element of this device consists of two different types of metal fixed together. When heated they bend; the longer the element, the more movement there will be at the end of the bar.

A long strip is coiled into a spiral to make the instrument compact and sensitive. One end is fixed whilst the other is attached to a pointer that moves over a circular scale graduated in degrees. This instrument is robust but has the disadvantage of not responding quickly to rapidly changing temperatures.

Bourdon gauge thermometer

The bourdon gauge thermometer is in fact a device for measuring pressure and is attached to a sensing element containing a small tube of mercury. Slight variations in temperature lead to changes in volume or pressure in the sensing fluid. The bourdon gauge, which is calibrated for temperature, picks up these changes.

Electrical techniques

There are three main electrical techniques for measuring temperature: the thermocouple, the thermistor and the resistance thermometer.

Thermocouple (Fig. 4.9)

When the junction between two different metals is heated, an electromotive force (EMF) is produced: heat energy is converted to electrical energy. This is the thermoelectric or Seebeck effect, and the arrangement of metals is called a thermocouple. The metals often used are copper and constantan, the latter being an alloy of copper and nickel.

In order to measure temperature, it is necessary to maintain the temperature of one junction at a constant value so that the other can be used to determine the required temperature, provided the EMF of the thermocouple is measured.

Thermistor

A thermistor is a semiconducting element consisting of a small bead made of either manganese, nickel or cobalt oxide. Thermistors have a very small thermal capacity and can respond to a change of temperature in as little as 0.2 s.

As thermistors are highly sensitive, they are well suited for measuring small changes, for example within the pulmonary artery during thermal dilution procedures for measuring cardiac output (see Ch. 6).

The disadvantage of thermistors is that as they age they increase their resistance. They therefore lose sensitivity and accuracy over a few months.

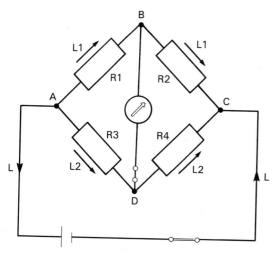

Figure 4.10 The Wheatstone bridge circuit.

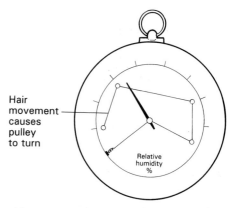

Figure 4.11 A hair hygrometer.

Platinum resistance thermometer

The working of this thermometer is based on the electrical resistance of a metal increasing linearly with a rise in temperature. It consists of a temperature-sensitive platinum wire resistor, a Wheatstone bridge circuit (Fig. 4.10) containing a number of coils, and an ammeter to measure current, which can be calibrated to indicate temperature. For medical use, the chief disadvantage of these resistance thermometers has been the physical size of the coil in the Wheatstone bridge circuit and a slow response time.

Although rectal and oesophageal thermometers have been produced commercially, smaller probes are not readily available. (See Ch. 6 for the clinical application of the measurement of body temperature.)

HUMIDITY

The mass of water vapour present in a given volume of air is called the humidity. Humidity is expressed in two ways:

1. *absolute humidity*, which is the mass of water vapour present in a given volume of air;
2. *relative humidity*, the ratio of the mass of water vapour in a given volume of air to the mass

required to saturate the same volume at the same temperature.

The values of absolute humidity are milligrams per litre (mg/L). The amount of water vapour that is present in a given volume of air is limited by temperature.

MEASUREMENT OF HUMIDITY

All the instruments available measure relative humidity: they are called hygrometers. There are two types of instrument: wet-and-dry-bulb hygrometers, and hair hygrometers.

Wet-and-dry-bulb hygrometers consist of two thermometers. Around the bulb of one is a muslin bag constantly supplied with water by a wick and reservoir. As the water evaporates, it cools the bulb down and a lower temperature is recorded. When the air is dry, evaporation takes place more quickly and the temperature drop is greater. When the air is saturated, no evaporation takes place and both thermometers read the same. Tables are supplied with this instrument, and the relative humidity can be determined from the dry-bulb temperature and the difference between the wet-bulb and dry-bulb readings.

Hair hygrometers (Fig. 4.11) give a direct reading of relative humidity. They work on the principle that a hair gets longer as the humidity rises, and the hair length controls a pointer moving over a scale. This instrument is simple to use and can be accurate if its working is restricted to humidities between 15% and 85%.

Another instrument, Regnault's hygrometer, is available which measures humidity accurately. It consists of a silver tube containing ether. Air is blown down the ether to cool it, thus initiating condensation on the shiny outside surface of the tube. The temperature at which condensation occurs is noted and called the dew point. This dew point represents the temperature at which the ambient air is fully saturated. Relative humidity is calculated from the dew point as follows:

$$\text{Relative humidity} = \frac{\text{Actual vapour pressure}}{\text{Saturated vapour pressure}}$$

$$= \frac{\text{Saturated vapour pressure at dew point}}{\text{Saturated vapour pressure at ambient temperature}}$$

From the dew point noted, and saturated vapour pressure which can be derived from tables, both relative and absolute humidities can be calculated at the temperature required.

IMPORTANCE OF HUMIDITY

Normally, when a patient breathes through his nose, the inspired air is warmed to body temperature and saturated with water vapour, to a level of $34\,\text{g/m}^3$ at 34°C, before entering the trachea. During anaesthesia, when the nose is bypassed by an endotracheal or tracheostomy tube, dry air enters the trachea. The secretions present in the trachea may dry out, and their mucous plugs tend to block the respiratory tract. At the completion of surgery, it may become difficult for the patient to cough up these secretions, and the anaesthetist has to aspirate them via an endotracheal tube.

Similarly, in the intensive care unit, if a patient is ventilated for prolonged periods, he receives dry inspired gases that inhibit the action of the cilia lining the tracheal mucous membranes. Eventually, these cilia disappear, and the lining of the trachea becomes keratinized.

For these reasons, humidification of inspired gases using various devices is recommended (see Ch. 6).

The atmosphere of the operating theatre, in which there is usually air conditioning, should be kept at a suitable level of relative humidity. This should be between 50% and 70%. A high humidity results in a most uncomfortable and tiring atmosphere for the theatre staff, and a very low humidity can increase the risk of explosion due to a build-up of static electricity.

MAGNETISM

The study of magnetism is one of the oldest areas of investigation in physics. A magnet has the property of attracting iron and steel (and special alloys of iron) and, to a lesser degree, cobalt and nickel. These substances are known as magnetic or ferromagnetic materials, and all other substances are non-magnetic.

When a magnet is dipped in a pile of iron filings and removed, it is seen that most filings cling to the ends of the magnet and very few to the middle. These ends are called the poles of the magnet. When these magnets are suspended in a paper stirrup, they first rotate freely and then settle down pointing in a north–south direction.

The law of magnetism is that unlike poles attract, and like poles repel. This can be demonstrated by bringing two different poles together. Repulsion is a definite test for a magnet. The method of identifying a magnet from an unmagnetized bar of iron is by bringing the pole of a known magnet to each end in turn of the iron bar. With an unmagnetized bar, there will be attraction at both ends, but with a magnet there will be attraction at one end (unlike poles) and repulsion at the other (like poles).

ELECTROSTATICS

It has been known since ancient times that certain substances when rubbed with fur or cloth attract light objects to them. Amber (Gk *elektron*), which is a yellow glass-like solid, exhibits this property but nowadays plastics are used in a similar way.

After a piece of plastic has been rubbed against a sleeve, it will pick up small pieces of paper. Substances such as amber or plastic, when rubbed, are said to be charged or electrified with electricity. As the charge stays on these amber rods or plastic and does not move, this kind of electricity is called static electricity, and the study of this area is called electrostatics.

Just as there is a magnetic field round a magnet, so there is an electric field round a charged body or between two charges. The electric field found between two metal plates is uniform except at the edges. Such a field is used in the cathode-ray oscilloscope to deflect electrons, this instrument being used to display an electrocardiogram trace, which can be photographed directly with a timed exposure.

The ability to store a charge is not limited to amber rods, plastics or capacitors. It can build up on the surface of any object insulated from its surroundings. In the case of a bobbin in the variable-orifice flowmeter of an anaesthetic machine (see Ch. 6), friction can result in electrons being removed from the bobbin surface when it rises, rotating against the wall of the flowmeter. Thus the opposite electric charges on the wall and bobbin can exert a force of attraction, causing the bobbin to stick. A temporary solution to this is to coat the inside of the tube with stannic oxide; a permanent solution is to use some other conductive material in the manufacture of flowmeters.

Similarly, insulators may develop static charge on their surface with risks of sparks, which can be dangerous in the presence of an inflammable anaesthetic agent.

ELECTRICITY

The word current means a movement or flow; an electric current is a flow of electrically charged particles.

There needs to be a source of electricity to, for example, light a lamp. This source could be either a dynamo or a battery. The route whereby the lamp is connected to a battery via a switch is called a simple circuit. For an electric current to flow, there must be a complete pathway without any gaps.

There are two types of electric current:

1. direct current (DC), in which a steady flow of electrons occurs in only one direction along a wire; a common example is a battery or a thermocouple;
2. alternating current (AC), in which electrons flow first in one and then in the opposite direction along a wire.

CONDUCTORS AND INSULATORS

Substances that allow electricity to flow through them are called conductors; materials that do not allow a current to flow through them are called insulators. Most wires used for making electrical connections are covered with a layer of insulating material so that if two wires touch they will not cause a short-circuit. Metals are good conductors, whilst non-metallic substances such as rubber and plastic are good insulators.

Conduction of electricity in metals

The atoms of metals are in a regular sequence, being held together by electrical forces. The electrons are loosely held in the outer layer and shared between the atoms. As the ends of a metallic conductor are connected to a battery, the negatively charged electrons move towards the positive end; this movement of electrons is called an electric current. As each electron carries a negative charge, an electric current is thus a movement of charge.

In addition to conductors and insulators, there are certain substances that contain fewer free electrons than conductors. These are called semiconductors.

MEASUREMENT OF CURRENT

The ampère (A) is the unit of current in the SI system, and the instrument used to measure the amount of electric current is the ammeter. An ammeter is connected in a circuit in such a way that current to be measured flows through it.

Whenever an electric current flows in a wire, a magnetic field exists around the wire. Thus when a wire carrying an electric current is placed in a magnetic field, there is a force on the wire that tends to move the wire in a direction perpendicular to both the electric current and the magnetic field. A *galvanometer* is an instrument that works on the principle of this interaction between an electric current and a magnetic field.

In a galvanometer, a coil of wire is suspended on a jewelled bearing in a magnetic field. The current to be measured passes through this coil, the interaction between the magnetic field and electric current causing the coil to rotate. The rotating force on the coil is balanced by a hair spring. The deflection of the coil is proportional to the electric current passing through the coil, which is indicated by a pointer moving over a scale. In operating theatres, many recorders and display devices are based on the principle of the galvanometer.

EFFECTS OF AN ELECTRIC CURRENT

When an electric current flows in a conductor, it produces certain changes in the space around the conductor and in the conductor itself; it has a heating effect, a chemical effect and a magnetic effect.

Heating effect

As electricity is a form of energy, it has the capacity to change into other forms of energy, such as heat. When the current supplying a domestic electric radiator is switched on, the coil of wire called the element in the radiator becomes red hot. In the element, electric energy is being converted into heat energy.

Fuses are a safety device for ensuring that the current in any particular circuit does not rise above a certain level and either cause the element to overheat and start a fire, or damage the equipment. A fuse consists of a thin piece of tinned copper wire. It is carried in a three-pin plug that connects appliances to the mains supply of

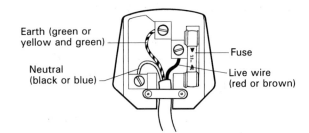

Figure 4.12 A fused three-pin plug.

electricity. A fused three-pin plug (Fig. 4.12) consists of a live (brown) wire that carries the current, an earth (green and yellow wire) and a neutral (blue) wire with a fuse. It is important that the correct value of fuse should be used, so that when a safe value of the current is exceeded, the fuse wire melts and breaks the circuit.

Chemical effect

Certain solutions of acids, alkalis (such as caustic soda) and salts (such as common salt) conduct electricity. Water is a poor conductor of electricity. Liquids that conduct electricity are called electrolytes. When an electric current is passed through an electrolyte, a chemical change takes place, which is termed electrolysis. The apparatus in which electrolysis occurs is called a voltameter.

The electrode at which current enters the liquid is called the anode, and the electrode at which current leaves the liquid is called the cathode.

Magnetic effect

As electric current flows, it produces a magnetic field. The path of the current sets the pattern of the magnetic field, which in turn depends on the shape of the conductor that carries the current. Thus, the magnetic field produced by a current flowing in a straight wire is different from that produced by a flat coil or a solenoid.

Any source of electricity that converts one form of energy into electric energy has an electromotive force (EMF), which measures the ability to drive a current through a circuit. It is measured by a voltmeter. The unit of electromotive force is the volt (V).

Some other terms should be noted here.

Charge. A current is the rate of flow of charge. The unit of charge is the coulomb (C), which is the quantity of charge involved when a current of 1 ampère flows for 1 s.

Current is the flow of electrons carrying a charge. The unit of current is the ampère (A). It represents a flow of 6.24×10^{18} electrons/s past a fixed point.

The potential difference determines whether or not a current will flow and, if so, in which direction. The unit of potential difference between two points when 1 J of energy is required to transfer 1 C of charge from one point to another is the volt (V).

Resistance is the opposition offered by a conductor to the flow of current. The unit if resistance is the ohm (Ω). A conductor has a resistance of 1 Ω when a potential difference of 1 V across its ends produces a current of 1 A.

Ohm's law states that 'the current (I) flowing through a conductor is directly proportional to the potential difference (V) across its ends provided the temperature is constant':

$$I \, \alpha \, V \text{ or } \frac{V}{I} = \text{Constant}$$

The constant quantity V/I is the resistance of the conductor. A conductor has a high resistance if the ratio V/I is large: only a small current can pass through it. If the ratio V/I is small, a large current can flow through, so the resistance of that conductor must be small.

PROPERTIES OF COMMON ELECTRICAL COMPONENTS

Figure 4.13 shows the standard symbols for some common electrical components used in the daily routine.

Alternating current (AC) is a current that changes its direction and magnitude at regular

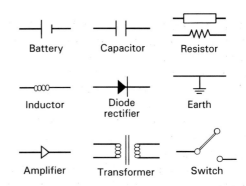

Figure 4.13 Standard electrical symbols.

intervals. The current grows to a peak volume, diminishes to zero, grows to a maximum in the opposite direction and then decreases to zero again.

Alternating current produces a heating effect, so it can be used for heating and lighting. It can also be used to make an electromagnet, although the polarity is constantly changing. One of the advantages of AC is that it can be 'transformed', i.e. the voltage can be altered using a transformer (see below).

Capacitance measures the ability of an object to hold electric charge, charge being a measure of the amount of electricity. As stated above, the unit of charge is the coulomb (C), which is the quantity of electric charge passing a particular point when a current of 1 A flows for 1 s:

Coulomb (C) = amperes (A) × seconds (s)

If two conductors are separated by an insulator, the resulting capacitor develops the property of storing electrons when a potential difference is applied to its terminals.

A transformer consists of an iron core with two coils of wire wound round it. The coil connected to the AC input is called the primary coil, and the coil connected to the galvanometer is the secondary coil. When the primary current is switched on and off, a current is induced in the secondary coil, but the current only flows in the secondary coil when the primary current is changing. If a primary coil is connected to a source of AC (which is regularly changing its direction of flow), there will be an induced current in the secondary coil. This current in the secondary coil will be changing in the same way and at the same rate as the primary alternating current.

The transformer is used to change voltage; thus, low voltages are supplied to laboratories, and high voltages are used for television sets and radios.

ELECTRICAL COMPONENTS USED IN MEDICAL EQUIPMENT

A potential difference exists between the surface of a cell and the underlying cytoplasm. A nerve fibre is a part of a cell, and an impulse travels along it when a wave of depolarization occurs (see Ch. 1). Similarly, a wave of depolarization occurs in muscle fibres before they contract. These waves of electrical change are also transmitted through the tissues overlying the nerve fibres and muscles, and the signals can be detected by appropriate electrodes placed on the skin, which display the signals as an electrocardiogram (ECG), electromyogram (EMG) or electroencephalogram (EEG).

The graphs that are derived from these recordings consist of complex wave patterns plotted as voltage against time. These complex wave patterns can be analysed and grouped using Fourier analysis.

Fourier analysis. In the 19th century, Fourier showed that, however complex a waveform is, it can be analysed as the composite of a number of simple waveforms. These simple waveforms have a shape similar to that of the AC mains voltage and are called sinusoids or simple harmonic waveforms.

Electrocardiogram (ECG). As the sine waves of different frequencies are added, they result in a complex ECG waveform. As described earlier, the potentials from the heart are transmitted through the tissues and can be detected by electrodes, thus giving rise to an ECG trace. The appearance of an ECG depends on the positioning of the electrodes on the surface of the body, the recordings being the difference in potential between two electrodes.

The frequency range for an ECG is about 0.5–80.0 Hz.

Electromyogram (EMG). The potentials from muscular contraction are picked up by surface electrodes. The potentials generated are large with sharp spikes, thus indicating that analysis of this wave will result in a large frequency distribution of sine waves.

Electroencephalogram (EEG). The changes in potential that occur in the cerebrum and brainstem can be picked up by electrodes placed over a patient's scalp. The EEG tracing consists of various waves – β, B, S, δ. The frequency distribution of these waves is small, being in the range 1–60 Hz.

All the above signals (ECG, EMG and EEG) should be displayed on a screen and if possible recorded on a recording device. To do this, three devices – an input transducer, amplifier and a display device – are required. These devices are regarded as a series of black boxes. It is important that electrical signals such as voltage, current and frequency from the output of one black box match the input of the next black box in the system. If these three black boxes are well matched, they can be connected together to give a good monitoring device (Fig. 4.14). The amplifier used should have a high input impedance, which is the total resistance to alternating circuits (see below).

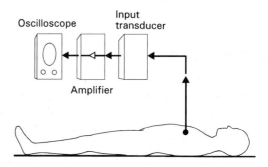

Figure 4.14 The black box concept.

Impedance

Circuits consisting of resistors, inductors and capacitors possess a resistance to the flow of electric current, which in turn depends on the frequency of the current flowing. The term used for this resistance is impedance. Its unit of measurement is the ohm (Ω).

For picking up EEG signals, whose voltage and electrode impedance are small, amplifiers should be provided with an input impedance of around $10\,000\,000\,\Omega$ (10 mega ohms). For ECG and EMG amplification, the input impedances required are still in the mega ohm range even though they are smaller.

Band width

To produce a perfect reproduction of an input signal, all the frequencies contained in it should be equally amplified. There is always a range of frequencies within which the degree of amplification is reasonably constant but outside which there is attenuation of the output signal. The acceptable band width of an amplifier is the range of frequencies in which there is less than 50% relative loss.

The band width of an amplifier should cover the range of frequencies relevant for picking up a signal. For an ECG machine, a flat band width from 0.14 to 50 Hz is required, whereas for an EEG machine the band width extends from 0.5 to 100 Hz. An EMG recorder requires a flat response from 20 Hz to 10 kHz (kilohertz), which will enable it to record the high frequencies contained in the signal.

Amplifiers that pick up ECG signals should have long time constants.

Time constant

This is the length of time that a change of 100% should take if the initial rate of change is maintained. In one time constant, 63% of the final value is completed. In two time constants, 63% of the remaining difference is completed, i.e. 63% + (63/100 × 37)% = 86%. In three time constants 86% + (63/100 × 14)% = 95%.

The time constant of an ECG amplifier is fixed, usually at 3 s, which means that if the trace is displaced, it will return to its baseline position in 9 s. EEG recorders have short time constants of 0.03, 0.1, 0.3 and 1 s.

The gain of amplifiers can be correctly adjusted with the aid of calibration voltages. An ECG machine, when calibrated, will produce a 1 cm deflection of the trace with a 1 mV input; similarly, an EEG machine produces a 1 cm deflection of the trace with a 0.1 mV input.

Display of signals

The biological potentials (ECG, EEG, EMG) can be displayed in two forms: analogue and digital recordings.

Analogue. This type of display allows a lever to move over a scale, which can provide a clear visual indication of the size of a signal. The recorders based on the analogue principle are:

1. *Galvanometers* (see p. 110). These recorders have certain disadvantages; for example, there is no permanent record or tracing, and the inertia of the coil and needle prevents the display of rapidly changing signals. Thus, monitors based on the principle of galvanometers are used for displaying slowly changing signals such as patients' pulse rates or temperatures.

These recorders can be modified to provide a continuous record. One method uses a galvanometer needle with a heated tip, so that a record may be produced on heat-sensitive paper. Another method conducts ink through a capillary to a writing point at the end of the galvanometer needle.

2. *Potentiometric recorders.* A potentiometer, as the name suggests, compares potential differences. It consists of a length of uniform resistance wire, to the end of which a difference of potential is applied so that a steady current flows.

These recorders have a limited frequency response. They are used for longer-term recordings such as patients' temperatures. They can also provide overlapping tracings.

Digital. A digital meter displays values as a set of figures. Such types of meter are used to record pulse rates.

Oscilloscope

When this instrument is used to display signals, the trace can be photographed directly with a timed exposure. Note that:

- cathode = negative charge
- anode = positive charge.

The cathode ray oscilloscope (CRO) consists of:

- an electron gun, which produces a beam of electrons from a heated cathode;
- a deflecting plate, which can deflect the beam from side to side and up and down;
- a fluorescent screen, on which the electrons produce a line or spot of light.

All these components are present in a highly evacuated glass tube, and the electrons are produced by an indirectly heated cathode.

The outside controls of a CRO typically consist of:

1. an off/on switch;
2. x-shift and y-shift controls to centre the spot on the screen;
3. a focus control;
4. x-gain and y-gain controls connected to the amplifiers between the input terminals and the deflector plates;
5. a time-base control, which applies a steadily changing voltage to the x-plates;
6. an AC/DC switch to use with alternating and direct current.

The electron beam produced by the hot cathode passes between the deflecting devices, one of which deflects the beam in the y-axis and the other on the x-axis. The beam then strikes a fluorescent screen, producing a tracing. A signal such as arterial blood pressure from an ECG transducer deflects the beam in the y-axis direction.

The oscillating circuit supplying the time-base produces a saw-tooth voltage. For an ECG signal, the sensitivity control of the CRO is adjusted to a 1 mV calibration signal, which thus gives a 1 cm vertical displacement of the trace.

The CRO is essentially a voltage-measuring apparatus, and whenever there is a potential difference between the deflecting plates, a deflection occurs. Its great advantage is the electron beam, which is the only moving part and shows minimal inertia. The beam responds instantly to any deflecting force and returns instantly to a zero position when the force is removed, thus making the CRO an apparatus with a very high-frequency response.

OTHER ELECTROMEDICAL EQUIPMENT

Defibrillator

This instrument is used for the treatment of ventricular fibrillation. In it, electric charge is stored in a capacitor and then released in a controlled fashion. Defibrillators are set according to the amount of energy stored, this energy depending on both the charge and the potential.

For treating a patient with ventricular fibrillation, electrodes are applied across the patient's chest, and, by means of switches, energy is released as a current that passes across the patient's chest and heart. This current produces a simultaneous depolarization of the entire heart, hopefully allowing a pacemaker cell to regain control of the heart's conducting system after the shock.

Defibrillators are also provided with lower-energy settings suitable for use with internal cardiac electrodes in a patient with an open chest or when shocking the patient out of atrial (as opposed to ventricular) fibrillation.

Some makes of defibrillator are designed for a synchronized mode, the principle being that the energy must be supplied at the correct time in the cardiac cycle, i.e. simultaneously with the R wave on the ECG. If the delivery of energy is mis-timed, it can cause ventricular fibrillation. This type of defibrillator is used in the treatment of atrial dysrhythmias.

Pacemaker

Patients with heart block and fainting attacks (syncope) as a result of slow ventricular rates are prescribed cardiac pacemakers.

Placement of electrodes when using a pacemaker

The myocardium can be stimulated by placing two electrodes on the heart (bipolar leads) or a single electrode on the heart and a second electrode on another part of the body (unipolar leads).

A typical theatre or bedside pacemaker with a catheter electrode provides a rate ranging from 30 to 150 beats per minute. These cardiac pacemakers can be either a demand type or a fixed type:

1. *Demand type.* The output from the pacemaker is inhibited if a spontaneous R wave is detected. If this expected beat is not found, the pacemaker delivers a pacing pulse. Similarly, if the spontaneous heart rate drops below a preset limit, the pacemaker will pace continuously at its default rate. Operating theatre personnel usually encounter this type of pacemaker inserted in patients following cardiac surgery.

2. *Fixed type.* As the name suggests, the pacemaker delivers a fixed pacing pulse to the heart.

Pacemakers can be inserted in the short term as an emergency procedure via either a transvenous or oesophageal route. Long-term pacing is carried out using:

- External pacemakers, which consist of wire running from the pacemaker box to an electrode situated on the surface of the heart. These are used post-cardiac surgery or as a temporary measure before an implantable pacemaker is fitted.
- An internal or implanted pacemaker, consisting of an electrode passed via a subclavian vein into the heart and the pacemaker being implanted in the abdomen, below the breast, or in the infraclavicular region. The connecting wire between the electrode and the implanted box runs subcutaneously.

Diathermy (Fig. 4.15)

Diathermy is the passage of a high-frequency electric current through the tissues, heat being produced as a result. It is used in surgery to coagulate blood and to cut through body tissues.

Current density is the amount of current passed per unit area. It is necessary to be familiar with this term in order to understand the principles of diathermy.

Unipolar diathermy equipment consists of an active part, which is the electrode used by the surgeon, and a plate that is applied to the patient's skin, usually on the thigh (patient plate). When diathermy is used, a current flows from the electrode, through the patient and out through the patient plate. This is safe because diathermy currents are of very high frequency.

The degree of burning produced by diathermy depends on the current density. When the current flows through the electrode used by the

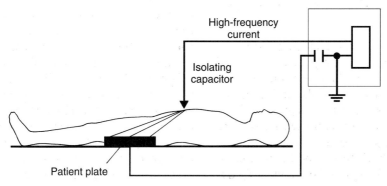

Figure 4.15 Diathermy.

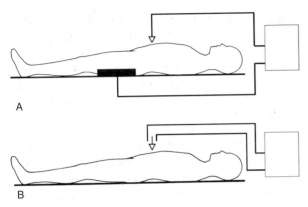

A

B

Figure 4.16   Bipolar and unipolar diathermy.

surgeon, it is focused on a very small area, thus leading to local heating and burning owing to a high current density. The exit point of the circuit, flowing through the patient plate, does not cause any burning because the patient plate has a large area (low current density). If the area of contact is reduced owing to improper application of the plate, the current density is considerably increased, with a risk of burning the patient. If the patient plate falls off the patient, the diathermy current flows to earth through any point at which the patient is touching an earth metal source, for example metal parts of the theatre table.

In certain diathermy sets, there are facilities for a bipolar system (Fig. 4.16) in which the current passes from one blade of the forceps to another. The current does not pass through any part of the patient's body other than that grasped by the forceps, and the circuit is earth-free. This type of bipolar lead is used for coagulation of tiny blood vessels and small pieces of tissue and thus finds a suitable place in neurosurgical and ophthalmic procedures. It is also used during surgery on patients with implanted pacemakers, as current flowing through the patient from a unipolar lead to the plate may interfere with the pacemaker.

Current strength used in diathermy. Normally, if AC from the mains electrical supply (60 Hz) passes through a patient, complications such as muscle contraction, cardiac dysrhythmias or cardiac arrest occur. However, if AC of a frequency

above 10 kHz passes through the body, these effects are not seen. This principle is used in the manufacture of a diathermy machine.

Diathermy units are basically of three types:

1. *Spark-gap generators* employ a current frequency of 0.4 MHz. They produce a damped wave that is used for coagulating tissues.
2. *Valve oscillators* employ a current frequency of between 1 and 1.5 MHz, and produce a sine waveform current that is used for cutting tissues.
3. *Transistorized diathermy sets* produce both a cutting and a coagulation current, although the latter effect is not as satisfactory as that produced by spark-gap generators.

Modern diathermy apparatus used in operating theatres is designed to produce both a coagulating and a cutting effect.

Accidents due to faulty use of diathermy sets

These can be either electrical burns to the patient, or fires or explosions caused by the use of diathermy in the presence of inflammable vapours.

Electrical burns can result from the following:

1. If the foot switch of the diathermy is accidentally pressed when the forceps are in contact with part of the patient's body not to be operated on, burns can occur. This hazard is usually prevented by keeping the forceps in an insulated container when not in use. Many diathermy sets are equipped with a buzzer that sounds when the foot switch is depressed.

2. A poor contact between the plate and the patient can cause burns, either at the diathermy plate site or at any site where the patient is in contact with earthed metal, for example the operating table. Modern diathermy sets are equipped with an audible warning system to alert if the plate is not making a good contact or is not plugged in, or if the electrical continuity is broken.

Fire and explosions can occur in the presence of an inflammable liquid or vapour. Modern anaesthetic vapours are not explosive in ordinary circumstances, but high concentrations of oxygen and agents used to clean skin prior to an operation, such as ethyl alcohol and isopropyl alcohol, can be dangerous. The drapes can trap oxygen and alcohol and can spectacularly burst into flames on contact with an active electrode or a faulty mains lead or floor switch.

Caution. Surgical diathermy should not be used on patients using a cardiac pacemaker as unwanted signals from the diathermy can cause false triggering of the pacemaker (see above).

INTERFERENCE WITH ELECTROMEDICAL EQUIPMENT

All the equipment necessary for measuring biological potentials (i.e. ECG, EMG and EEG) has a major problem with interference or 'noise'. This could be due to noise originating in the patient, his surroundings or the instrument itself.

Ideally, all instruments should have a high signal-to-noise ratio. This means that interference should be reduced to a minimum by eliminating its source or by the use of a differential amplifier. This is an amplifier that measures the potential difference between two sources and eliminates interference from the mains supply.

The noise originating from an instrument is reduced by good design, adequate screening and the use of high-quality components. The major sources of 'noise' are the patient or his surroundings:

1. *Interference from the patient.* The EEG signal detected from the scalp has a potential difference of 50 V, whereas the ECG signal has a potential difference of 0.5–2.0 mV. The EMG has a much larger potential than the EEG and ECG signals, so it can submerge the other two signals. This is avoided by the use of differential amplifiers.

2. *Interference from the patient's surroundings.* These could be due to electromagnetic induction or electrostatic induction.

Electromagnetic induction. When a current flows, it generates a magnetic field around and through the patient and any apparatus connected to him.

This form of interference is seen in the vicinity of wires carrying AC from the mains supply.

The magnetic field is developed in the loops of wire with their own voltage, thus causing interference. This type of interference can be minimized by keeping the wires together twisted around one another.

Electrostatic induction. If a cable from the mains supply lies close to the input lead of an amplifier or a patient, it will induce an electrostatic charge in the lead or the patient. Interference will be seen because the mains cable or the lead acts as one plate of a capacitor that superimposes on the signal from the patient.

This interference can be decreased by increasing the distance between the leads of an amplifier and the mains supply cable, or by decreasing the resistance of the patient–lead combination.

SAFETY PRECAUTIONS WITH MONITORING APPARATUS

When a number of monitoring instruments with mains supply are connected, it is essential to make sure that the patient does not receive a dangerous electric shock. The operating rooms should be supplied with an earth-free mains supply. The isolated mains supply should not come into contact with an earthed object, because if it does a small leakage current will flow. The maximum leakage current allowed is 5 mA RMS (RMS = root mean square), which can be detected by an earth-leakage current detector. If this leakage current exceeds the maximum, the faulty condition should be detected and a fault warning indicator alarm should be set off.

RADIOACTIVE SUBSTANCES

ATOMS AND ISOTOPES

An atom consists of a nucleus containing positively charged protons and uncharged neutrons. This nucleus is surrounded by negatively charged electrons in an orbit.

An element consists of atoms containing the same number of protons (the atomic number). For example, carbon has six protons, whereas hydrogen has one proton. The neutrons contribute towards the stability of the nucleus. Atoms containing the same number of protons but with different numbers of neutrons are called isotopes. A number of elements have stable isotopes that do not disintegrate spontaneously. However, there are other isotopes that are unstable, their nuclei breaking down in a number of ways; these are said to be radioactive.

Types of radiation following atomic disintegration

When an atom disintegrates, it may be accompanied by the emission of energy, particles or both. There are three types of radiation:

1. *Alpha radiation*. Its emission results in the formation of an element with an atomic number two less and an atomic weight four less than the original element. Alpha particles are easily absorbed and, as they are doubly charged, can be extremely harmful biologically if retained in a tissue.

2. *Beta radiation*. In this type of nuclear disintegration a neutron breaks down into a proton and an electron, the electron being ejected as a beta particle. Beta particles emerge with a wide range of energies and are slowed down by collision with electrons of any atom which they encounter. The electrons are easily absorbed and transfer their energy if administered internally.

3. *Gamma radiation* is a shortwave type of electromagnetic radiation, similar to light waves and X-radiation.

METHODS OF DETECTING RADIATION

There are two main methods of detecting radiation: scintillation detectors and Geiger-Müller counters.

Scintillation detectors. When radiation reacts with certain materials, it produces small flashes of light. These materials are called scintillators or phosphors.

Gamma radiation can be detected by using a detector made up of a crystal of sodium iodide, which produces a small flash of light when in contact with the rays.

Beta rays can be detected by these methods, but as the penetrating power of these rays is less, this technique is ineffective.

Geiger-Müller counters. The principle of this equipment is that radiation causes inert gases to ionize. When a voltage is applied to the gas contained between two electrodes, ionization of gas occurs, producing free electrons and positively charged gas ions, which tend to migrate under the influence of an electric field to produce an electrical signal. Geiger counters are sensitive to beta radiation but relatively insensitive to gamma radiation.

Units of measurement – the becquerel

A given quantity of radioactive substance is presumed to have an activity of 1 becquerel (Bq) if one disintegration of a nucleus takes place on average every second. The basic unit used was the curie (C), which was defined in terms of the absolute rate of disintegration. A substance that underwent 3.7×10^{10} disintegrations per second contained 1 curie of activity.

Half-life

The rate of decay of radioactive material is measured by the half-life. This is the time required for half the radioactive atoms present to disintegrate.

USES OF RADIOACTIVE ISOTOPES

Isotopes are used for both diagnostic and therapeutic purposes.

Diagnostic

Radioactive isotopes can be used for diagnostic purposes in two forms: imaging and non-imaging.

Imaging techniques. These use gamma rays emitted from an isotope, and the distribution of these rays in the body can be detected using a gamma camera.

A commonly used isotope is technetium-99m, technetium-99m labelled red blood cells or albumin being used for vascular imaging and assessing cardiac activity. Technetium-99m pertechnetate is used in brain and thyroid scans.

Non-imaging techniques. Fibrinogen labelled with radioactive iodine-125 is used to detect deep vein thrombosis. This labelled fibrinogen is injected i.v. and, should a clot begin to form, fibrinogen (from the normal clotting factors) begins to concentrate within the clot. A part of this fibrinogen in the clot is the injected radioactive fibrinogen, which emits gamma rays. A scintillation counter detects a high level of radioactivity just above the formed blood clot.

Blood flow into and/or out of a body organ such as the liver or kidney can be measured if a radioisotope is used as an indicator.

Therapeutic

Radiation may be given by means of either an internal or an external source in the treatment of tumours. For example, a sealed caesium-137 capsule is implanted in the uterus for uterine tumours. As an external source, the most common radioactive material used is a sealed capsule of cobalt-60.

RADIATION HAZARDS AND SAFETY

All radioactive substances and X-rays can cause tissue damage and chromosomal abnormalities. Hence it is essential to limit exposure to a minimum. An individual can be exposed to radiation either from outside (i.e. her surroundings) or from radioactive elements within the body.

Exposure to external radiation can be minimized by keeping radioactive sources in containers that absorb radiation. As alpha particles travel only a few centimetres in air, it is essential to contain them in specialized containers. Beta particles

travel a distance of a few metres in air before they are absorbed. As beta particles also produce X-rays, it is safer to provide a protective shield for staff, made of Perspex, a material with a low density. A dense material such as lead is used as a shield against gamma rays, which travel long distances. Lead also tends to absorb X-rays, so it is added (during manufacture) to aprons to be worn by staff exposed to radiation.

The dose of radiation received is directly proportional to the square of the distance away of the source; thus the risk of exposure can be considerably reduced by moving further from the source of radiation.

As the fetus is at specific risk from radiation, women of child-bearing age should be X-rayed only in the first 10 days of their menstrual cycle (i.e. before ovulation and to exclude conception).

Personnel who are constantly exposed to X-rays should wear a photographic film badge to monitor the total radiation dose received. The badge consists of a small piece of photographic film behind several filters, through which the dose of radiation received passes.

Each hospital has a radiation control officer who is consulted before radioactive compounds are used.

HAZARDS IN THE OPERATING THEATRE

The source of power for most anaesthetic apparatus and monitoring equipment is AC current. In the UK, electrical power is supplied at a frequency of 50 Hz. It is essential to be aware of the principles behind the mains supply to the hospital and the operating theatre.

The hospital site receives electrical power as a three-phase 11 000 V supply. A local transformer transforms this power into three 240 V supplies. Each 240 V supply is 120° out of phase with the other two, so it is obvious that interconnected electrical devices should not receive power from different phases. Hence all the wiring outlets of the operating theatre should be connected to the same phase supply. The current used in electro-

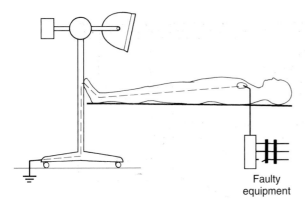

Figure 4.17 The safety of electromedical equipment.

medical equipment passes between a live 240 V wire and the neutral.

Electromedical equipment connected to the mains consists of a live component called 'load', which is covered by an insulated 'earthed' metal casing. This earth is important for the safety of the equipment (Fig. 4.17). If the insulation deteriorates, a connection is established between the load and the earthed metal casing, and current produced as a result of this connection is called 'leakage current'. If this is high, the line current will exceed the rating of the fuse, making it blow and thus breaking the circuit.

The fuse protects the equipment from the effects of large leakage currents, but if the earth connection becomes faulty, a dangerous situation develops. The current does not flow because of loss of the earth connection, the fusing does not blow and the metal casing (Fig. 4.17) remains at the same potential as the leakage source. In this situation, if a person standing on an antistatic floor touches the case, current passes through him to the earth and mains, giving him a painful shock. However, if he touches this case with a wet hand, he will receive a dangerous electrocuting current.

PROTECTION AGAINST ELECTRIC SHOCK

Electromedical equipment can be divided into three classes by the degree of protection needed to protect against the risk of electric shock:

1. *Class I equipment*. In this type of equipment, any conducting part that can touch a user, such as the metal case of an instrument, is connected to an earth wire, which becomes the third wire connected via the plug to the mains supply socket.

2. *Class II equipment*. In this type of equipment (also called double-insulated equipment), parts that can be touched easily are protected by two layers of insulation. An earth wire is not required.

3. *Class III equipment*. In this type of equipment, there are no potentials exceeding 24 V AC. Thus, it does not produce an electric shock, although it can still produce a microshock.

Risks of shock with earthed equipment

If the patient is allowed to be in contact with Class I type equipment in theatre, there is a risk that he will be electrocuted. In older diathermy machines, the patient's plate acted as a possible connection between the earth and the patient, increasing the risk of electrocution in the event of an electrical fault occurring in any equipment to which he was attached.

Microshock. If an electric current passes through the myocardium, it can cause ventricular fibrillation as a result of electric shock. If an electric current passes from a hand to the feet, the current flows not only through the heart but also through the rest of the body, so that the total current flow through the heart is a fraction of 24 mA that may pass from the hand to the feet. It is that fraction of the current passing through the myocardium, or the current density in the region of the myocardium, which determines whether ventricular fibrillation will occur.

If there is a faulty intracardiac catheter passing from the monitoring equipment into the heart (Fig. 4.18), and if this catheter touches the wall of the heart, an electric current flowing along the catheter will pass through a very small area of the heart. In such a case, a current of 150 µA can produce the same current density in a portion of the myocardium as that produced by 24 mA flowing from a hand to the feet, and ventricular

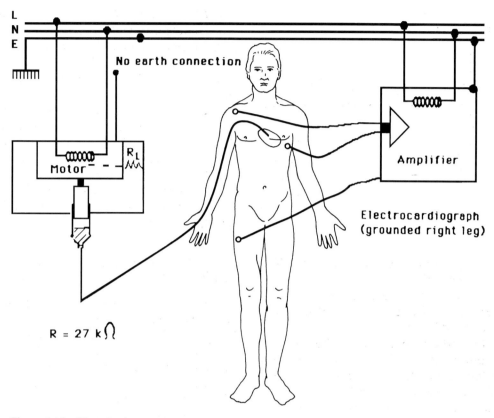

Figure 4.18   Microshock.

fibrillation can occur. This phenomenon is known as a microshock.

Microshock can occur in patients who have an intracardiac pacemaker with an external lead.

ULTRASOUND

This is used as a diagnostic tool when X-rays are contraindicated, as in pregnancy, or when they give poor images, such as those of soft tissues. Ultrasound instruments using the Doppler principle were introduced in 1958. The Doppler technique allows repeated measurements of the same patient without causing any harm. It is used to measure the blood flow (e.g. in a limb) and differentiate between a solid or cystic swelling.

Principles of ultrasound

The human ear can detect sound waves of a frequency between 20 and 20 000 Hz. Any sound waves generated above this level (i.e. above 20 000 Hz), which are inaudible to the human ear, are called ultrasound. In diagnostic instruments, the frequency of ultrasound employed is between 1 and 10 MHz.

In some instruments, ultrasound can be produced as a narrow continuous beam with a set direction at the target organ, whereas in others it can be produced as a series of short bursts.

Ultrasound is generated and detected by transducers made up of crystals with a piezo-electric effect: when crystals made up of quartz or rochelle salt (potassium or sodium tartarate) are pressurized, an electric charge appears on their surface (both positive and negative).

Display of ultrasound signals

As ultrasound signals have a short duration, they are continuously displayed on a cathode ray oscilloscope. The types of scanning techniques available are:

1. *A-scan* (A-mode or amplitude scan). This is simple, although expensive. It is used to differentiate between solid and cystic lesions (e.g. in the kidney) and for obtaining accurate measurements such as identifying the midline of the brain when there is a suspected mass in the cranium.

2. *B-scan* (B-mode or brightness scan). B-scanning is used in obstetrics to detect multiple pregnancies, fetal size and abnormality, and the size of the placenta. In cardiology, it is used to detect the mobility of cardiac muscle and heart valves.

Clinical uses of ultrasound and the Doppler technique

Ultrasound and the Doppler technique are used in the following situations:

- in the indirect measurement of systolic and diastolic blood pressure in operating theatres, using arteriosonde;
- to detect air embolism during neurosurgery;
- to detect fetal heart movements during labour;
- to detect the patency of a peripheral blood vessel after a suspected embolism.

LASER PHYSICS

Laser is an acronym for **L**ight **A**mplification by **S**timulated **E**mission of **R**adiation.

Visual light is electromagnetic radiation, as are radio waves and X-rays. These different electromagnetic radiations occur at very different wavelengths. The wavelength for visible light ranges from 385 to 760 nm; shorter wavelengths are ultra-violet, longer are infra-red light.

Laser light differs from ordinary light in three ways:

1. It is highly monochromatic. Laser light consists of photons that are well defined, with a very narrow band of wavelengths, whereas ordinary light contains a wide spectrum of wavelengths.

2. It is coherent, which means that the electromagnetic fields of all the photons in the laser beam oscillate synchronously in an identical phase. In ordinary light, the electromagnetic fields are phased randomly, even at the same wavelength.

3. Directed beams of laser light are collimated, i.e. they have minimal dispersion. The light remains in a narrow, collimated beam, whereas ordinary light beams spread out in all directions from a source point.

These three characteristics allow lasers to generate intense beams of light, to sense and to deliver intense energy to small target sites.

HARDWARE FOR LASER SYSTEMS

The essential components of a laser system include:

- a lasing medium that holds the atoms whose electrons create the laser light;
- resonating mirrors to boost lasing efficiency;
- an energy source to excite or 'pump' the lasing atoms into producing laser light.

The different types of lasers used in clinical practice employ a variety of lasing media and energy pumps. Some use a gaseous lasing medium such as carbon dioxide, argon, krypton or helium–neon, and are pumped by electric discharge through the gas. Gas lasers may produce either a continuous or an intermittently pulsed beam output.

Other lasers use solid rods or laser–passive material containing small quantities of ionic impurities, known as dopants, that are the actual lasing material. Dopants commonly used for their laser potential include chromium (as in the ruby laser), neodymium (Nd) or holmium (Ho). A synthetic gem crystal known as YAG (yttrium–aluminium–garnet) is commonly used as a passive hose matrix. Solid lasers are usually pumped by high-energy photons from a xenon flash lamp, and therefore produce a pulsed beam (see also Table 4.4).

Some medically relevant lasing media and their output wavelengths are listed in Table 4.5.

Frequency doublers convert laser light to a different wavelength, thus enhancing therapeutic flexibility. A beam of laser light passed through a crystal of potassium–titanyl–phosphate (KTP) will emerge with a wavelength double the frequency. In medical practice, KTP is most often used with Nd-YAG lasers.

A light guide directs the laser beam to the surgical site. Once the laser beam is delivered near the surgical site, it is either focused on the site by the lens of an operating microscope, or the shape of the beam can be intentionally altered by passing it through a contact probe directly on the tissue to be lasered.

An operating microscope can accurately aim a laser by directing a low-powered visible beam, usually from a low-powered helium–neon gas laser, through the same optical path as the surgical laser.

Table 4.4 Properties of laser

Property	N_2O	CO_2	O_2
Boiling point	−88.6°C	–	−183.1°C
Critical temperature	36.4°C	31.04°C	−118.4°C
Molecular weight*	44.01	44.00	32.00

*Molecular weight is the sum of the atomic weights of the atoms of which an element is composed.

Table 4.5 Laser media wavelengths

Laser medium	Colour	Wavelength (nm)
Carbon dioxide	Far infra-red	10 600
Holmium YAG	Infra-red	2 060
Neodymium YAG	Near infra-red	1 064
Ruby	Red	694
Krypton	Red	647
Helium–neon	Red	632
Argon	Blue	488
Krypton–fluoride	Ultra-violet	248
Argon–fluoride	Ultra-violet	193

FURTHER READING

Apfelberg D B 1987 Evaluation and installation of surgical laser systems. Springer-Verlag, New York
Lucas D J 1988 A concise 'O' level physics. Edward Arnold, London
Muncaster R 1995 'A' level physics, 4th edn. Stanley Thornes, Cheltenham, Glos
Parbrook G D, Davis P D, Kenny G N S 1995 Basic physics and measurement in anaesthesia, 4th edn. Butterworth Heinemann, Oxford
Scurr C, Feldman S, Soni N 1990 Scientific foundations of anaesthesia, 4th edn. Heinemann Medical, Oxford
Wilson J, Hawkes J F B 1987 Lasers: principles and applications. Prentice Hall, New York

5

Patient care and theatre technique

In every hospital, during the simplest operation or the most complicated, nurses and operating department personnel (ODPs) should understand their roles within the organizational structure of the operating theatre to be effective members of the surgical team. The role and relationships of each member of the team should be clarified in order to achieve a safe environment for the care of the patient. In addition to members of the medical profession (i.e. surgeons and anaesthetists), charge nurses/nursing officers, theatre sisters, staff nurses, technicians and ancillary staff form part of the theatre team.

The time spent by patients in the operating theatre is relatively short (but important) compared with the length of their overall stay in hospital. The responsibility of theatre personnel lies in maintaining the safety, comfort and welfare of the patient from the time he arrives in the operating theatre until the time he departs.

PSYCHOLOGICAL SUPPORT

Patients presenting for surgery are usually highly anxious about the surgery and its outcome. The patient may give the nurse either verbal or non-verbal clues about his anxiety during the preoperative visit. Patients may also be scared, disorganized and dependent, with a feeling of loss, and may have maladaptive behaviour.

From the time the patient arrives in the operating room until the induction of anaesthesia, he or she needs psychological support. On arrival, the patient should first be transferred to quiet surroundings. The operating department nurse or ODP with a friendly, caring, supportive attitude can make a patient calm and relaxed. Nurses planning care for the patient should cater for both psychological and physiological needs. The nurse provides psychological support, combining sensitivity, empathy and courtesy. Touch, for example holding the patient's arm, may aid in this reassurance. Holding areas in the operating department or anaesthetic room give excellent opportunities for nurses and ODPs to offer psychological support to day-stay surgery patients.

On arrival in the operating department, the patient should be greeted by a nurse or ODP who is warm and friendly. The nurse calls the patient by name and checks his or her identity, the procedure to be performed and the surgical consent form. The patient also needs to see the surgeon prior to the induction of anaesthesia to allay any anxiety and to ask any further questions. The nurse, ODP and anaesthetist continue to describe, as and when necessary, what is happening until the administration of anaesthesia.

Conversation at the scrub sink should be kept to a minimum, and laughter and joking give the patient the impression that the surgery is not taken seriously.

Teenagers presenting for surgery tend to behave inconsistently, some being brave and others anxious. Teenagers having abortions or anaesthesia for caesarean sections need to be given special emotional support. Nurses and ODPs can help by giving support and showing acceptance and a non-judgmental attitude.

Children under 4 years of age presenting for surgery may find the experience traumatic. Many anaesthetists are happy to have a parent in the anaesthetic room during induction, but this should be checked beforehand. If the parent is present during induction, it is the job of some member of the team *other than the anaesthetic assistant* to accompany the parent out of theatre once the child is asleep. In some hospitals, school-age children are either shown a video or taken into the theatre the day before surgery.

A child is allowed to sit up, be held or lie on the anaesthetic trolley while anaesthesia is being induced, and as anaesthesia progresses, restraints may be necessary. Most older children are offered a choice of i.v. induction (with EMLA preparation on the dorsum of the hand) or inhalational induction, with various devices attached to the face mask to make it acceptable to the child.

PATIENTS UNDERGOING SURGERY UNDER LOCAL ANAESTHESIA

If a patient is having a procedure under local anaesthesia, the nurse or ODP explains the procedure as and when necessary without disturbing the surgery. Movements in the operating room should be kept to a minimum, with due precaution taken to prevent dropping of supplies, instruments or equipment. While attaching ECG electrodes, blood pressure cuffs, diathermy pads, pulse oximeter probes or oxygen tubing, the nurse should explain the procedure and how it affects the patient.

Patients are apprehensive about what will happen, and the operating department nurse or ODP needs to monitor the patients' anxiety level.

Throughout the surgical procedure, the nurse should offer support by:

- accepting patients' dependency;
- demonstrating warmth and friendliness;
- showing empathy.

While the patient is undergoing surgery, the nurse should make sure that he or she is comfortable by checking the pillows and drapes.

In the present hospital system, because of the number of patients being treated, attention paid to patients' needs is sometimes scant. Theatre personnel play a vital role in ensuring that every patient arriving in the theatre is treated as an individual and not identified by the operation. This will enable the patient to adjust to a strange environment while trying to retain dignity in the process.

In some operating theatres, patients' aids or prostheses are not allowed, which can cause discomfort, embarrassment and confusion. For example, an edentulous (toothless) patient may not be able to speak without his dentures; patients with hearing aids may not be able to understand pre- and postoperative commands; some patients may be wearing wigs due to premature baldness; and some ethnic minority patients (Sikhs) do not like having their turbans removed because of their religious beliefs. Hence concessions need to be made regarding these factors in order to maintain patients' dignity and safety, and respect their religious beliefs.

In the operating theatre, the nurse who receives the patient from the ward will explain the entire operation, so kind, friendly attention is of great importance. In addition to caring for their patients' physical needs, attending to their emotional needs will help many patients to remember their time in theatre more pleasantly.

PREOPERATIVE PREPARATION OF THE PATIENT

Preoperative visiting

Preoperative visiting of patients undergoing surgery has been a standard practice in a number of hospitals in the UK. Such a visit is invaluable to build a rapport with the patient, relieve anxiety and provide an explanation of the perioperative period.

With advances in day-stay surgery and a shortage of beds, a number of patients, both adults and children, arrive only on the day of surgery, which prevents nurses visiting them. However, there is a considerable scope for nurses to make preoperative visits to patients undergoing major surgery, and new methods of reaching day-care patients perhaps need be evolved.

Elective surgery

Patients scheduled for elective surgery are normally admitted at least the day before the operation following a preoperative assessment in the outpatient clinic by either a nurse or a doctor. This allows patients to undergo haematological,

biochemical, radiological and any other appropriate investigation. If the patient is anaemic, he may receive a blood transfusion to bring his haemoglobin concentration up to an adequate level. If a diabetic patient (receiving long-acting insulin treatment) is admitted, her blood sugar will be controlled by changing the regimen to short-acting insulin, with repeated blood sugar estimation.

A patient who is adequately prepared for surgery can be assessed the day before the operation by the anaesthetist and prescribed a premedication.

Starvation

Adults. A recent editorial commented that patients scheduled for either day-case or inpatient surgery may take, if they wish, clear fluids (such as water, sugar water, apple juice and black tea) by mouth up to 3 hours before surgery (Sutherland et al 1986). This allows for alterations in the list and should not lead to cancellation of surgery. An adequate time (6 hours) must be allowed for solid foods to be emptied from the stomach before elective surgery. A number of studies have shown that there is no difference in gastric fluid volume or pH between those patients who were allowed to drink until 3 hours preoperatively and those who fasted from midnight.

In emergency surgery, any factor which might reduce gastric volume (e.g. metoclopramide) or acidity (sodium citrate), or dilute solid material, should be tried, as this could prevent either respiratory obstruction or Mendelson's syndrome, should pulmonary aspiration occur. 'Rapid sequence induction' of general anaesthesia, with cricoid pressure, awake tracheal intubation if indicated, or the use of H_2 receptor blockers (see p. 79) or antacids for emergency anaesthesia in patients 'with a full stomach', remains the standard of care.

Children. A review article suggested that children undergoing elective surgery should be allowed free clear fluids (see above) until 2 hours before the scheduled time of surgery (Bates & Broome 1986). This article also proposed that children requiring emergency surgery should avoid all food and drink for at least 6 hours before operation.

Anaesthetic management should proceed as if the child had a full stomach.

The potential benefits of reduced thirst, better perioperative experience, improved compliance and reduced hypoglycaemia are important from the point of view of both the child and his parents.

Emergency surgery

Patients present for emergency surgery at short notice. Some of them are very sick, not adequately starved, dehydrated and hypovolaemic due to bleeding (e.g. from a ruptured ectopic pregnancy or ruptured aortic aneurysm). The aim of doctors and resuscitation staff in these situations is to rehydrate the patient, make sure blood and blood products are available (see p. 178), and transport the patient immediately to theatre so that appropriate surgical procedures can be carried out.

If the patient is being resuscitated in the anaesthetic room, the role of the nurse is to observe the patient closely. The theatre technician's role is to help the anaesthetists in resuscitating the patient and in administering the anaesthetic.

Starvation

Patients who have eaten within 4 hours of injury, pregnant women and patients with intestinal obstruction are potentially in danger because their gastric emptying time is delayed. Patients with a full stomach can soil their lungs by aspiration if they vomit during induction of anaesthesia or in the immediate postoperative period, because the swallowing reflexes are either absent or inadequate. The methods used to empty the stomach are described on page 206.

Safety period for anaesthesia

In patients who have abdominal pathology or who have been injured, there is no definite safety period for the induction of anaesthesia with regards to gastric contents, regurgitation, etc. Hence, in spite of a minimum 4-hour interval after eating, if the patient arrives for an anaesthetic, the role of a theatre technician is to apply cricoid pressure during the induction of anaesthesia and intubation (see p. 208 for details of cricoid pressure application).

Nursing models in the operating theatre

Day-stay surgery has become popular, with an increased throughput of patients in the operating theatre, and nursing models have been developing in this area.

A care plan has been devised as a link between the nurses on the wards and those in theatre responsible for the patient. This nursing documentation shows what care has been planned for each patient, informs nursing staff involved in delivering care, is used to record changes in the patient's condition or case and helps to maintain continuity of care.

A number of models based on the work of Roper and Orem have been devised in ward situations and operating theatre environments. There are a number of arguments for and against the developments of these models. The arguments put forward in favour of nursing models based on Orem suggest that care can take the form of:

- a preoperative visit, when patient assessment and education can take place;
- the patient's care being handed over to the nurse in theatre, when the patient cannot engage in self-care activities;
- in the recovery area, the nurse extending the care when the patient cannot maintain his or her airway.

Some argue that directing nursing attention toward a theory base has led people to lose sight of the real goals of nursing.

Reception of the patient

All patients arriving in theatre should have someone in constant attendance; they should *never* be left alone on a trolley. The patient should be welcomed by the operating room nurse with a relaxed, well-modulated tone of voice. A short period of conversation, including an introduction to the operating theatre, is reassuring.

Identification of the patient

Patient identification is absolutely essential in order to avoid the possibility of carrying out the wrong operation on the wrong person. The nurse in the reception area of the operating theatre should ask the patient's name. The patient is correctly identified, and his identification band should correspond with the case notes and operating list with respect to his registration number, name, etc. The site of operation (e.g. amputation of the right leg) should be checked and identified with a marker by the surgeon before the patient arrives in theatre.

The patient should not be transferred into the anaesthetic room until the nurse is certain that he has been correctly identified. The nurse should also make sure that relevant X-rays and laboratory reports have accompanied the patient and that blood (if likely to be needed) is cross-matched and readily available in theatre. Special care with identifying procedures is necessary when the patient is confused or speaks little English.

Protecting the patient's possessions

Prostheses, such as contact lenses and dentures, should be removed before the patient leaves the ward. As discussed earlier, hearing aids, and occasionally dentures, should be allowed into theatre until the patient is anaesthetized. If dentures or prostheses are removed after the induction of anaesthesia, they should be looked after by the anaesthetic nurse until the patient recovers from his anaesthetic. If the patient has crowned or loose teeth, they should be mentioned in the notes and to the anaesthetist once again before the induction of anaesthesia.

Patient transfer

In many UK hospitals, patients are transferred from the reception area to the anaesthetic room, but certain hospitals in the UK, and many hospitals around the world, lack this facility; hence the patient is brought directly into the operating room on a trolley and then transferred to the table.

For elective surgery, the patient is usually anaesthetized on a theatre trolley, but in some emergency cases (e.g. aneurysms, ectopic pregnancies, intestinal obstruction and caesarean sections), patients are, despite the availability of the anaesthetic room, anaesthetized on the table in the operation room. This allows the patient's abdomen to be explored immediately if he or she becomes hypotensive during induction of anaesthesia (e.g. in aneurysms or ectopic pregnancy), or the table can be tilted head down if the patient is seen to regurgitate.

Regardless of where the patients are anaesthetized or transferred, they should be encouraged to move by their own effort, provided they are not heavily sedated. It is safer if one person stabilizes the trolley while another person stands on the opposite side of the table to receive the patient. If the patient is too drowsy, owing to premedication, he or she must be lifted correctly by at least four people: one supporting the head and shoulders, one lifting the feet and legs, and one on each side to lift the trunk. The lifting effort should be coordinated by the person who has control of the patient's head. All drains, i.v. lines and urinary catheters should accompany the patient on his move. For the protection of both patient and personnel, it is advisable to have enough people to lift the patient to the table, otherwise accidents and strained backs can result. In many hospitals, rollers and lifter sheets are used. Once the patient is placed on the table, he should be carefully observed until he is anaesthetized to prevent his falling.

Anaesthetic management

The patient, after being identified and made comfortable, is anaesthetized using either a general or a regional anaesthetic technique (see p. 159).

Positioning the patient

After administration of the anaesthetic, the patient is positioned as required for the surgical procedure. The ideal position allows good access to the operating site, does not hinder respiration and circulation, does not cause injury to nerves and blood vessels (see p. 203) and allows adequate monitoring.

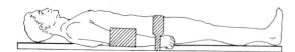

Figure 5.1   The supine position.

All operating theatre personnel should be accustomed to the working conditions of the operating table. They should be able to manipulate the controls, make and break, and lock and unlock the table.

Measures before positioning

The patient should be moved gently after administration of the anaesthetic; rapid turning or moving the extremities can cause dislocations and fractures. The head and neck are usually supported by the anaesthetist to prevent injury and accidental extubation. The patient's clothing is removed before positioning, and afterwards parts of the body other than the surgical site are covered with aluminium foil to prevent accidental hypothermia.

Usually, one arm is secured to a padded armboard so that an i.v. infusion can be given during the operation. The angle of abduction should not be more than 90°, i.e. at right angles to the body. If the arm is severely abducted, the brachial plexus will be stretched, causing paralysis of the nerves in that arm. The elbow should be protected with cotton wool to prevent pressure on the ulnar nerve (which lies on the medial side of the elbow joint) from a hard surface. If the patient is placed in a lithotomy position (see below), the knee joint should be protected on the lateral side from being rubbed against the stirrups to prevent injury to the lateral popliteal nerve. If this nerve is damaged, foot drop can result.

Supine (dorsal) (Fig. 5.1)

The patient lies flat on his or her back, both arms being secured at the sides with palms down, or one arm extended on an armboard for i.v. therapy. The patient's heels are supported with either a pillow or a sandbag, and the legs are positioned uncrossed.

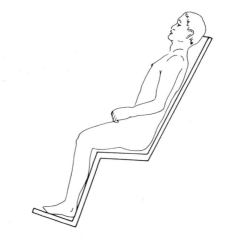

Figure 5.2   The sitting position.

Patients are anaesthetized in this position routinely for abdominal, some thoracic and thoracoabdominal operations and some operations on the hip and lower extremities.

A few modifications are made to this position for good surgical access, for example for surgery on the face and neck, the head is stabilized in a 'doughnut'. For shoulder and thyroid operations, a small sandbag or rolled sheet is placed under the shoulder. For operations involving an upper extremity, for example the breast, the arm on the affected side is placed on an armboard at right angles to the body. For operations on the groin or varicose veins, the knees are slightly flexed over a pillow, with the thighs externally rotated.

Sitting (Fig. 5.2)

Initially, the patient lies supine with the knees over the lower break of the table, a padded footboard supporting the feet. The foot of the table is lowered, with slight flexion of the knees. The upper section of the table is raised to a full sitting position, the head being supported on a headrest. The arms rest on a large pillow in the lap, the shoulders and thighs being strapped to the table.

This position is used for craniotomies and some facial operations.

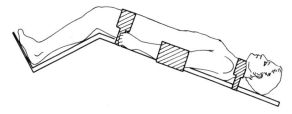

Figure 5.3 The Trendelenburg position.

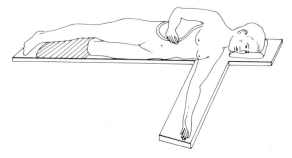

Figure 5.4 The lateral position.

Prone

The patient is turned onto the abdomen, with rolled sheets or pillows placed under the chest and pelvis, thus facilitating free movement of the diaphragm during respiration. The arms are secured alongside the body. The feet and the ankles rest on a pillow to prevent pressure on the toes, a safety strap being placed below the knees.

This position is used for operations on the posterior chest and legs. A slight modification, adjusting the mattress so that the patient's lumbar area is over the upper break in the table, is suitable for laminectomy.

The trolley on which the patient came to theatre should always be readily available when a patient is operated on in the prone position. This allows the patient to be rapidly turned onto his or her back again in the event of an emergency.

Trendelenburg (Fig. 5.3)

The patient is placed on the table in a supine position with the knees directly over the lower break of the table. The foot of the table is lowered to flex the knees, and the table tilted to lower the head. A knee strap helps to prevent the patient sliding towards the head of the table.

This position is used for operations on the pelvis or lower abdomen where it is essential to obtain better exposure by letting the abdominal viscera fall into the upper abdomen.

Reverse Trendelenburg

With the patient in the supine position, the table is tilted upwards to raise the head and lower the feet. A padded footboard is used to prevent the patient sliding.

This position is used for thyroidectomy to decrease the blood supply to the operative site, thus facilitating surgery.

Lithotomy

The patient is placed on the table in a supine position. A polyethylene pad is placed at the lower end of the table (to prevent the mattress being soaked with blood, etc.), and the patient is moved onto the pad so that the buttocks extend slightly past the lower break in the table. The legs are put into stirrups. It is essential to lift and flex both legs simultaneously to prevent lower back strain for the patient when either leg is placed in the stirrup. Similarly, the legs should be removed from the stirrups simultaneously. Strap stirrups are commonly used and preventative measures should be taken using paddings to prevent direct contact between metal and the patient's legs at any point.

After the foot section of the table is lowered, a footboard may be attached to provide a ledge for the surgeon. The arms are secured across the patient's abdomen by folding the gown over them and tucking it under the body. During perineal operations, a better surgical access can be achieved in male patients by gently pulling the genitalia onto the lower abdomen and strapping them with an adhesive plaster.

This position is used for cystoscopy and vaginal, perineal and rectal operations.

Lateral (Fig. 5.4)

The patient is turned onto the unaffected side, with the back near the edge of the table. The arm

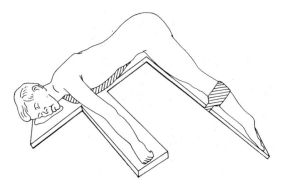

Figure 5.5 The jack-knife position.

on the affected side is placed on an armrest in slight flexion and minimal abduction. Cotton wool or padding below the elbow joint prevents compression of the ulnar nerve, and minimal abduction prevents stretching of the brachial plexus. The unaffected arm is placed on an armboard for venous access or positioned across the chest with a folded sheet in between. A sandbag is placed below the chest to support and elevate it. The lower leg is flexed, and the upper leg remains straight; a large pillow between the legs relieves the pressure of one leg on the other. Braces are attached to the table, the short one at the patient's back, the long one in front. A safety strap over the hip provides stability.

This basic position can be modified for operations on the chest, kidney and ureters. For operations on the kidney, the mattress is adjusted so that the kidney area is over the kidney elevator. The table is flexed at the upper break, and the kidney rest is raised to spread the space between the lower ribs and the iliac crest.

Jack-knife (Fig. 5.5)

The patient is placed in a prone position with the hips over the upper break in the table and the safety strap below the knees. The foot of the table is lowered, and the arms are placed on armboards at right angles to the body, or placed on either side of the head with padded support under the elbows. The chest and pelvis are supported on sandbags and the entire table tilted head down so that the hips are elevated.

This position is used for haemorrhoidectomy and excision of pilonidal sinuses. The theatre trolley should be readily available (see above).

OPERATING THEATRE ENVIRONMENT

Design, ventilation and the control of pollution and traffic all need to be considered.

Design

A proper design of the operating theatre allows a one-way flow of traffic and prevents the return flow of contaminants into the clean area. Separate rooms are allocated for use as shown in Box 5.1.

Box 5.1 Rooms and areas in the operating theatre

- Anaesthetic room
- Scrub-up area
- Sterile supply area
- Dirty utility area
- Sterilizing room
- Unsterile stock and heavy equipment area
- Plaster room
- Recovery room
- Medical, nursing and technicians' lounge rooms
- Dark rooms for processing X-rays
- Staff changing rooms
- Cleaners' room

Lighting and power. Fluorescent lighting is best for general illumination, with provision for emergency back-up. In patient areas, white light is preferred as blue light can make the patient appear cyanosed.

Overhead lights. These are specially designed, shadowless lights made up of tungsten lamps and incandescent bulbs, with heat filters that act as reflectors to prevent overheating of patients and theatre staff. The lights can be dimmed or increased by turning a knob. They have autoclavable handle covers so that the surgeon can adjust the position of the light on the operating site.

Ventilation

Air movements and air conditioning in the operating theatre are regulated so that the patient

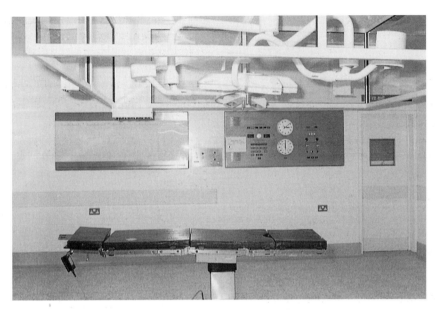

Figure 5.6 The Charnley tent.

and theatre staff are comfortable. Air flow in the operating room is directed from clean to less clean areas. The method of ventilation used to remove bacteria (in the air) in the operating theatre is described below.

Plenum ventilation. A positive pressure is applied to force a downward displacement of fine filtered air from ceiling level. The air is filtered, humidified and either warmed or cooled.

Humidity prevents bacterial growth and the build-up of static electricity. Relative humidity (see p. 107) is maintained at between 50 and 55%. Heat and water loss can occur in small babies during prolonged operations in cool air conditioning; hence the humidity needs to be adjusted.

Air change

1. *Pressurization.* Each operating room should have an air change rate of approximately 20 times per hour. Air supply and exhausts are adjusted in such a way that the operating room and the adjacent clean areas are at positive pressure in relation to the surrounding areas.

2. *Doors.* The doors should be kept closed at all times to maintain the correct pressure in the operating room and surrounding rooms.

3. *Exhaust.* Exhaust vents are positioned in such a way that bacteria and dust particles do not get distributed into the atmosphere.

4. *Laminar flow ventilation.* This ventilation provides 100 changes of air per hour with bacteria-free air in the operating theatre. It is a highly efficient but expensive method of removing bacteria. Laminar flow is used in cardiac surgery and hip replacement surgery to control infection. Patients lose water and heat more rapidly in such an environment.

5. *Recirculation of air.* A certain amount of the exhaust air is filtered to remove bacteria and is then reintroduced. This is a less expensive means of ventilation.

6. *Charnley down-flow clean-air enclosure* (Fig. 5.6). This allows the patient and the operating team to be in an enclosure isolated from other people in the operating room. The flow of air produces a positive movement in a determined route, with 300 changes of air per hour. The air is taken from outside the hospital into the enclosure. The surgeon and the team inside the enclosure wear special clothing using a 'body exhaust' system: a vacuum is used to remove bacteria, dust particles and expired air from the inside of their gowns.

Control of pollution and traffic

Anaesthetic gases are scavenged from the expiratory valve of the anaesthetic apparatus to the atmosphere via tubing.

Traffic of personnel is restricted in the operating theatre, and there should be a limited number of people in the operating room during surgery. The important factors that need to be considered when planning traffic controls are the movement of staff and patients, the removal of linen and contaminated waste, and the delivery of supplies.

If visitors arrive in the theatre complex, they should be taken to the changing rooms and shown how to don the appropriate clothing.

PREPARATION BY THE THEATRE PERSONNEL

Before beginning any surgical procedure, the following points need to be strictly followed:

1. *Personal hygiene.* All theatre personnel should have a bath or shower and change their underwear daily. Hands should be washed frequently and nails cut.
2. *Operating theatre clothing.* Theatre personnel must change into theatre clothes, wear caps that cover all their hair, and wear antistatic, rubber-soled shoes. Jewellery must not be worn in the operating room. A mask is tied securely around the nose and mouth to allow the air to filter through the mask and not escape around the sides. Masks should be thrown away after each use and not worn around the neck.

Aseptic technique

Staff in the operating theatre should make sure that they maintain asepsis to limit the risk of contamination of a surgical wound. The main principles of an aseptic technique are:

1. All instruments used in the theatre must be sterile.
2. Sterile and non-sterile instruments must be kept apart.
3. Correct sterile scrubbing, gowning and gloving procedures must be followed.

4. The patient's skin must be prepared properly.
5. The patient must be draped with an aseptic technique.
6. An unsterile person should always face the sterile field, never lean over a sterile trolley and never walk between sterile trolleys and the operating table.

Surgical scrubbing

The surgical hand scrub is essential to remove bacteria and dirt from the hands and arms, and to provide an antiseptic cover on the skin preventing the growth of bacteria.

A brush is used to remove visible soil from the fingernails and between the fingers. Brush dispensers, from which sterile scrub-brushes are dispensed, are attached to the wall of a scrub-up area. A number of antiseptic agents, such as povidone iodine (Betadine), chlorhexidine (Hibitane) and hexachlorophane (pHisohex), are available. In each operating area there is a separate 'scrub-up' zone outside the operating room.

The first scrub of the day lasts for 5 minutes and is described below:

1. The hands and arms are rinsed under running water.
2. Antiseptic agent is squeezed into the palm of the hand, and the hands and arms are washed to the elbows for 2 minutes.
3. The lather is rinsed off with running water.
4. The fingers and fingernails are scrubbed with a brush for 1 minute.
5. The hands are rinsed.
6. The procedure of washing the hands and arms for 2 minutes is repeated.
7. Following a rinse, the hands and arms are elevated away from the body.
8. The hands and arms are dried using a sterile towel before donning the gown and gloves.

Wearing gown and gloves (Fig. 5.7)

Each hospital has a different technique but a common procedure is:

1. The gown is lifted upwards, holding it at the neck end.

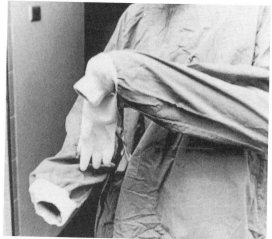

A Unexposed left hand holds the right-hand glove, thumb faces upwards.

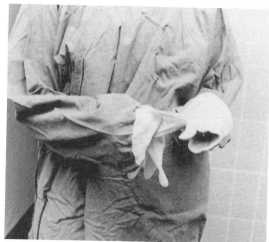

B Cuff of the glove is grasped in the left hand and slid over the right hand.

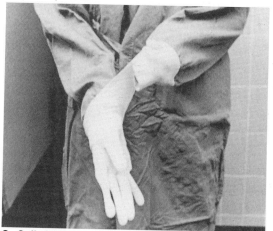

C Cuff of the glove is stretched over the stockinette cuff of the sleeve.

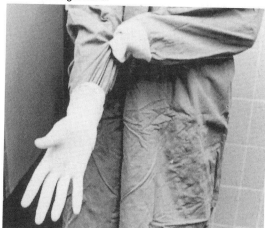

D Stockinette cuff of the sleeve is positioned over the wrist.

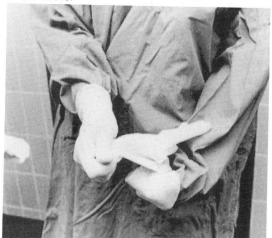

E Repeat the technique for left hand.

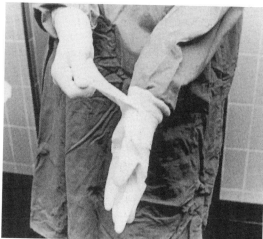

F Completing the closed method of gloving.

Figure 5.7 Gloving technique (from Kaczmarowski N 1982 Patient care in the operating room, Pitman).

2. The scrubbed person touches only the inside of the gown, as the outside of the gown is sterile.
3. The gown is worn by sliding the arms into the armholes.
4. The hands are left within the sleeves of the gown to allow gloves to be put on.
5. The hands and fingers are kept within the cuff of the gown, and the right glove is picked up with the left hand.
6. The palm of the glove is put against the palm of the right hand with the thumbs together and the fingers of the glove pointing to the right elbow.
7. The folded edge of the cuff of the glove is grasped in the left hand and inverted over the right hand. The glove is pulled on at the same time over the wrist area. The same procedure is repeated for the left hand.

After putting on gown and gloves, the scrubbed person, assisted by another 'sterile' person, ties the gown at the front. A sterile person should never turn his back to the sterile trolley and should keep his hands above waist level. The arms are never folded and sterile people pass back to back.

When discarding the gown and gloves, the gown is removed first, then the gloves.

Patient preparation

Skin preparation. Preoperative skin preparation removes bacteria and dirt from the skin and provides an antiseptic cover on the skin surface. On the ward, the skin area is shaved according to the type of surgery. The surgeon in the operating theatre prepares the patient's skin with a swab attached to sponge-holding forceps dipped into antibacterial skin solution. The various antiseptic solutions used are mentioned above.

Draping (Fig. 5.8). Sterile drapes are used to provide a safe barrier between sterile and non-sterile parts of the body, thus preventing cross-infection and contamination of the surgical wound. Drapes may be disposable or reusable, their use depending on the operating room policy and the surgeon's preference.

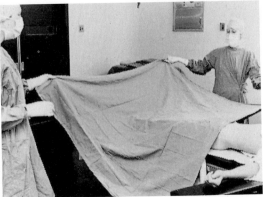

A Placing the first sterile drape over the lower part of the patient's body for an abdominal operation.

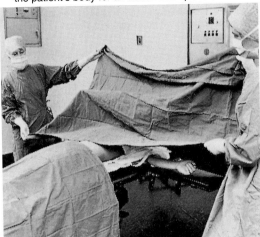

B Placing the second sterile drape.

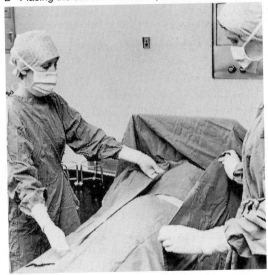

C Placing the sterile side drapes.

Figure 5.8 Sterile draping (from Kaczmarowski N 1982 Patient care in the operating room, Pitman).

Draping is carried out by two 'sterile' people. The sterile drapes are placed over the patient, allowing only the operative site to be exposed. For an abdominal operation, the patient is draped from the incision site to the foot of the operating table. The next drape is arranged from the incision site to the head of the operating table. The side drapes are then placed to provide a sterile surgical field. A split (fenestrated) sheet may be used to cover the initial drapes for added protection. An anaesthetic screen is used to separate the sterile surgical area from the non-sterile anaesthetic area and to hold the drapes away from the patient's face. It is covered by the drape extending from the incision site to the head.

Swabs, sponges, instruments and needles

It is extremely important to count the various pieces of surgical equipment before and after surgery, and to inform the surgeon at the end of surgery that the count is correct. During each case, a circulating nurse counts the swabs with the scrub nurse and writes the number correctly on the swab board. Before the closure of the peritoneum, the scrub nurse and the circulating nurse check the board to ascertain the total number of swabs in use, along with the swabs on the instrument trolley and the ones the surgeon is using. When the check is complete, the scrub nurse informs the surgeon that the swab count is correct. If the count is not correct, the surgeon is informed and a search made until the missing swabs are found. The wound is not closed until the swab count is correct. Before skin closure, a third count is made. Where there is a discrepancy in the swab count and swabs are not found, even after X-ray of the patient, the senior nurse must be informed. The red tags off each bundle of swabs must be kept and checked to ensure that the swabs recorded tally with the number of tags.

Instrument check. Each scrub nurse is responsible for checking all her instruments before, during and after every operation. Particular attention is paid to any loose blades and screws on retractors.

Special instrument set. Arterial clamps should be checked and recorded on a board. The time of application and removal of arterial clamps should be recorded. At the end of each operation, the scrub nurse must sign the card that is in the instrument tray and check that the patient's name label is on the card; the circulating nurse witnesses her signature.

Needles and tapes must be counted before and after an operation.

Atraumatic sutures are placed on a discard-a-pad and the cut-off end of the suture packet placed on the pad, with the used needle alongside.

Procedure for application of a diathermy pad

Operating theatre personnel ensure that the diathermy pad is in satisfactory working order before the list begins. The scrub nurse checks the lead and forceps. After positioning the patient on the theatre table, operating theatre personnel check the site where the diathermy pad is to be placed to make sure that the skin is clear (with no abrasions or redness). The diathermy pad is placed smoothly on the skin, without wrinkles or air bubbles, and bandaged firmly, but not tightly, in position. At the end of surgery, the diathermy pad is removed and the site checked for any signs of redness. If any are seen, the surgeon is informed immediately, an accident form is completed and the senior theatre nurse advised of the incident.

Tourniquet

A tourniquet is applied to make the operative site bloodless, for example arthroscopy for upper limb surgery and foot surgery. The tourniquet consists of a cuff and a pressure gauge (Fig. 5.9). The tourniquet pressure is usually 50–150 mmHg greater than the patient's systolic blood pressure. When a tourniquet is applied, the time of application is recorded with the patient's name on the tourniquet board; the time is recorded again when the tourniquet is released. This is important as surgeons will put these times in the patient's notes after surgery. The surgeon should be reminded after each half an hour of tourniquet time during surgery.

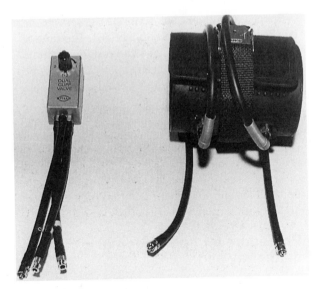

Figure 5.9 Dual-cuff tourniquet.

The sister in charge should check that the tourniquet has been removed before the patient leaves the theatre.

Frozen section specimens

During surgery, the surgeon may take a piece of suspected tissue (e.g. suspected breast cancer) and send it for a frozen section biopsy. The laboratory technician is informed by the medical staff, before they start surgery, of details of the patient who is to have a frozen section operation and the time at which the specimen will be available from theatre. A pathology form is completed in advance.

When the section is taken, the tissue is put in a dry sterile container and sent immediately to the pathology department. The result of the pathological examination is telephoned to theatre, and the medical staff take the message.

Specimen collection for histology and bacteriology

The scrub nurse finds out from the surgeon whether any tissue removed from the operative site is to be sent for laboratory examination.

Histology specimens. The specimen is put in a container and covered with formal saline. Two patient name labels are removed from the patient's notes by the circulating nurse who, after checking with the sister, puts one label on the container and one on the histology form. The medical staff complete the form. The specimen book is completed by the circulating nurse and the specimen sent to the laboratory.

Bacteriology specimens. The same procedure is carried out as for histology specimens but the specimen is not covered with formal saline: it is left dry in its sterile container.

Procedures for hepatitis B-positive patients undergoing surgery

Preparation of theatre. All unnecessary furniture and equipment is removed from the theatre and, wherever possible, disposable equipment is used. The circulating staff wear plastic aprons/disposable gowns and gloves. The scrub team wear disposable plastic aprons under disposable gowns, and all staff wear goggles.

During surgery. The used swabs are placed in bags labelled 'Infected material' and removed immediately for collection. All the used instruments and anaesthetic equipment are placed in a BIOHAZARD bag and sent to the sterilization unit for autoclaving. If linen is used, it should be placed in special linen bags and removed for collection. All equipment and furniture is cleaned with hypochlorite solution, and specimens are placed in adequately sized containers with the lids fully secured. The specimen container is placed in a sealed plastic bag and sent to the pathology laboratory with a form clearly stating that the specimen is from a hepatitis B-positive (Australia antigen-positive) patient.

Any injury to staff, no matter how trivial, is reported to the senior theatre nurse, and the member of staff is sent to the occupational health department.

The same procedure is followed for AIDS patients; further details can be found on page 95.

Methicillin-resistant *Staphylococcus aureus* infections (MRSA) and the operating theatre

The term MRSA implies resistance to the commonly used antibiotic flucloxacillin. Another antibiotic, methicillin, is used to detect this resistance in the laboratory.

Mode of transmission

MRSA is transmitted by the hands of health-care workers in the hospital. In addition to carriers of MRSA who are heavily colonized, inanimate objects such as the operating table, attachments and supports in the theatre have been identified as a route of transmission.

MRSA infections

MRSA infection can occur in bones, joints, wounds, the urinary tract and the lungs.

In the operating theatre, MRSA infections can occur via the skin incision.

Implications for operating theatre staff

- All theatre staff should be aware of any MRSA patient on the operating list.
- Patients with MRSA should be scheduled at the end of the list.
- Patients with MRSA should be recovered in the operating theatre.
- Correct handwashing between patients should be a standard practice for good infection control.
- Apron and gloves should be worn by theatre staff caring for the MRSA patient.
- Staff who become colonized should remain off work until complete clearance has been confirmed by screening.

Control of Substances Hazardous to Health (COSHH) Regulations

The COSHH Regulations protect individuals at work from hazardous substances in the workplace including:

- substances labelled corrosive, irritant, harmful, toxic or very toxic;
- pesticides and other chemicals;
- products or byproducts (dust, fumes, etc.);
- microorganisms (viruses, bacteria, etc.);
- carcinogens (cancer-causing agents).

COSHH Regulations cover most places, such as manufacturers, service industries, farms, utilities, construction sites and laboratories. These regulations are important in identifying hazardous substances, how to guard against them and how to keep the workplace healthy and safe. It is important to assess:

- which substances people are likely to be exposed to every day;
- how substances are handled and stored;
- whether death, illness and injury could result from a single exposure, from a short exposure or from long-term exposure;
- whether a substance could be swallowed, inhaled or absorbed through the skin;
- whether employees, contractors, visitors and others are at risk.

Various steps can be taken to prevent or control exposure. The employer may:

- remove a substance from use;
- change a work practice;
- use a less hazardous substance;
- use a less hazardous form of the same substance;
- use ventilation or exhaust extraction;
- isolate or enclose the area;
- reduce the length or level of exposure;
- use other types of control measure.

For airborne substances with designated MELs (maximum exposure limits), exposure must be reduced to as low a level as possible (below the MEL). For airborne substances with given OESs (occupational exposure standards), exposure should be reduced as far as possible (below the OES). For other airborne substances, exposure must be reduced so that health is not endangered.

The duties of the employer under the COSHH Regulations are:

1. to review regularly to ensure that new equipment, material, etc. has not created new health risks;
2. to maintain, examine and test equipment to ensure that it is in good working order, and to change and replace it as necessary;
3. to provide information about health risks, and to give training in the use of control measures and protective equipment;
4. to monitor and record exposure in some cases, to ensure that control measures are effective;
5. to arrange health surveillance in the form of regular medical check-ups, and to maintain health records;
6. to supply, in addition, protective equipment;
7. to instigate other measures, for example setting up separate washing and eating areas, providing facilities for washing contaminated clothing and making sure that control measures and protective equipment are being used properly.

The duties of the employee are :

- to take part in training programmes;
- to practise safe habits;
- to read container labels;
- to report any hazard or defect to the supervisor;
- to use personal protective equipment properly;
- to store equipment and tools properly;
- to take part in health surveillance;
- to use control measures properly;
- always to practise safe work habits;
- to know first-aid and emergency procedures;
- to practise good personal hygiene;
- to ask the supervisor if any questions arise.

Risk management in operating theatres

Risk management is defined as the systematic identification, assessment and reduction of risks to patients and staff, and the prevention and avoidance of untoward incidents and events.

The operating theatre is a highly technical area, complicated by the size of the team and intricate equipment. Areas of risk in the operating theatre are given in Box 5.2.

Box 5.2   Areas of risk in theatre

- The wrong patient
- The wrong operation or the wrong site or side
- Lack of written consent
- An extension of surgery not covered by the patient's consent
- A drug or transfusion error
- Patient injury due to incorrect patient positioning or while moving the patient
- Burns, fire or explosions
- Retained swabs, needles and instruments
- Injury secondary to the improper use of equipment or to faulty equipment
- Unplanned equipment disconnection that has a potential for patient injury
- Cardiorespiratory arrest during surgery not caused by those risks already listed

---

Communication. It is essential that there is effective communication between the patient and theatre staff.

Patient identification. The patient is identified in the operating theatre by the ward nurse, theatre nurse, anaesthetist and surgeon by checking the patient's name and identification bracelet, and the side, site and name of the proposed operative procedure.

Patient monitoring. The patient is monitored during the perioperative period in accordance with the minimal monitoring standards recommended by the Association of Anaesthetists of Great Britain and Ireland (see the Appendix).

Consent. Consent is a legal concept that requires that the patient or his or her legal guardian be advised of and understand the risks, expected benefits and postoperative lifestyle/health status, and the involvement of junior doctors in the procedure.

'Informed consent' implies that the patient has been given enough information of the real (common) and material (life-threatening or disabling) risks of their surgery and anaesthesia versus the expected (probable) outcome that their consent can be said to be properly 'informed'.

The language used in explanation should be non-technical and easily understood.

Patient positioning/movement. It is important to take adequate precautions when positioning or moving an unconscious patient in theatre. It is necessary to avoid:

- damage to peripheral nerves (see p. 203);
- mechanical damage to the cardiovascular and respiratory systems;
- mechanical trauma;
- inadvertent disconnection of breathing systems, i.v. drains, urinary catheters and other attached equipment.

Care needs to be taken in positioning and placing instruments and diathermy equipment. Some well-lit part of the patient should be visible to the anaesthetist, even if it is only the surgical field. This allows direct visual examination of the patient's colour.

Theatre counts. It is essential to have established policies and procedures concerning instrument, swab and needle counts, including appropriate documentation. The same theatre staff should be present throughout the procedure to provide continuity and safety; switching of staff should be kept to a minimum. Theatre nurses should not allow outside distraction to interfere with their duty to report correct counts.

Members of the nursing staff can be found liable for incorrect counts even if the surgeon has overall responsibility and delegates the task of counting.

Surgical equipment. All surgical equipment in use should meet the current standards and be adequately serviced to provide safe care to patients. All safety checks and infection control measures need to be documented, including all initial and ongoing checks on the safety aspects and use of the equipment.

Health and safety aspects

Lifting and handling

Further to European Commission directives, the 'Codes of practice for the handling of patients' were set up by the Royal College of Nursing in 1993. These regulations apply to any handling operation that may cause injury at work. Such operations include not only the lifting of loads, but also lowering, pushing, pulling, carrying or moving them, whether by hand or by other bodily force.

Equipment and working practices

1. It is the duty of an employer providing work equipment to ensure that it is suitable and properly maintained and that certain specified risks are addressed.
2. In order to safeguard that new equipment is properly used and its working understood, regular demonstrations and training programmes need to be set up.
3. The Personal Protective Equipment (PPE) at Work Regulations cover equipment and the clothing worn by employees while at work.

The employer's key duties, as stated in the 1992 Regulations, cover equipment and clothing used at work to protect employees against risk to their health and safety.

Needlestick injuries

Needles that are carelessly discarded are always a cause for concern and a dangerous source of injury and infection. It is important that all sharps and needles are placed in the puncture-proof containers provided. To prevent personal needlestick injuries, it is essential that needles should be discarded in the bins provided and not put back into their sheaths.

Control of Substances Hazardous to Health (COSHH) Regulations

The regulations set out under COSHH (see above) outline measures that employers and employees have to take in handling substances considered to be hazardous to health, and the Health and Safety at Work Act of 1974 provides the legal structure by which a high standard of health and safety at work can be encouraged. The employer is responsible for assessing the risk to his employees in handling hazardous substances.

When considering the use of chemical substances such as glutaraldehyde in the operating theatre, it is essential that protective clothing and appropriate waste disposal systems are provided to control the risk of sensitization. Glutaraldehyde is the most effective and commonly used solution for the cold disinfection of endoscopes, but it has been known to have adverse effects on health. It is irritant and sensitizing, so strict precautions have to be taken to avoid inhalation and skin and eye contact. Thorough rinsing and automated processing are advised.

Death of a patient in theatre

In the event of the death of a patient in theatre, the sister in charge informs the senior theatre nurse, and the medical staff advise the ward sister. An oxygen mask and blankets are placed on the patient, who is transferred to the ward for the last offices. Last offices may also be performed by the theatre staff in theatre.

Accidents to staff

In the event of an accident occurring to a member of staff on duty, an accident form is completed by the sister in charge and the incident reported immediately to the senior nurse. Arrangements are made for the member of staff to go to the occupational health department for examination and treatment. All accident forms are forwarded to the senior theatre nurse.

Where a 'near miss' occurs, in which no-one is injured but an injury risk is identified, an incident form may be completed. These forms are reviewed and changes in policy, practice or equipment authorized as necessary, in order to avoid a repetition of the danger.

Scheduled drugs

The recovery nurse, in liaison with the anaesthetic sister/charge nurse, maintains stocks of scheduled drugs and lotions. Stocks are checked weekly to avoid over- or understocking. A member of the trained staff on night duty checks the pharmacy in the emergency theatre each morning.

THEATRE SAFEGUARDS

The Medical Defence Societies and the Royal College of Nursing, in association with the National Association of Theatre Nurses, have formulated guidelines for working in theatre, a summary of which is as follows:

- Label all patients admitted for surgery immediately on admission.
- Place identity bracelets on unconscious patients in the accident and emergency department.
- Day-bed patients should be admitted in the same way as inpatients.
- The nurse in charge of theatre, in agreement with the anaesthetist, sends for the patient.
- The senior ward nurse is responsible for checking that all patients going for surgery are properly labelled.
- The side and site of operation are marked with a skin marker by a surgeon.
- The patient is identified in the anaesthetic room by the full name and hospital number on the identity bracelet. An additional check is made against the theatre list. The consent form is also valuable in identifying the patient and the proposed operation.
- The nurse who sends for the patient, and the anaesthetist, are responsible for making sure that the correct patient has been brought into the anaesthetic room.
- The surgeon or his assistant should check that the patient's full name, hospital number, date of birth and nature of the operation, as set out on the operation list, correspond with the entries in the clinical notes and on the identity bracelet.
- The operation list is drawn up by the surgical team, indicating the nature and site of the proposed operation.
- The procedures or site are written in full. Abbreviations such as 'l' for left and 'r' for right are to be avoided.

- The site of the operation is marked by a member of the surgical team before the patient arrives in theatre.
- All swabs and packs to be used should be in bundles of five and should be counted again before the start of the operation.
- The swabs from previous operations must be removed. The circulating nurse or operating department assistant should count all the swabs and packs before any body cavity or joint space is closed.
- The circulating nurse or operating department assistant counts the swabs during the operation.
- Swabs used in the theatre should be radio-opaque. Non-radio-opaque swabs should not be given to the surgeon until after the wound is closed. The radio-opaque swabs should not be cut into pieces.
- When using powered tools and other similar instruments, it is important to check that attachments and fitments are neither faulty nor loose.
- Patients' notes should be marked with warnings of allergies to plaster, to skin-cleansing agents and drugs.
- Cross-matched blood should be checked and made available in theatre before the induction of anaesthesia.
- Care is taken during lifting and transferring anaesthetized patients between theatre trolleys and the operating table.
- In positioning the patient, nerves must be protected from pressure (see p. 203), particularly in thin patients.
- Eyelids should be closed with tape in an unconscious patient to prevent exposure and damage from foreign bodies.
- All pneumatic cuff pressure gauges and monitors should be checked regularly by qualified engineers. When a tourniquet is applied, the operating department assistant should make a note of the time and inform the surgeon (see p. 137).
- The surgeon and the nurse in charge of theatre should make sure that instruments heated during sterilization are cooled before being used on the patient.
- Staff should be familiar with the use of diathermy and other electrical equipment.
- Regular checks must be made to make sure that equipment has been maintained on the due dates.

FURTHER READING AND REFERENCES

Preoperative starvation

Phillips S, Daborn A K, Hatch D J 1994 Preoperative fasting for paediatric anaesthesia. British Journal of Anaesthetics 73: 529–536

Phillips S, Hutchinson S, Davidson T 1993 Preoperative drinking does not affect gastric contents. British Journal of Anaesthesia 70: 6–9

Scarr M, Maltby J R, Janu K, Sutherland L R 1989 Volume and acidity of residual gastric fluid after oral fluid ingestion before elective ambulatory surgery. Canadian Medical Association Journal 14: 1151–1154

Sturnin L 1993 How long should patients fast before surgery? Time for new guidelines. British Journal of Anaesthesia 70(1): 1–3

Sutherland A D, Stock J G, Davies J M 1986 Effects of preoperative fasting on morbidity and gastric contents in patients undergoing day stay surgery. British Journal of Anaesthesia 58: 876–878

Watson B G 1972 Blood glucose levels in children during surgery. British Journal of Anaesthesia 44: 712–714

Control of Substances Hazardous to Health (COSHH)

Control of Substances Hazardous to Health (COSHH) 1994 Approved codes of practice L5. HSE Books, London

Risk management

Hewitson G 1994 Ignorance is not bliss. Informed consent. British Journal of Theatre Nursing 4(9): 15–16

Medical Defence Union 1991 Risk management in anaesthesia. Medical Defence Union, London

Medical Defence Union 1993 Theatre safeguards, consent, anaesthetic risks and day unit surgery. Medical Defence Union, London

National Association of Theatre Nurses 1994 Quality assessment document. NATN, Harrogate

UKCC 1993 Standards for records and record keeping. UKCC, London

Wilson J 1995 Clinical risk management. British Journal of Theatre Nursing 4: 1115–1117

Health and safety

Gamble P, Aires P 1994 Caring for health and safety counts. British Journal of Theatre Nursing 4(9): 5–9

Health and Safety Executive 1992 Manual handling operations regulations. Health services sheet No. 2

Health and Safety Executive 1992 Personal protective equipment at work summary. Health services sheet No. 3

Royal College of Nursing 1993 Code of practice for the handling of patients. RCN, London

Methicillin-resistant Staphylococcus aureus *infection (MRSA)*
Ayliffe G, Lowbury E, Geddes A 1992 Control of hospital infection – a practical handbook, 3rd edn. Butterworth Heinemann, Oxford
Duckworth G 1993 Diagnosis and management of methicillin resistant *Staphylococcus aureus* infection. British Medical Journal 307: 1049–1052
Taylor M, Quick A 1994 MRSA in the operating department. British Journal of Theatre Nursing 3(10): 4–7

Nursing models in the operating theatre
Kendrick J 1990 Nursing models: enhancing or inhibiting practice. Nursing Standard 5(11): 39–40
Roper N 1976 Clinical reference in nurse education. Churchill Livingstone, Edinburgh
Roper N, Logan W, Tierney A 1965 The elements of nursing. Churchill Livingstone, Edinburgh
Stevens B J 1979 Nursing theory: analysis, applications and evaluation. Little, Brown, Boston

Psychological support
Bates T, Broome M 1986 Preparation of children for hospitalization and surgery: a review of literature. Journal of Pediatric Nursing 1: 230–239

Kneedler J A, Dodge G H 1994 Perioperative patient care. The nursing perspective, 3rd edn. Jones & Bartlett, London
Meeker B J 1989 Preoperative teaching: easing the patient's anxiety. AORN Journal 47(5): 1200–1212
Rothrock J 1992 Perioperative care planning. C V Mosby, St Louis
Wheeler B R 1988 Crisis intervention. AORN Journal 47(5): 1242–1248

Preoperative visiting
Burridge L 1993 Challenging the traditional view of preoperative visiting. British Journal of Theatre Nursing 3(4): 12–15
Caunt H 1992 Preoperative nursing interventions to relieve stress. British Journal of Theatre Nursing 1(4): 171–174
Hathaway D 1986 Effect of preoperative instruction on postoperative outcome: a meta analysis. Nursing Research 35(5): 269–274
Kalideen D 1991 The case for preoperative visiting. British Journal of Theatre Nursing 5: 19–20
Meeker B 1989 Preoperative teaching: easing the patients' anxiety. Today's OR Nurse 1980: 14–18
Nightingale K 1988 The ideal and the actual: preoperative revisited. NAT News 25(12): 12

6

Anaesthesia

Anaesthesia is divided into three phases: preoperative, intraoperative and postoperative.

PREOPERATIVE PERIOD

Each patient undergoing surgery is seen by the anaesthetist either a day before (if an inpatient) or on the day of the surgery (if a day-bed unit patient). The anaesthetist interviews the patient with regard to health, allergies, drug usage, alcohol, smoking, past anaesthetic experience, family problems with anaesthetics (e.g. death due to malignant hyperpyrexia during anaesthesia; following suxamethonium, prolonged muscle paralysis due to pseudocholinesterase deficiency) and any concurrent illness.

While talking to the patient, the anaesthetist assesses aspects of the patient's physical status, such as prominent teeth, a short neck or immobility of the neck, which may cause technical difficulties during anaesthesia (e.g. an inability to maintain airway following the induction of anaesthesia, or difficulty with intubation).

The airway is assessed using Mallampati's scoring system. The patient sits upright, with his or her head in the neutral position and opens the mouth, sticking the tongue out as far as it will go:

- Class I: soft palate, uvula and anterior and posterior tonsillar pillars are visualized.
- Class II: all the above except the tonsillar fauces can be seen.

- Class III: only the base of the uvula is visualized.
- Class IV: only the posterior portion of the hard palate can be seen.

Difficult intubation can be anticipated with Classes II and III. In Class IV, visualization of the vocal cords and even the epiglottis may be highly unlikely, so alternative measures need to be taken to overcome difficulty during intubation.

Another test that can be used to predict difficult intubation is the thyromental distance: if the distance from the thyroid cartilage to the mental prominence (chin) is less than 6 cm, difficulty in visualizing the vocal cords can be predicted.

The following investigations are carried out routinely in patients before surgery:

- haemoglobin estimation
- urine analysis.

In some centres, routine haemoglobin estimations are not carried out on fit children and adults. If the patient is of Afrocaribbean origin, a sickle-cell test is ordered and, if positive, haemoglobin electrophoresis is carried out.

Patients on antihypertensive drugs, diuretics or digoxin, or who have suffered from diarrhoea or vomiting, will have their serum urea and electrolytes measured.

A chest X-ray is indicated in patients who have cardiac or respiratory disease or who are over the age of 40 years. An electrocardiogram (ECG) is performed in patients who have cardiorespiratory disease or who are above the age of 40 years. Lung function tests and arterial blood gas analysis are carried out in those with lung disease.

X-rays of the neck (cervical region) are carried out in patients who have severe rheumatoid arthritis, or a neck or head injury, or in whom endotracheal intubation is anticipated to be difficult (e.g. a large thyroid goitre).

Physical status of the patient

The patient's preoperative physical condition is classified into five groups, based on the criteria laid down by the American Society of Anesthesiologists (ASA) (Box 6.1).

Box 6.1	ASA preoperative classification
ASA classification	*Physical status of patient*
1	Normal, healthy
2	Mild-to-moderate systemic disease, e.g. mild diabetes or anaemia
3	Severe systemic disease that limits activity but is not incapacitating, e.g. severe diabetes
4	Severe systemic disease that is life-threatening, e.g. severe cardiac, pulmonary or liver failure
5	Moribund patient with little chance of survival, e.g. with a ruptured aortic aneurysm
Emergency (E)	Any patient in one of the classes mentioned above who undergoes an emergency operation is considered to be at greater risk than a similar elective patient. The letter E is placed beside the number (e.g. 2E)

Premedication

All patients undergoing surgery are anxious about anaesthesia and the outcome of the operation, so it is important to visit them preoperatively to decrease their anxiety and fear. Many patients will also require anxiolytic drugs, of which benzodiazepines are the most commonly used.

The purposes of a premedication (any drug given just before an operation) are:

- as an anxiolytic, e.g. benzodiazepines;
- to continue a preoperative drug regimen, such as antihypertensives, antiasthmatic drugs, steroids and insulin;
- to reduce pain, e.g. opiates and EMLA skin cream in children;
- to reduce nausea, e.g. metoclopramide;
- to reduce the volume and acidity of the gastric contents, e.g. H_2 antagonist, sodium citrate and 5-HT3 antagonists;

- to prevent abnormal blood clotting, e.g. heparin;
- to decrease secretions, e.g. atropine.

Some of the commonly prescribed premedicant drugs are listed in Tables 6.1 and 6.2.

Metoclopramide (Maxolon) and droperidol are prescribed preoperatively to decrease the incidence of nausea and vomiting. Metoclopramide hastens gastric emptying.

Ranitidine (Zantac) 150 mg or cimetidine 200 mg is given orally 90 minutes before the operation to increase the pH of the gastric contents to above 2.5 and to decrease the gastric volume.

Atropine (0.3–0.6 mg) or glycopyrrolate (Robinul) 0.2–0.4 mg is given i.m. or i.v. to prevent the occurrence of bradycardia.

After adequate starvation and premedication (see p. 146) the patient is brought into the anaesthetic room. The type of anaesthesia, either general or regional, is selected based on the type of operation and the anaesthetist's choice. Before any local or general anaesthetic is given, the following must be available:

- suction;
- a tilting table;
- a source of oxygen;

Table 6.1 Commonly prescribed premedicant drugs for healthy adults

Drug (trade name)	Route of administration	Dosage	Remarks
Diazepam (Valium)	Oral	10–20 mg	Good anxiolytic
Lorazepam (Ativan)	Oral	2–4 mg	Prolonged action Anterograde amnesia*
Diazepam (Valium)	Oral	10 mg	Metoclopramide acts as an antiemetic and lowers the tone of lower oesophageal sphincter
Metoclopramide (Maxolon)	Oral	10 mg	
Temazepam	Oral	10–20 mg	Temazepam is used because of its short duration of action
Metoclopramide	Oral	10 mg	
Papaveretum (Omnopon)	i.m.	20 mg	Causes good sedation
Hyoscine (Scopolamine)	i.m.	0.4 mg	Causes good sedation

*Loss of memory for events since taking the drug.

Table 6.2 Commonly prescribed premedication for children

Weight of child	Drug	Dosage (/kg body weight)	Route	Timing (before op.)
Less than 10 kg	Chloral hydrate	50 mg	Oral	45 min
Above 10 kg	Triclofos	25 mg	Oral	60 min
10–15 kg	Diazepam	5 mg	Oral	90 min
	Droperidol (Droleptan)	2.5 mg	Oral	90 min
Above 15 kg	Diazepam	5 mg	Oral	90 min
	Droperidol	2.5 mg	Oral	90 min
Any age	Temazepam	0.5–1.0 mg	Oral	90 min

- some method of delivering positive pressure ventilation;
- resuscitation drugs and equipment.

INTRAOPERATIVE PERIOD

It is always essential for anaesthetists and theatre personnel to have an adequate knowledge of the anaesthetic machine and other equipment, which should be checked every time before use.

ANAESTHETIC MACHINE

The anaesthetic machine comprises: a supply of compressed gases; a method of metering and releasing the gases; a method of vapourizing volatile anaesthesia agents; equipment for delivering vapours and gases to the patient (breathing systems); a means of scavenging anaesthetic gases; and alarms to indicate the delivery of hypoxic mixtures.

Compressed gases

There are several general principles in the use of medical gas cylinders:

1. Medical gas cylinders are used to store compressed gas.
2. Cylinder sizes are designated according to letters, size A being the smallest. Size E is that most commonly used on anaesthetic machines.
3. All cylinders are colour coded according to which gas the cylinder contains (Table 6.3). This code is international and applies in all countries except the USA.
4. The pin-index safety system prevents attachment of the wrong gas cylinder to the yoke on the anaesthetic machine (which could allow a hypoxic mixture to be delivered). It consists of two pins projecting from the cylinder yoke on the machine, which correspond to two holes drilled into the cylinder valve on the gas cylinder.
5. Cylinders should be stored in cool, well-ventilated areas, well away from naked flames.
6. In the case of oxygen and other gases that do not normally liquefy, the cylinder gauge

Table 6.3   Colour coding of medical gas cylinders

Gas	Cylinder body colour	Cylinder shoulder colour
Oxygen	Black	White
Nitrous oxide	Blue	Blue
Enfonox (50% O_2/50% N_2O)	Blue	White and blue quarters
Air	Grey	White and black quarters
Carbon dioxide	Grey	Grey
Helium/oxygen	Black	White and brown quarters

accurately reflects the cylinder's fullness since the amount of gas is proportional to the pressure.

7. Nitrous oxide and carbon dioxide are liquefied gases, so the pressure gauges on their cylinders reflect the vapour pressure of the liquid gas and do not indicate the amount of liquefied gas remaining in the cylinder.

Oxygen

Oxygen (O_2) is supplied to the anaesthetic machine as a compressed gas in cylinders of various sizes or from a pipeline source. In large hospitals, pipeline oxygen comes from a liquid oxygen store. Liquid oxygen is stored at a temperature of −183°C at 10.5 bar in a giant thermos flask: a vacuum-insulated evaporator (VIE) (Fig. 6.1). Constant pressure is maintained by the transfer of gaseous oxygen into the pipeline system. In some hospitals, instead of a liquid oxygen store, the hospital pipeline is supplied by a double bank of large cylinders. In addition to oxygen, gases such as compressed air, nitrous oxide and Entonox are piped.

Oxygen is stored as a gas in compressed form at a pressure of $137 \times 10^3\,kPa$. It follows the principle of Boyle's law (see p. 103), and the pressure gauge gives a reliable indication of the proportion of the original contents still remaining.

The cylinders are made of molybdenum steel. They are checked at intervals by the manufacturer for defects, using the following tests:

- *Tensile test.* One out of every 100 cylinders manufactured is tested. Strips are cut and stretched; the 'yield point' should not be less than 15 tons/in².

- *Hydraulic or pressure test*. This is a water-jacket test. The filling ratio of a cylinder is the ratio of weight of gas in the cylinder to the weight of water the cylinder could hold.
- *Flattening impact and bend tests*. These tests are carried out on at least one out of every 100 cylinders made.

Oxygen cylinders supplied are colour coded black for the cylinder body, with white shoulders (see Appendix).

Nitrous oxide

Nitrous oxide (N_2O) is supplied in cylinders colour coded blue. It is liquid at room temperature when compressed, and exerts a pressure of 4.4×10^3 kPa at 15°C. The liquid nitrous oxide evaporates into the gaseous phase when it is released from the cylinder.

When all the liquid nitrous oxide evaporates, the nitrous oxide pressure gauge starts to fall, showing imminent emptying of the cylinder. The filling ratio of nitrous oxide cylinders is 0.75.

Entonox

A mixture of nitrous oxide and oxygen (50:50) supplied in cylinders colour coded blue with white segments on the shoulders, Entonox is stored at a pressure of 137×10^3 kPa at 15°C. The constituent gases in the cylinder will separate at −7°C. A cylinder whose gases have separated delivers initially a mixture rich in oxygen but then, as the cylinder empties, a mixture deficient in oxygen.

Before use, cylinders are stored horizontally at a temperature above 5°C for 24 hours. If the cylinders are required urgently, they should be stored at a temperature above 10°C for 2 hours and then inverted three times.

Carbon dioxide

This is a colourless gas supplied in cylinders painted grey. The filling ratio is 0.75 in tem-perate and 0.67 in tropical climates. Carbon dioxide occupies 90–95% of the cylinder in a liquid form.

Air

Supplied either via a pipeline or in cylinders painted grey with black and white shoulder quadrants, air is stored at 137×10^3 kPa.

Types of cylinder

There are five sizes of nitrous oxide cylinder (C, D, E, F and G) and six sizes of oxygen cylinder (C, D, E, F, G and J). The larger oxygen cylinders are fitted with a bull-nose valve, which can be connected to the pipeline manifold. The largest nitrous oxide cylinders (F and G) are fitted with a handwheel valve.

Piped gas supplies

For reasons of economy and to avoid frequent changing of gas cylinders in busy theatres, gases may be piped from a remote storage area. The central source of oxygen may be a liquid oxygen tank (Fig. 6.1) or a cylinder manifold. This storage area is outside the main hospital buildings because of the increased fire risk in all areas where oxygen is stored.

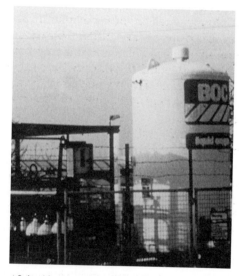

Figure 6.1 Liquid oxygen tank.

Table 6.4 Piped gas supplies

Gas	Hose colour	Wall socket colour
Oxygen	White	White
Nitrous oxide	Blue	Blue
Air	Black	Black
Suction	Yellow	Yellow

To avoid accidental misconnection of piped gases to the anaesthetic machine, all wall gas outlets are clearly labelled and colour coded (Table 6.4). The wall sockets and the probes for the anaesthetic machine pipes are gas specific and non-interchangeable (e.g. a nitrous oxide probe will not fit an oxygen socket). The anaesthetic machine hoses are colour coded.

Nitrous oxide

This is stored in a bank in the form of a cylinder manifold and piped to the operating theatres (Fig. 6.2). Each cylinder is connected to a pipeline by a coiled tube that passes to a central control box. The pressure gauges on the left and right sides of the box indicate the contents of the cylinder banks, and below are high-pressure valves that reduce the cylinder pressure of 137×10^3 kPa to approximately 10×10^3 kPa. There is a change-over valve that switches automatically from the in-use bank to the reserve bank of cylinders when the pressure falls below a certain value. Attached are two electrical warning devices activated by the valve, which switch on warning lights or audible alarms at a control box and remote points to indicate the need to change the empty bank of cylinders. At the outlet of the change-over valve is a second-stage valve to reduce the pressure from 10×10^3 kPa to 4.1×10^3 kPa, the normal pipeline pressure.

Air

Air is supplied to the theatres through pipelines. They can be provided from a manifold of cylinders or a central compressor plant.

A centralized vacuum system is installed along with oxygen, nitrous oxide and air. It consists of a pump, a large receiver and a filter unit. Air from the theatres is drawn into drainage traps and

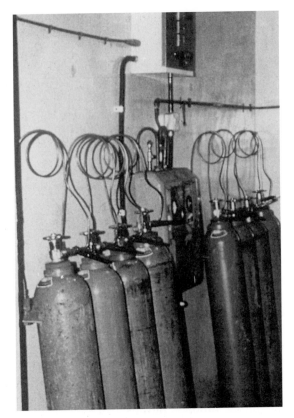

Figure 6.2 Manifold of nitrous oxide cylinders.

bacterial filters to dry and clean it. The air then passes through a constant suction, which maintains a vacuum of around 53 kPa (400 mmHg) below the standard atmospheric pressure of 101.3 kPa (760 mmHg). The exhaust gases from the pump pass through a silencer before being discharged from air intakes or an active scavenging system.

Suction apparatus

This is connected to the vacuum pipeline. The apparatus consists of a collector jar, a filter, a float, a vacuum inlet and a diaphragm. Suction units provide a maximum flow of 40 L/min at a vacuum of 53 kPa.

Schraeder valves

In the UK, all piped supplies to operating theatres finish in special terminal units with a non-inter-

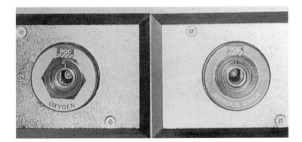

Figure 6.3 Schraeder outlet.

changeable coupling called a Schraeder valve. The Schraeder outlet (Fig. 6.3) is labelled and colour coded, and contains an internal non-return valve that seals the gas supply until the probe is plugged in.

Pin-index system (Fig. 6.4)

This is designed to prevent incorrect placement of a cylinder into the wrong yoke. Two pins located in the yoke should fit into corresponding holes drilled into the cylinder neck. The design of these pins and corresponding holes is unique for each gas. The pin-index system applies to small gas cylinders mounted on anaesthetic machines.

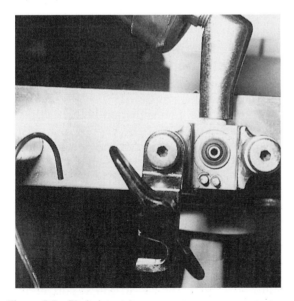

Figure 6.4 Pin-index system.

Pressure regulators (reducing valves)
(Fig. 6.5)

In the anaesthetic machine, it is important to provide a controlled and steady low pressure (0.53 bar) from a high-pressure source such as a cylinder. This is carried out by a pressure regulator.

Flow restrictors and working pressures

The anaesthetic machines work at pipeline pressures (60 p.s.i., 4 bar). To prevent sudden rises in pressures at the downstream end of the machine, flow restrictors are introduced into the gas line before the delicate needle valve. The flow restrictor protects the machine rather than the patient.

Pressure gauges

Pressure gauges are attached to the anaesthetic machines in two places, one at the gas inlet side to indicate the pressure in the gas cylinders or pipelines, and the other in the patient circuit. The gauge in the patient circuit indicates the airway pressure.

Oxygen pressure failure safety valves

All anaesthetic machines have an oxygen pressure safety (fail-safe) system. The fail-safe system consists of a master pressure regulator, which controls slave pressure regulators present in the

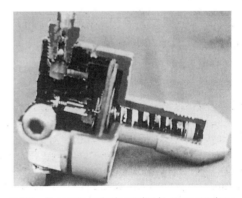

Figure 6.5 Pressure-reducing valve in cross-section.

nitrous oxide line. It is situated between the gas inlet of the anaesthetic machine and the device that controls and measures gas flow. The regulator valve shuts off the nitrous oxide if the pressure in the oxygen line falls below a preset value.

Methods of metering and releasing the gases

The gas is directed to the flow delivery unit from the gas supply via the fail-safe system. There are two ways for delivering and controlling the gas mixture: a gas-mixing system and a gas-proportioning system.

Most anaesthetic machines use a gas-mixing technique, in which the flow rate of each gas is independently controlled and measured by a delivery unit. In most machines, the delivery unit is made up of a needle valve and a variable orifice flowmeter. The needle valve acts as a flow controller and a means of turning gas on and off. In a gas-proportioning system, the gases delivered are set to a definite ratio.

Flowmeters (Fig. 6.6)

The most common flowmeter used in the anaesthetic machine is a tapered glass tube (a rotameter) containing a bobbin, which indicates the flow rate on a scale engraved on the tapered glass tube. Gas is introduced at the bottom of the rotameter tube; as the flow increases, the bobbin rises.

Flow-control (needle) valves

The needle valve is placed at the bottom of the corresponding flow tube. It has an on/off function in addition to regulating the gas flow rate.

High-flow oxygen flush

It is sometimes necessary during anaesthesia to fill the breathing system with oxygen at a higher rate than the rotameter can deliver. This situation arises when there is a leak between the face mask and the patient's face, or in an emergency. Oxygen is delivered at a high pressure (20–45 p.s.i.) at the rate of 30–70 L/min.

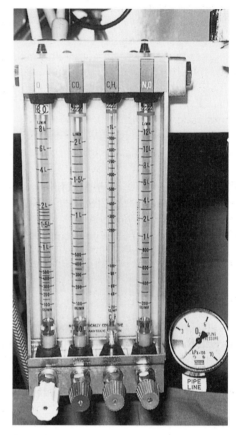

Figure 6.6 Flowmeters. Conical shaped with flow control (needle) valves at the bottom, which regulate the flow of gases.

Method of vaporizing the volatile anaesthetic agent

Vaporizers

A vaporizer is a device that adds the necessary concentration of anaesthetic vapour to a stream of carrier gas (usually oxygen and nitrous oxide).

The saturated vapour pressure (SVP) (see p. 102) of a volatile anaesthetic such as halothane at room temperature is many times higher than that necessary to produce anaesthesia, so the vaporizer mixes gas passing through a vaporizing chamber with gas containing no vapour to produce a final mixture of the appropriate concentration. This is carried out by splitting the flow of gas to the vaporizer into two streams: one passes through the chamber containing the volatile anaesthesia agent and the other bypasses the chamber. These streams reunite and are delivered to the patient. The resistance to gas flow that occurs, especially at the flow-splitting valve, requires that the carrier gas be delivered to the vaporizer under pressure.

Plenum vaporizer (Fig. 6.7). A Boyle's bottle is a typical example of the Plenum vaporizer. In this vaporizer, the liquid anaesthetic is kept in a glass bottle, and a part of the gas flowing through the bypass is controlled by a rotary valve. The problems associated with this type of vaporizer are that the saturation of the gas leaving the chamber depends on the flow rate and, as the anaesthetic agent vaporizes, the temperature falls, which in turn lowers the SVP of the agent, thus decreasing the concentration of vapour delivered to the patient.

The development of flow- and temperature-compensated vaporizers has solved the problem of flow-rate dependence and temperature fall.

Flow-rate dependence. This is overcome and full saturation achieved effectively by placing fabric wicks or metal in the vaporizing chamber, one end of which dips into the anaesthetic liquid while the other projects into the chamber. This method is used in most vaporizers, for example the Abingdon and Fluotec vaporizers.

Temperature compensation. Modern vaporizers are made of metal, which has good thermal conductivity and which therefore allows heat to be transferred from the surroundings to the vaporizing chamber, minimizing the fall in temperature that occurs during vaporization. This system is not perfect, and some cooling will still occur. This problem is solved by changing the splitting ratio of the carrier gas as the temperature changes, so that more gas flows through the vaporizing chamber as the temperature falls. The vaporizer thus gives a steady concentration of anaesthetic agent. The temperature-controlled valve that adjusts the splitting ratio is a strip made of two metals, with different coefficients of thermal expansion, which are joined together to form a bimetallic strip. As the temperature changes, the shape of the two-metal strip alters so that it bends or straightens, increasing or decreasing the gas flow through the chamber. This mechanism is seen in the Tec series 3 to 5 vaporizers (Figs 6.8 and 6.9).

Desflurane (Tec 6) vaporizer. Desflurane liquid is held within the vaporizing chamber and heated to 39°C by two 100 W electric heater elements. Two further heater elements warm the upper part of the vaporizer to prevent condensation. When the operating temperature has been reached, the upper part of the vaporizing chamber contains desflurane vapour under pressure, and solenoid-operated locks on the concentration dial and vaporizing chamber outflows are released. Fresh gas from the

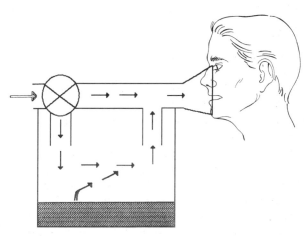

Figure 6.7   Plenum vaporizer.

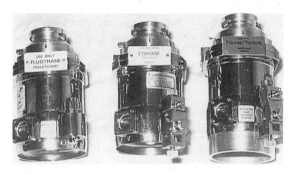

Figure 6.8   Mark 3 vaporizers. Left to right: halothane, enflurane and isoflurane.

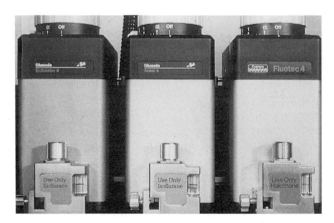

Figure 6.9   Mark 4 vaporizers. Left to right: enflurane, isoflurane and halothane.

flowmeters enters the vaporizer and passes through a fixed flow-restrictor, to generate back-pressure, sensed by two independent pressure sensors. Desflurane vapour passes through a shut-off valve – a pressure-regulating valve – to the concentration selection dial. The pressure of the vapour is detected by these pressure sensors and, by control of the pressure-regulating valve, the pressure may be matched to the back-pressure generated by the fresh gas flows. The concentration selector has a dial-release bar on the back, which is compressed when initially setting a desired concentration. The dial is graduated in increments of 1% between 0 and 10% and in increments of 2% between 10 and 18%.

Vaporizer position and controls. On the anaesthetic machine, the vaporizer is placed between the flowmeter block and the emergency oxygen flush control. This prevents the high flow of oxygen being delivered through the vaporizer.

Care of vaporizers. According to the manufacturer's recommendation, the vaporizer needs to be serviced every year. Halothane vaporizers are drained and refilled at regular intervals (weekly) to prevent the accumulation of preservatives such as thymol in the vaporizing chamber.

It is essential to fill vaporizers with the correct anaesthetic liquid and to prevent their accidental filling with the wrong liquid. A safety system is available, which consists of filter tubes and caps that fit only the appropriate bottles of anaesthetic and vapourizers.

Equipment for delivering vapours and gases

Anaesthetic breathing systems

'Breathing system' and 'circuit' refer to an assembly of tubes and valves through which the patient breathes. The components of a breathing system are:

1. *Tubing*. Most breathing systems are now disposable and made of plastic. The tubing has flexible corrugated walls so that it can bend into acute angles without kinking.

2. *Rubber reservoir bag*. This is a compliant bag that allows the accumulation of gas during expiration so that a reservoir for peak flows is available for the next inspiration. The other uses of this bag are as a visual monitor in the spontaneously breathing patient and to facilitate manually ventilating the apnoeic patient.

3. *Valves*. The anaesthetic circuits may contain either non-breathing, unidirectional breathing or adjustable pressure-limiting (APL) valves. Non-breathing valves are attached close to the patient. The valve discs and springs are light, to reduce resistance.

In the circle absorber system (see p. 156) three valves exist: two unidirectional breathing valves and the adjustable pressure-limiting valve.

In 1954, W. W. Mapleson classified anaesthetic breathing systems into five groups: A, B, C, D and E. These are classed as semi-closed systems, in which partial rebreathing may occur.

Mapleson A (Fig. 6.10). The most commonly used version is the Magill circuit. It is effective in patients breathing spontaneously and is not ideal for intermittent positive-pressure ventilation (IPPV). A modification of the Mapleson A circuit is the LACK circuit (Fig. 6.11), which consists of a long tubing that lies inside a corrugated tube, making up a co-axial circuit. Expiration occurs through the inner tubing, and inspiration through the outer tubing.

A fresh gas flow rate equivalent to the patient's total minute volume is required in these circuits.

Mapleson B and C. These systems are more efficient than the Mapleson A during IPPV. The Mapleson C circuit (Fig. 6.12) is usually seen in the recovery room.

Mapleson D. The Bain co-axial system (Fig. 6.13) is the most common version of Mapleson D. In this system, the fresh gases pass through the inner tubing to the patient, and expired gases pass through the outer tubing. During spontaneous ventilation, the fresh gas flow should be about 2.5 times the minute volume of the patient. For IPPV, a fresh gas flow of 75–80 ml/kg/min is adequate.

Mapleson E. Also known as Ayres T-piece, this is used in babies and children less than 25 kg body weight. The fresh gas flow should be 2.5–3.0 times the minute volume (minimum

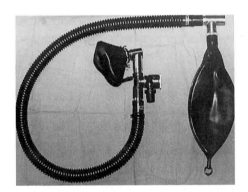

Figure 6.10   Magill circuit (Mapleson A system).

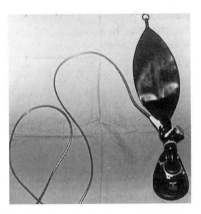

Figure 6.12   Mapleson C circuit (seen in the recovery room).

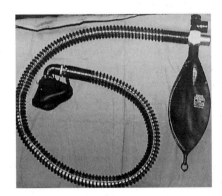

Figure 6.11   LACK circuit (note the non-breathing valve away from the patient).

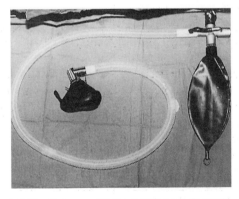

Figure 6.13   Bain co-axial circuit (Mapleson D circuit).

4 L/min). The Ayres T-piece can be used for IPPV, by intermittently occluding the end of the reservoir tube with the thumb.

Mapleson F. This was added by Jackson-Rees as a modification of Ayres T-piece (an open-ended bag being added to the end of the reservoir limb). It provides a method for carrying out IPPV. The bag's movement is a useful monitor in the spontaneously breathing child.

Humphrey A, D and E circuits. These circuits can be effectively used in adults and children, their principles being similar to the Mapleson A, D and E systems.

Circle absorber system (Fig. 6.14). This consists of an inspiratory hose, an expiratory hose, a soda lime canister, two unidirectional valves, a reservoir bag on the end of a third hose, pressure relief valves and an inflow tube.

In this system, carbon dioxide in the inhaled gas is removed chemically using soda lime or baralyme. Soda lime consists of: calcium hydroxide, $Ca(OH)_2$; sodium hydroxide, NaOH; potassium hydroxide, KOH; and silica; with a moisture content of 14–19%. It is firmly packed in the canister, avoiding any gaps that could lead to channelling of gases and inadequate carbon dioxide absorption.

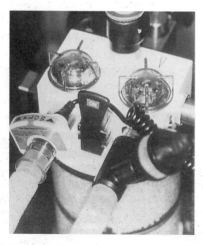

Figure 6.14   Soda lime absorber (also called a circle absorber).

Absorption of carbon dioxide (CO_2) occurs by the following chemical reactions:

$$CO_2 + 2NaOH \rightarrow Na_2CO_3 + H_2O + Heat$$
$$Na_2CO_3 + Ca(OH)_2 \rightarrow 2NaOH + CaCO_3$$

When the soda lime is becoming exhausted, the indicator, for example durasorb, changes its colour from pink to white. Trichloroethylene (Trilene) is not used in soda lime absorber as toxic substances such as phosgene, dichloracetylene and carbon monoxide are produced if the vapour comes into contact with hot soda lime granules. Sevoflurane also forms toxic compounds in the presence of soda lime.

Ventilators

The principle of operation of the ventilator is described by its functional analysis, i.e. how it works during each phase of the respiratory cycle: inspiration, change-over from inspiration to expiration, expiration, and change-over from expiration to inspiration.

Inspiration

Ventilators produce inspiration by delivering a predetermined pressure (pressure generators) or predetermined flow of gas (flow generators) to the patient.

Pressure generators. In this type of ventilator, for example the Manley (Fig. 6.15), the machine delivers gases to the patient at a constant pressure. If there is an increased resistance to the flow, due to bronchospasm or kinking of the tube, the gases will not be delivered to the patient.

Flow generators. These types of ventilator deliver gases to the patient at a constant flow irrespective of the changing compliance and resistance of the lungs. An example is the Oxford Penlon ventilator (Fig. 6.16), in which the flow of gases is initiated by a piston compressing the bellows.

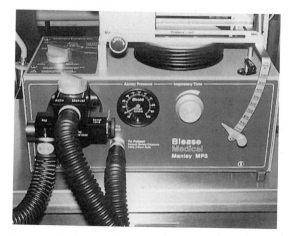

Figure 6.15   Manley ventilator.

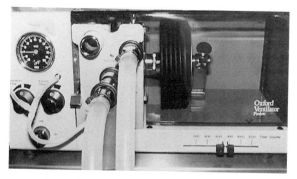

Figure 6.16   Oxford ventilator.

Change-over from inspiration to expiration

This can occur either by volume-cycling (when the predetermined volume is delivered), time-cycling or pressure-cycling.

Expiration

The patient is allowed to exhale to atmospheric pressure. Some ventilators can provide positive end-expiratory pressure (PEEP), above atmospheric, to reduce the danger of alveolar collapse.

Change-over from expiration to inspiration

This can occur either by volume-cycling, time-cycling or pressure-cycling.

Scavenging of anaesthetic gases

The pollution of atmospheric air in the operating theatres occurs from anaesthetic gas discharged from the ventilators, breathing circuits, leaks from equipment, and spillage that occurs when filling the anaesthetic vapourizers. Because prolonged exposure to anaesthetic agents could theoretically have an adverse effect on the staff working in the operating theatre and recovery room, scavenging of waste gas is recommended.

Scavenging of anaesthetic gases can be achieved using:

1. *Active systems* (Fig. 6.17). This means that active suction is applied near to the expiratory part of the anaesthetic breathing system to remove waste gases. The exhaust is able to accommodate 75 L/min continuous flow, with a peak of 130 L/min.

2. *Passive systems*. These allow the venting of patients' expired gas from the anaesthetic system to the outside atmosphere or to a ventilation extract duct. It is important to avoid long lengths of tubing, as this may increase the resistance to exhalation and thus injure the patient.

Alarms

Anaesthetic machines are provided with an oxygen-failure warning device, a gas-powered whistle activated by a decrease in oxygen pressure. The oxygen failure alarm does not rely on any gas other than the machine's oxygen flow, nor does it need any battery or electrical power. As the oxygen in the machine fails, the whistle blows and a valve in the machine

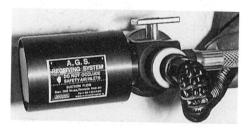

Figure 6.17   Active scavenging system.

opens. This valve simultaneously switches off the nitrous oxide and opens the machine to air, so that the patient should at least receive 21% oxygen (the concentration of oxygen present in air).

Humidification of gases

Unlike atmospheric air, all cylinder and pipeline gases are dry. Patients breathing these dry gases may lose a significant amount of water in humidifying them. During prolonged procedures, it is preferable to prevent this excess water loss by humidifying the anaesthetic gases.

In the operating theatre, inspired gases are most commonly humidified using a condenser humidifier, also called an artificial nose (Fig. 6.18). This humidifier conserves the water that would otherwise be lost on expiration. When the warm, moist expired gases pass through the condenser, they cool and the water condenses on the filter; on inspiration, dry gases are drawn through the moist filter and humidified. For fuller humidification, an active system is necessary, for example a water bath (Fig. 6.19).

Testing anaesthetic machines

Before commencing the anaesthetic, the anaesthetist must check the anaesthetic machine. First, before starting the tests, the machine is disconnected from all piped medical gas supplies, the oxygen and nitrous oxide cylinders being turned off. Then the following procedure is carried out:

1. Check that full cylinders of oxygen and nitrous oxide are properly attached to the yokes on the anaesthetic machine and that the cylinders are turned off.
2. Open the oxygen and nitrous oxide flowmeter valves; no flow should be seen.
3. Turn on the oxygen cylinder: the oxygen flowmeter should register a flow. If the nitrous oxide flowmeter registers a flow, reject the machine.
4. Turn on the nitrous oxide cylinder and check that the nitrous oxide flowmeter

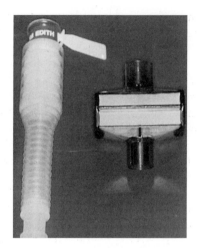

Figure 6.18   Edith humidifier and condenser.

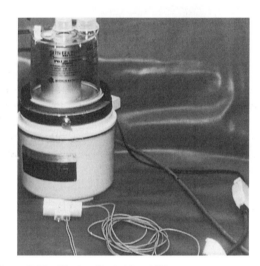

Figure 6.19   Fischer-Peykel humidifier.

registers a flow. If the oxygen flowmeter registers a flow, reject the machine.
5. Set the oxygen failure warning device in operation.
6. Turn off the oxygen cylinder and check that the oxygen failure warning device works.
7. Insert the oxygen probe of the hose into the piped oxygen supply connection at the wall (the terminal unit). This must cancel the noise of the oxygen failure alarm. Apply the 'tug test' to this connection.

8. Turn off the nitrous oxide cylinder. See if there is any change in the oxygen flowmeter bobbin setting as the nitrous oxide flowmeter bobbin falls. If the oxygen flowmeter bobbin shows any change, reject the machine.
9. Insert the nitrous oxide probe from the anaesthetic machine into the piped nitrous oxide supply connection at the wall (the terminal unit). Apply the 'tug test' to this connection.
10. To complete the check, test for leaks by occluding the outlet from the machine until the pressure relief valve on the back-bar is seen or heard to operate. The anaesthetic machine is now ready for use.
11. Test the circuit to be used for leaks and the correct function of any valves.

Checking the Bain circuit

The end of the little finger or the plunger of a 2 ml syringe is used to occlude momentarily the spout of the inner tube of the Bain circuit while gas is passing through the tube. Sounds indicate whether this manoeuvre is causing a build-up of pressure and confirms that the inner tube is intact.

PREPARING FOR ANAESTHESIA

Before the patient receives an anaesthetic, it is important to complete this checklist:

- correct patient, correct procedure, including which side of the body;
- the type of anaesthetic to be given: general or regional;
- the drugs and equipment needed for anaesthesia and monitoring;
- intravenous fluids and blood for transfusion;
- postoperative care and recovery facilities.

At the beginning of the operating list, the anaesthetist checks the anaesthetic machine (see p. 158) and the equipment to be used.

The equipment that an ideal trolley for endotracheal intubation should carry is listed in Box 6.2.

Box 6.2   Endotracheal intubation equipment

- Endotracheal tubes of correct size and a smaller size
- Two laryngoscopes, small blade and long blade (there must be two laryngoscopes in case the first one suddenly fails)
- Endotracheal tube connector
- Gum elastic bougies and wire stilette
- Cuff-inflating syringe
- Magill forceps
- Artery forceps
- Bandage or tape to secure the endotracheal tube
- Catheter mount
- Local anaesthetic spray (4% lignocaine)
- Tube of lubricant
- Face masks and breathing circuit
- Throat pack

When administering anaesthesia, it is important to fulfil a triad of anaesthesia, analgesia and muscular relaxation.

INDUCTION OF ANAESTHESIA

A patient can be induced by either an i.v. or an inhalational technique.

Intravenous induction

Intravenous induction is suitable for all routine surgical cases and is particularly important during emergency surgery where there is a high risk of regurgitation of gastric contents.

All the drugs necessary for anaesthesia are prepared and the syringes labelled with the name of the drug and its concentration. An i.v. cannula is inserted into the back of the hand, or a large-bore cannula (14G or 16G) is inserted in the forearm vein for transfusion of blood and fluids. Before inserting a large-bore cannula, the skin is infiltrated with 1–2 ml 1% plain lignocaine. In children, EMLA cream applied to the skin 1 hour preoperatively will numb the skin to allow 'ouchless' venepuncture.

In an emergency, before commencing induction, preoxygenation is carried out by the administration of 100% oxygen via a face mask.

The common induction agents, along with their dosages, are given in Box 6.3. The details of induction agents are described on page 60.

Box 6.3	Common induction agents
Thiopentone (Pentothal)	3–5 mg/kg body weight
Methohexitone ((Brietal)	1.0–1.5 mg/kg
Etomidate (Hypnomidate)	0.2–0.3 mg/kg
Propofol (Diprivan)	1.5–2.0 mg/kg
Ketamine (Ketalar)	2 mg/kg i.v.
	10 mg/kg i.m.

After attaching the patient to the ECG and blood pressure monitor, induction is commenced. Induction occurs within one arm–brain circulation time (12–30 s), and anaesthesia is maintained with an inhalational agent (such as halothane, enflurane or isoflurane), oxygen (33%) and nitrous oxide (66%).

The complications that can occur during i.v. induction are:

- regurgitation and vomiting;
- injection outside the vein into the subcutaneous tissue;
- cardiovascular and respiratory depression;
- inadvertent arterial injection;
- reactions to individual drugs, such as hiccup (methohexitone) or involuntary movements (methohexitone, etomidate or propofol);
- anaphylaxis (a severe, life-threatening allergic reaction).

Inhalational induction

The indications for inhalational induction are:

- uncooperative or very young children;
- bronchopleural fistula;
- any condition in which intubation is predicted to be difficult, for example epiglottitis or foreign body.

A 'no-mask' technique using a cupped hand around the gas delivery tube is used in young children. As the child falls asleep, the hand, and later on the mask, is gradually brought closer to the face until the patient is completely unconscious. Initially, high concentrations of halothane (1–4%), enflurane (1–4%) or isoflurane are used; once the patient goes to sleep, the concentrations are decreased.

Anaesthesia is maintained by firmly placing the mask on the face as consciousness is lost. Once anaesthesia is established, either an oropharyngeal (Guedel) or a nasopharyngeal airway, a laryngeal mask or an endotracheal tube can be inserted.

An inhalational induction may take much longer than an i.v. one. The problems that can occur with inhalational induction are salivation, airway obstruction, laryngeal spasm and hiccups. The high doses of volatile agent can cause raised intracranial pressure in patients at risk of this, for example those with a head injury.

MAINTENANCE OF ANAESTHESIA

Anaesthesia can be continued using inhalational agents (oxygen, nitrous oxide and volatile agents), total i.v. infusion anaesthesia (propofol infusion with an air/oxygen mixture), or a combination of the two.

The patient may breathe spontaneously or by ventilation controlled with an endotracheal tube and muscle relaxants. If a patient is breathing spontaneously, a face mask, with a Guedel or nasopharyngeal airway (Fig. 6.20), or a laryngeal mask is used. In some procedures (dental and ENT), the patient is paralysed with suxamethonium and an endotracheal tube is inserted. Once the patient recovers from suxamethonium, he or she breathes spontaneously through the endotracheal tube.

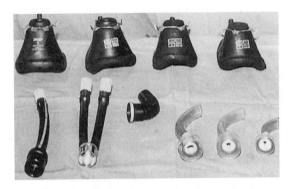

Figure 6.20 Face masks, catheter mounts, angle piece and Guedel oropharyngeal airway.

Endotracheal intubation

The indications for endotracheal intubation are:

- to provide a patent airway in a difficult mask airway;
- to prevent aspiration of stomach contents into the lungs;
- to facilitate positive-pressure ventilation;
- in any operative position other than the supine;
- with an operative site near or involving the upper airway.

Before beginning anaesthesia, the anaesthetist confirms that endotracheal tubes of the appropriate type, size and length are available, and checks the cuff of the tube and both laryngoscopes.

Endotracheal tubes (Fig. 6.21)

In the majority of hospitals, plastic (e.g. Portex or Mallinckrodt) tubes are used. In patients who are undergoing surgery in unusual positions (such as prone or sitting), an armoured tube is used, whereas in plastic surgery preformed RAE tubes are used. In thoracic surgery, a double-lumen (e.g. Robertshaw) tube is used (Fig. 6.22). For the sizes and lengths of tubes, see the Appendix.

An appropriate connector is required between the endotracheal tube and the anaesthetic circuit. A catheter mount connects the endotracheal connector to the breathing circuit.

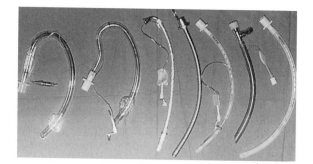

Figure 6.21 Endotracheal tubes. Left to right: RAE tube, preformed (for plastic surgery), tube with aluminium foil, metal tube, microlaryngoscopy tube, armoured and uncuffed tube.

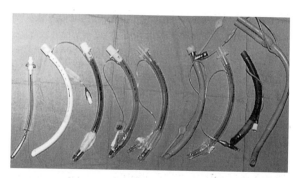

Figure 6.22 Endotracheal tubes and airways. Left to right: nasopharyngeal airway, uncuffed endotracheal tube, sizes 8 and 9 high-volume, low-pressure cuffed tubes, red rubber tube, Hi-Lo endotracheal tube, armoured tube and Robertshaw tube.

Laryngeal masks

The laryngeal mask airway (LMA) is a device that fills the gap in management of airway between the use of the face mask and endotracheal intubation. The LMA was developed in 1981 by Dr A. Brain and became commercially available in the UK in 1988.

Physical appearance

The LMA is made of soft silicone rubber and comes in seven sizes (Table 6.5). A typical size 4 device consists of a 12 mm internal diameter (ID) internally ridged tube or shaft fused at a 30° angle to a distal, elliptical, spoon-shaped mask with an inflatable rim, resembling a miniature face mask. The cuff is inflated via a pilot balloon. The shaft opens into the concavity of the ellipse via a fenestrated aperture with three orifices to prevent the epiglottis from falling back and blocking the lumen. A black line runs longitudinally along

Table 6.5 Laryngeal mask airways

Mask size	Patient weight (kg)	Cuff volume (ml)
1	<6.5	4
2	6.5–20	10
2½	20–30	14
3	30–70	20
3 ST	30–70	20
4	>70	30
5	>70	45

the posterior curvature of the shaft to aid in orientating the tube in situ. LMA modifications such as flexometallic tubes are available for use in maxillofacial surgery.

Technical aspects of the LMA

The LMA is a reusable device and must be checked carefully for faults. Before each use, the LMA is checked for breaks, and the cuff is deflated with its anterior face firmly applied against a hard surface. The posterior surface is lubricated. After the induction dose of propofol and fentanyl (50–75 µg) has been administered, the LMA is inserted with the patient's neck flexed and head extended. The jaw is allowed to fall open or is held open by a member of the operating department staff. There are a number of variations in the way in which the LMA is inserted. Once the LMA is inserted, the tube is advanced in one smooth movement until a resistance is felt as the upper oesophageal sphincter is engaged.

Once the mask portion is in place, the cuff is inflated with the correct volume of air (Table 6.5), which causes an outward movement of the tube with a forward movement of the thyroid and cricoid cartilages. The longitudinal black line on the shaft of the tube should lie in the midline against the upper lip. Any deviation indicates misplacement of the cuff and partial airway obstruction. The 15 mm proximal connector is attached to the anaesthetic circuit and either spontaneous respiration or IPPV is commenced.

Securing the LMA in position

The LMA is secured with either a tape or a ribbon. Some anaesthetists use a bite-block to prevent the patient from biting and obstructing or damaging the expensive LMA.

Removal

The LMA is kept inflated until the protective reflexes return.

Sterilization and cleaning

The LMA should be washed with water and a mild detergent as soon as possible after extubation. The device should then be autoclaved at 121–134°C for at least 3 minutes.

Risk of aspiration

The LMA is contraindicated if a risk of aspiration of gastric contents exists (a full stomach), unless other techniques for securing the airway have failed.

According to manufacturers, the risk of aspiration using the LMA can be minimized if:

- the cuffs are routinely tested for defects before operation;
- lubrication of the anterior surface of the LMA is avoided;
- the LMA is inserted with an adequate depth of anaesthesia;
- adequate anaesthetic depth is maintained throughout surgery;
- one avoids disturbing the patient during the emergence from anaesthesia;
- the cuff is kept inflated until the patient is awake.

The difficult airway

The LMA has a role in supporting airways that are difficult to manage and as an aid to blind and fibreoptic intubation in both elective and emergency situations. It is possible to pass a fibreoptic bronchoscope through the LMA into the trachea. A 6.0 mm cuffed tracheal tube premounted on the fibreoptic bronchoscope can be advanced through the LMA.

The LMA in cardiopulmonary resuscitation

In difficult airways, paramedics have used LMAs during resuscitation. The role of the LMA in cardiopulmonary resuscitation is being evaluated, and it may become available, although standard teaching still recommends the use of a cuffed endotracheal tube.

Obstetric anaesthesia

The LMA has been proved to be life saving in caesarean sections when tracheal intubation or ventilation with a face mask has been unsuccessful.

Cricoid pressure

It has been shown that in failed intubation (in obstetric anaesthesia), insertion of the LMA is difficult when cricoid pressure is applied. However, the transient release of cricoid pressure allows the insertion of the LMA and subsequent intubation through it.

Paediatric anaesthesia

It has been recommended that LMA should be used only in spontaneously breathing children. IPPV with the LMA should be avoided because, even with correct positioning of the LMA, inflation of the stomach is still possible if airway inflation pressure exceeds the LMA cuff real pressure (a leak at about 20 cmH$_2$O is usually found).

A study carried out at the Hospital for Sick Children in London concluded that the LMA is useful in spontaneously breathing children, and it should be inserted at an adequate depth of anaesthesia and firmly secured. It also suggested premedication used an antisialogogue (e.g. atropine).

Other situations in which the LMA has been used include:

- head and neck surgery;
- ophthalmic surgery;
- for repeated dressings in burn patients;
- in professional singers (to prevent damage to the vocal cords);
- in magnetic resonance imaging in children; the valve on the standard LMA contains a metal spring that may interfere with the MRI scan, so especially adapted LMAs are available.

The advantages and disadvantages of the LMA are shown in Box 6.4.

Box 6.4 Advantages and disadvantages of the LMA

Advantages

- Technique of insertion can be easily learnt
- Low incidence of sore throat
- Frees the anaesthetist's hands for monitoring and record-keeping
- Minimal cardiovascular response to the insertion of the LMA
- Better tolerated than an endotracheal tube at a lighter level of anaesthesia
- Decreased atmosphere pollution with anaesthetic gases (because scavenging is easier than during face mask anaesthesia)
- Less risk of oesophageal or endobronchial intubation
- Useful role in management of difficult intubations

Disadvantages

- Aspiration of gastric contents can occur during use
- Cuff herniation after overinflation or repeated autoclaving may lead to difficulty in placement of the LMA
- Coughing and laryngospasm when inserted during too light a plane of anaesthesia
- Difficult positioning in the presence of enlarged tonsils
- Diffusion of nitrous oxide in the LMA cuff over a prolonged period, causing expansion of the cuff and airway obstruction
- Bruising of the uvula after repeated attempts at insertion

Contraindications to the use of LMAs

These are:

- an inability to extend the neck or open the mouth above 1.5 cm (as in rheumatoid arthritis, ankylosing spondylitis or cervical spine instability);
- airway obstruction at or below the level of larynx;
- pharyngeal pathology (e.g. abscess or haematoma);
- morbid obesity;
- an increased risk of regurgitation (e.g. hiatus hernia, pregnancy, a full stomach or intestinal ileus).

Laryngoscopes

There are two basic blades: curved and straight. The tip of the curved blade (Macintosh) is inserted anterior to the epiglottis in the vallecula and, by lifting, exposes the larynx and vocal cords. The straight blade (Magill) is used in children whose epiglottis is floppy. The blade is passed posterior to the epiglottis and lifts it anteriorly, exposing the larynx.

Other laryngoscope blades available are the Polio blade, left-handed blade, blade with a prism and McCoy blade. These are used in difficult intubation if a fibreoptic laryngoscope (Fig. 6.23) is not available.

Endotracheal intubation can be performed with the patient awake and under local anaesthesia, or with the patient asleep after inhalational or i.v. induction. Intubation may be carried out blindly or under direct vision using a laryngoscope or fibreoptic bronchoscope.

While it is not absolutely necessary for a muscle relaxant to be given, intubation is usually easier if it is. The muscle relaxants used for intubation are suxamethonium (1.5 mg/kg) in emergency surgery or when it is intended that the patient be allowed to breathe spontaneously through the tube. A small dose of nondepolarizing muscle relaxant is given before the injection of suxamethonium to minimize postoperative muscle pains in young, fit patients.

Conduct of laryngoscopy

After injecting the induction agent and the muscle relaxant, the patient's head and neck are positioned. The neck is flexed and the head extended with a pillow as a support. This brings the oral, pharyngeal and tracheal axes into line (Fig. 6.24). The laryngoscope is introduced into the right side of the mouth, moving the tongue to the left. The blade passes over the whole tongue, and the laryngoscope is lifted upwards and forwards, avoiding using the teeth as a lever. (The teeth can be protected with a plastic guard.) With a curved blade, the tip of the laryngoscope passes into the vallecula, and lifting the handle exposes the vocal cords. With a straight blade, the tip is passed posterior to the epiglottis, which is lifted anteriorly, and the vocal cords are visualized.

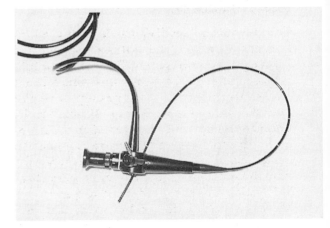

Figure 6.23 Fibreoptic laryngoscope.

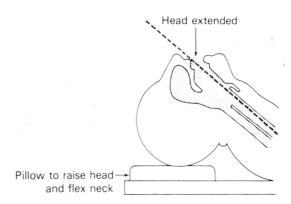

Figure 6.24 Positioning for laryngoscopy.

After visualizing the vocal cords, the appropriately sized tube is passed from the right side of the mouth. Sometimes the assistant may have to apply external pressure on the thyroid cartilage to bring the larynx into view. On other occasions, a semi-rigid stillete (gum elastic bougie) is used to provide the correct degree of curvature of the endotracheal tube to allow intubation. Once in place, the endotracheal tube cuff is inflated to prevent an audible gas leak on inflation. The position of the tube is checked by listening to both sides of the chest with a stethoscope (auscultation) to prevent right bronchial intubation.

Some anaesthetists prefer to spray the vocal cords with 4% lignocaine or to have the tubes lubricated with lignocaine jelly.

Nasal intubation

This is carried out for ENT and dental operations. A slightly smaller tube (8.0 mm for men and 7.0 mm for women) is used. This lubricated tube is passed through the right nostril and, when it reaches the pharynx, a laryngoscopy is carried out. The tube is passed into the trachea by grasping the tip with Magill intubating forceps or by manipulation of the proximal tube. In dental operations, a moist gauze throat pack is introduced into the pharynx after intubation. This pack is meant to hold blood and secretions above the cuff of the endotracheal tube and reduce the risk of tracheal soiling or aspiration. A 'tail' of the pack is left protruding from the mouth and the anaesthetist makes a note to remove it at the end of the operation.

Difficult intubation

Difficulty in intubation may be expected or unexpected. As described on page 145, in the preoperative visit the anaesthetist assesses the patient's airway and, if difficulty is expected, precautions are taken in the form of using a fibreoptic laryngoscope, awake intubation with local analgesia, and retrograde intubation using an epidural catheter and a Tuohy needle passed through the cricothyroid membrane into the mouth.

If the difficult intubation is unexpected, the anaesthetist uses bougies and manipulates the cricoid pressure; if the patient cannot be intubated in spite of this, he follows a 'failed intubation drill' (see p. 191).

Complications of endotracheal intubation

The immediate complications of intubation are trauma to the lips, teeth or dental crowns, jaw dislocation, and trauma to the larynx and vocal cords. If a red rubber tube is used, the cuff exerts a high pressure on the tracheal mucosa, which can be damaging. Hence, plastic tubes with high-volume and low-pressure cuffs are used.

There may also be misplacement of the tube: it may be either too far in, when it will (usually) be in the right main bronchus, or it may not be in the lungs at all (oesophageal intubation). In a bronchial intubation, one side of the chest will not be ventilated (there will be no air entry to that lung on auscultation) and will eventually collapse. In oesophageal intubation, neither lung will be ventilated (no air entering the lungs, the chest not rising with ventilation, there being no end-tidal carbon dioxide trace, and air entry being heard over the stomach), and the patient will rapidly become hypoxic. The tube must be removed and the patient ventilated by mask until pink before any further attempt at intubation is made.

ANALGESIA

The patient who is anaesthetized (nitrous oxide, oxygen and a volatile agent) is given an analgesic intraoperatively in the form of opiates or non-opiates, or local block. The opiates will be alfentanil (Rapifen), fentanyl (Sublimaze), phenoperidine (Operidine), pethidine, nalbuphine (Nubain), morphine, diamorphine or a combination of these. It can be given as i.m. or i.v. boluses or as an i.v. infusion (see p. 58 for dosages). The analgesia can be extended into the postoperative period (see p. 231).

The non-opiate analgesic commonly used is diclofenac (Voltarol) 1 mg/kg i.m.

Analgesia can also be given as nerve blocks, or as epidural or spinal local anaesthetics (see p. 234). Opiates can also be given through epidurals or in spinals; however, care must be taken that only preservative-free drugs are used as the preservative in some opiates may be toxic if placed directly on nerves.

MUSCULAR RELAXATION

Muscle relaxants allow the use of lighter planes of anaesthesia and the preservation of autonomic reflexes. Muscle relaxants (with IPPV) are used for major intracranial, thoracic and abdominal operations. They are used as follows.

If a difficult intubation is expected or in an emergency, suxamethonium is given after the induction of anaesthesia. Once the effects of suxamethonium wear off, a non-depolarizing muscle relaxant is given. The choice ranges from atracurium (Tracrium) and vecuronium (Norcuron), to pancuronium (Pavulon) and tubocurarine (Tubarine). The first two drugs can be given as an infusion. The dosages can be found on page 74. IPPV is maintained by a ventilator that delivers the appropriate minute and tidal volume.

During anaesthesia, the following points are checked:

- *Awareness.* Because the patient is paralysed, he or she will not be able to move even if awake or in pain. If the patient is inadequately anaesthetized ('light'), he may show signs such as crying (lacrimation), sweating, hypertension, tachycardia and pupillary dilatation.
- *Adequate ventilation.* If the patient is inadequately ventilated, he or she may have raised carbon dioxide levels, which cause excessive oozing from the wound, tachycardia, hypertension and ventricular dysrhythmias.
- *Adequate muscle relaxation.* If the muscle relaxant is wearing off, the muscle tone increases and the ventilator airway pressure increases. A peripheral nerve stimulator (see Fig. 6.29 on p. 170) can detect the degree of muscular paralysis.

END OF SURGERY

At the end of surgery, the residual neuro-muscular block is reversed with atropine (0.02 mg/kg) and neostigmine (0.05 mg/kg). In patients with cardiac disease, glycopyrrolate (Robinul) is used instead of atropine to antagonize the muscarinic side-effects of neostigmine because glycopyrrolate causes less tachycardia (which may be bad for the heart) than atropine.

Extubation

When spontaneous breathing is resumed, tracheo-bronchial suction is carried out and extubation carried out in a lateral position (in patients with a full stomach), or supine or in a sitting position (for obese patients). The tube is removed during inspiration when the larynx dilates, the cuff is deflated and the tube withdrawn. At this stage, if a throat pack was inserted, it is removed before the tube is taken out.

Emergence

Once extubation takes place, the patient receives 100% oxygen via a face mask and is then moved to the recovery area when ready.

MONITORING DURING ANAESTHESIA

A monitor is 'one who warns', or something that gives warning or reminds. A monitor used during the course of an anaesthetic will measure, display or record the information provided. Some monitors give an alarm if the measured values during anaesthesia fall outside previously defined limits.

It is important to monitor a patient from the time of induction until discharge from the re-covery area. In a fully equipped hospital, monitors are found in the anaesthetic room as well as the operating theatre. If this is not the case, provision should be made to wheel the monitoring equip-ment into the anaesthetic room or to anaesthetize the patient in the operating theatre.

The anaesthetist is an important monitor, who can care for the patient during anaesthesia, and the instruments used by the anaesthetist act to:

- warn about changes in the state of the patient;
- help the anaesthetist in the maintenance of physiological balance;
- warn about the changes in the function of anaesthetic equipment, including the supply of gases and vapours.

Monitoring can be carried out with or without equipment.

Without equipment

The anaesthetist can observe:

- pupillary size for hypoxia or depth of anaesthesia;

- the breathing pattern, rate, rhythm and depth;
- the heart rate and peripheral perfusion by feeling the radial pulse;
- a cold clammy skin, which indicates poor perfusion;
- the rotameters, vapourizer settings and reservoir bag on the anaesthetic machine;
- the movements of the ventilator and thus gain warning about disconnection, obstruction or the return of spontaneous breathing.

With equipment

All the body systems can be monitored during anaesthesia. The common monitoring, as carried out in everyday working surroundings, is briefly described below.

Cardiovascular system

Electrocardiogram

Three-lead bipolar ECG monitors are used, of which lead II is popular. With the ECG monitors, heart rate and dysrhythmias can be detected. A CM5 lead (lead placed on the 5th intercostal region near the manubrium sterni of the chest) can detect myocardial ischaemia.

Arterial blood pressure

Blood pressure can be monitored non-invasively or invasively.

Non-invasive monitoring. In routine surgical cases, blood pressure is monitored non-invasively using an oscillotonometer or an automated oscillotonometer, for example the Dinamap.

In an oscillotonometer, the principles of the aneroid pressure gauge are used. It has two cuffs: the upper cuff measures the pressure around the upper arm; the lower cuff measures the pressure differential between the cuffs in order to detect the flow of blood from under the upper cuff. The disadvantage of a non-automated oscillotonometer is that it cannot measure the blood pressure when it is low.

An automated oscillotonometer (e.g. Dinamap) consists of a single cuff connected to a display and control box. Inside the box, one length of the tubing is connected to a pump that inflates the cuff and a bleed valve that deflates the cuff. The output from the pressure transducer is connected to either an AC-coupled or DC-coupled amplifier. This output of the DC amplifier produces a voltage indicating the pressure in the cuff. The AC-coupled amplifier detects oscillations due to blood passing under the cuff. The first oscillations in the cuff are taken as systolic pressure, the largest pulsations as mean blood pressure and the smallest pulsations as diastolic pressure.

The Ohmeda Finapres is a continuous, non-invasive blood pressure monitor. It works on principles similar to those of Dinamap, but the cuff is placed around a finger and its volume is measured photometrically.

Other instruments available are the Arteriosonde, which uses the Doppler ultrasound principle, and the Infrasonade, which uses ultrasonic principles for detecting arterial wall motion.

Invasive monitoring. Direct measurement of blood pressure provides continuous, beat-to-beat blood pressure readings. It requires the use of a catheter placed in an artery, associated tubing, a pressure transducer and an electronic processor (Fig. 6.25). Invasive pressure transducers need to be internally zeroed, and transducers are kept at the level of the right atrium during measurement.

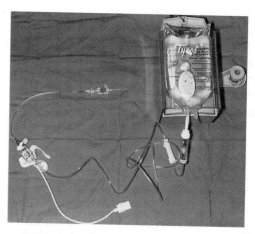

Figure 6.25 Catheter-transducer system.

The system is affected by the connecting tube between the arterial cannula and the transducer.

Terms used are 'underdamping' or 'overdamping'. An 'underdamped' trace shows catheter 'whip' with overshooting of systolic and diastolic pressures. This occurs due to excessive length of tubing, which can be corrected using a shorter tube. An 'overdamped' trace shows lowered systolic and higher diastolic pressure, with an accurate mean arterial pressure. This is due to air bubbles in the tubing, which need to be removed to give accurate results. The indications for direct intra-arterial monitoring are:

1. cardiac, aortic and carotid surgery;
2. aneurysmal repair in the brain;
3. thoracic surgery, requiring one-lung ventilation;
4. the controlled hypotensive technique (induced hypotension; see p. 194).

The arterial sites used are the radial, ulnar, brachial, axillary, femoral or dorsalis pedis. When the radial artery is cannulated, Allen's test is performed before the insertion of the cannula to detect the adequacy of collateral blood flow from the ulnar artery.

A number of transducers are available. The catheter-transducer system is filled with heparinized saline. Heparin 500 IU is added to 500 ml of normal saline, which is connected to the catheter-transducer system after being pressurized by a bag. The pressure in the bag is maintained at 50 mmHg greater than the systolic pressure. The flush releases 1–3 ml/h of saline into the cannula to keep it patent.

Central venous pressure

Central venous pressure (CVP) is the pressure in the right atrium and reflects the volume entering it (preload). The CVP is normally less than 6 mmHg in the spontaneously breathing patient.

A central venous catheter can be inserted either through the internal or the external jugular vein in the neck, or via the subclavian or cephalic vein. Either a single-lumen or a triple-lumen catheter is inserted. A guide wire is passed into the vein after localization; the catheter is passed over it and the wire is removed (the Seldinger technique).

The indications for CVP monitoring are:

1. assessment of blood volume, especially where large intraoperative fluid shifts are expected or the patient is brought to theatre in shock;
2. to give inotropic drugs, as most inotropes cannot be given through peripheral veins;
3. with difficult peripheral venous access;
4. in cases where there is a risk of air embolism (see p. 190);
5. when a large line is needed for rapid volume replacement.

An unusually high CVP reading may indicate increased circulating blood volume, pulmonary hypertension, pneumothorax, heart failure or valvular heart disease. A very low CVP reading can indicate hypovolaemia. The CVP trace will show cyclical variation with the heart beat and respiration, and will tend to read higher during the inspiratory phase of IPPV or when PEEP is used. During spontaneous breathing, the CVP reading will be lower during inspiration. This is because the CVP reflects not only the pressures inside the right atrium but also the intrathoracic pressures.

The complications associated with central venous cannulation are pneumothorax, air embolism, carotid artery puncture and thoracic duct injury (when cannulation is carried out on the left side).

The waves seen in the CVP are an 'a' wave due to atrial contraction, a 'c' wave due to bulging of the tricuspid valve into the right atrium, and a 'v' wave due to the right atrial filling.

Pulmonary artery pressure monitoring

Pulmonary artery pressure (PAP) monitoring devices were made popular by Swan and Ganz in the 1970s using multilumen, balloon-tipped, radio-opaque catheters. These are passed via the internal jugular vein or subclavian vein, passing through the right atrium and right ventricle into the pulmonary artery (Fig. 6.26). A pulmonary artery balloon-flotation catheter is shown in Figure 6.27.

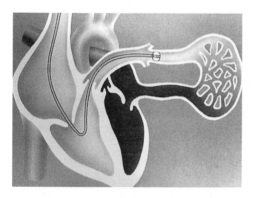

Figure 6.26 A multilumen balloon-tipped flotation catheter, which has been passed through the right atrium and right ventricle into the pulmonary artery.

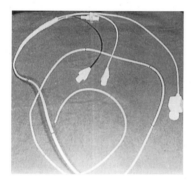

Figure 6.27 A typical pulmonary artery balloon-flotation catheter.

The indications for PAP monitoring are:

1. any condition where right heart performance (CVP) may not reflect left heart performance (PAP), for example acute myocardial infarction, shock, valve disease, and cardiac surgery;
2. to measure cardiac output, for example in shock or inotrope therapy;
3. to measure mixed venous oxygen, as in shock patients;
4. as a route to give rapid volume infusions or inotropes (the pulmonary introducer is 8 G).

The PAP catheter is connected to a pressure-transducer system via tubing containing heparinized saline. The internal jugular vein or subclavian vein is located and a dilator sheath introduced over a guide wire (the Seldinger technique). The PAP catheter is introduced once the sheath and wire have been removed through a protective sheath. As the PAP catheter passes through various chambers of the heart, the pressure tracing changes (Fig. 6.28). Once the catheter is in the pulmonary artery, the balloon is inflated to get a wedge pressure reading. The pulmonary capillary wedge pressure (PCWP) reflects the pressure in the left atrium (left ventricular preload).

Complications associated with the insertion of a PAP catheter are similar to those of CVP insertion. In addition, it is possible to clear the pulmonary artery or, if the balloon is left inflated for too long, to infarct (kill) a segment of lung.

The pressures in various chambers of the heart are listed in Table 6.6.

Cardiac output measurement

Cardiac output is most often measured by thermodilution using a pulmonary artery catheter (see above). Other methods available are dye dilution or the use of a flowmeter.

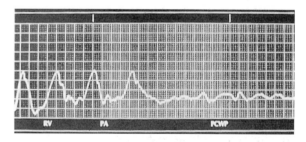

Figure 6.28 Tracings when the PAP catheter passes through various chambers of the heart. RV, right ventricle; PA, pulmonary artery; PCWP, pulmonary capillary wedge pressure.

Table 6.6 Pressures in the heart

	Systolic pressure (mmHg)	Diastolic pressure (mmHg)	Mean pressure (mmHg)
Right atrium	–	–	–2 to +6
Right ventricle	15–30	0–5	5–15
Pulmonary artery	20–25	10–15	0–12
Left atrium	–	–	0–12
Left ventricle	100–140	60–90	70–105

Respiratory system

Pulmonary ventilation

This can be effectively monitored as described below.

Movement of the chest wall. Impedance plethysmography and inductance plethysmographs are used for research purposes.

Movement of air in and out of the lungs. It can be detected using: (1) a Fleisch tube respirometer, which has a fixed-orifice principle; water vapour condensation gives inaccurate results; or (2) a Wright respirometer, a simple instrument that uses the turbine principle. The other example in this category is the Magtrak, which is an electronic form of the Wright respirometer.

Airway pressure. Measurement with either an aneroid gauge or an electric manometer is the most effective way of detecting a disconnection or leak in the patient circuit in a patient receiving IPPV. Most airway pressure monitors also alarm if the airway pressure is too high. (Incorrect ventilator settings, kinked tubing or asthma may all cause abnormally high airway pressures.)

Composition of respired gases

1. *Oxygen concentration of the inspired gas.* This can be measured using oxygen analysers with either fuel cells, polarographs or paramagnetic analysers.

2. *Carbon dioxide concentration in the expired gas* (end-tidal). This measures the adequacy of ventilation during anaesthesia. The values of carbon dioxide seen on a capnograph, a carbon dioxide monitor, are an indirect measure of the arterial partial pressure of carbon dioxide (P_{CO_2}).

A sudden fall in end-tidal P_{CO_2} may be due to apnoea, cardiac arrest, pulmonary embolus or air embolism (see p. 190). The capnograph is also useful in detecting the correct placement of an endotracheal tube.

3. *Mass spectrometry.* This powerful machine, when used, analyses up to eight gases and vapours simultaneously. Mass spectrometers are only available in large centres and act as a research tool.

4. *Anaesthetic gases and vapours.* All volatile anaesthetic agents have absorption bands in the infra-red spectrum. Instruments such as Datex Normocap and Engström Emma use this principle. The instruments detect all the anaesthetic vapours.

5. *Arterial blood gases.* In major surgical procedures, such as cardiac or thoracic surgery, arterial blood gases are estimated at regular intervals (see p. 251).

6. *Pulse oximetry.* This shows the percentage oxygen saturation of the blood. It works on the principle of transmission and absorption of light of various wavelengths across tissue (usually a finger). This device has become highly popular and is seen in anaesthetic rooms, operating theatres and recovery areas.

7. *Measurement of transcutaneous* P_{CO_2} *and* P_{O_2}. By applying carbon dioxide- and oxygen-sensitive electrodes to the skin, indirect measurements of arterial gases can be made.

Neuromuscular junction

The degree of neuromuscular block using muscle relaxants can be effectively measured using a peripheral nerve stimulator (Fig. 6.29). The electrodes are applied on the skin at the wrist (ulnar nerve), lateral aspect of the knee (lateral popliteal nerve) or face (facial nerve). There are three types of stimulus that can be applied:

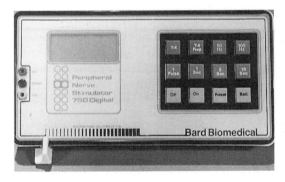

Figure 6.29 Peripheral nerve stimulator.

- *Single impulse*. This can be used to detect whether the patient has recovered from a single dose of suxamethonium following intubation.
- *Tetany*. This involves stimulating at 50–100 Hz; post-tetanic facilitation is defined as stimulating the nerve with 50 Hz for 1 s followed by a single twitch. If the patient has any residual paralysis due to a non-depolarizing relaxant, the height of the response to a single twitch will be higher than the tetany.
- *Train of four*. Four stimuli at 0.5 Hz are given over a period of 2 s. In a patient with a non-depolarizing muscular block, the twitches will be successively reduced.

Measurement of temperature

Body temperatures (core and peripheral) are measured using thermistors or thermocouples (p. 106) in operating theatres. Temperature probes are inserted in the oesophagus (to measure core temperature) or nasopharynx (brain temperature), or are attached to the toe (peripheral temperature).

Measurement of blood loss

Blood loss can be measured by observing the degree of bleeding, weighing the swabs (1 ml of blood = 1 g) and measuring the volume of blood collected in the suction bottle. As a rough guide, if a swab is lightly stained, blood loss is 5 ml, if moderately stained, 10 ml, and if heavily stained, 15 ml. Three abdominal packs heavily soaked can contain about 500 ml.

Other ways of measuring blood loss are calorimetric and haemoglobin extraction dilution methods.

Measurement of urinary output

Urinary output can be measured using an indwelling urinary catheter in prolonged surgery or where severe blood loss is anticipated. Roughly, the amount of urine excreted per hour should be 0.5–1.0 ml/kg body weight.

Cerebral function and monitoring the depth of anaesthesia

To detect cerebral hypoxia, an EEG is valuable, while a cerebral function analysing monitor (CFAM) can be used to assess the depth of anaesthesia. These monitors are rare outside neurosurgical institutes and research centres.

REGIONAL ANAESTHESIA

History

Cocaine was the first local anaesthetic agent introduced into medical practice by Koller in 1884. Uhlmann and Merscher introduced nupercaine in 1929, and lignocaine was synthesized in 1943 by Lundquist and Lofigren. (See p. 73 for the mode of action of local anaesthetic agents.)

Although there are a number of regional techniques, only those which are carried out frequently are described here.

General considerations

Before commencing regional techniques, it is essential to check that equipment for resuscitation is ready (anaesthetic machine, drugs such as thiopentone, suxamethonium, midazolam and ephedrine, and endotracheal tubes) and that an indwelling i.v. cannula is inserted in the vein.

Blocks of the upper extremity

Brachial plexus block (BPB)

Anatomy. The brachial plexus is formed from the anterior primary divisions of C5, C6, C7, C8 and T1. It forms the motor and sensory nerve supply to the arm (see p. 17 for details).

Indication: The BPB is carried out for blocking the upper extremity and shoulder.

Technique: The brachial plexus can be blocked by one of the following methods.

Interscalene approach. The patient lies supine with head rotated to the side opposite to the block. The cricoid cartilage (C6) is felt and the finger moved laterally until the interscalene groove is felt posterior to the sternomastoid muscle at this level. A 2.5 cm needle is inserted in the groove, and once paraesthesia is elicited, approximately 20–30 ml 0.5% plain bupivacaine are injected. During injection, the anaesthetist repeatedly aspirates the syringe to check that the needle has not migrated into a blood vessel (blood in the syringe) or the epidural space (CSF in the syringe).

Supraclavicular approach. The aim of this approach is to block the brachial plexus at the midclavicular point between the skin and the first rib. The patient lies supine with the head rotated to the side opposite to the block and the arm and shoulder depressed. A needle is inserted 1 cm above the midpoint of the clavicle, the direction of the needle being downwards, inwards and backwards. If paraesthesia is felt, the needle is stabilized and 30–40 ml 0.5% plain bupivacaine are injected after a negative aspiration for blood. It may take up to 20 minutes for the block to develop fully.

Axillary approach. In the axilla, the nerves of the brachial plexus and the axillary artery are enclosed in a fibrous neuromuscular fascial sheath. The aim of the axillary block is to inject the local anaesthetic around the axillary artery into the fibrous neurovascular sheath. The patient lies supine with the arm abducted at a right angle. The skin of the axilla is shaved and cleaned, and a weal of local anaesthetic raised at the highest point of the axilla at which arterial pulsation is felt. Through the weal, a 2.5 cm needle (blue needle) is inserted until a click is felt, which shows that the needle has entered the neurovascular sheath. After negative aspiration, 30 ml 0.5% plain bupivacaine or prilocaine are injected. It takes about 30 minutes for the block to be fully effective.

Advantages: In the interscalene and axillary approaches, the dangers of pneumothorax are remote. There is an obvious landmark for the axillary approach, i.e. the axillary artery.

Disadvantages: In the interscalene approach, there is a risk of injection into the cervical epidural space, the CSF or the vertebral artery.

In the supraclavicular approach there is a real risk of pneumothorax, puncture of the subclavian artery and local anaesthetic block of the phrenic nerve (thereby paralysing the diaphragm for the duration of the block).

Wrist block

Indication: It is carried out for blocking the digits during tendon repair. The median, ulnar and radial nerves supply the wrist.

Technique: Circular lines of intradermal and subcutaneous infiltration are carried out just above the wrist joint.

Total intravenous regional analgesia (TIVR) (Bier's block). This is the only technique in which local anaesthetic is deliberately injected into a blood vessel. TIVR consists of injection of a local anaesthetic into a vein of a limb that has been isolated from the general circulation by a tourniquet. The site of action of the drug is on the peripheral nerve endings.

Indication: It is carried out for operations on arms and also on legs.

Technique: A butterfly needle or a Venflon is inserted into a vein on the dorsum of the hand and firmly secured. The limb is drained of blood by elevation for 5 minutes or by using an Esmarch bandage. A double cuff is placed on the proximal part of the limb, and the upper cuff is inflated to a pressure a little above the systolic blood pressure before removing the Esmarch bandage. Approximately 40 ml 0.5% prilocaine (Citanest) is injected, and after 5 minutes the lower cuff is inflated and the upper one released to minimize cuff discomfort.

At the end of surgery, the cuff deflation should be carried out slowly. The tourniquet must be left inflated for at least 30 minutes after the local anaesthetic injection. Signs of local anaesthetic agent toxicity (see p. 73) can be seen if the cuff is deflated before this period passes. The patient is carefully observed for 10 minutes after the release of the cuff. Neither lignocaine nor bupivacaine should be used for TIVR, as both these drugs may cause toxicity even 30 minutes after injection.

Contraindications: The contraindications are sickle-cell disease, scleroderma and Raynaud's disease.

Precautions: The double cuff mechanism should always be tested before use. Resuscitation equipment must be at hand and only prilocaine used.

Blocks of the lower extremity

Femoral nerve block

This is carried out for pain relief following a fractured neck of femur.

Technique: A weal of local anaesthetic is raised, just below the inguinal ligament, a finger breadth lateral to the femoral artery. A needle is inserted for 3–4 cm and 20 ml 0.5% plain bupivacaine are injected, after negative aspiration for blood.

Sciatic nerve block

This is carried out for the reduction of fractures around the ankle and, in combination with femoral nerve block, for the ligation of varicose veins.

Technique: The patient lies on the sound side with the hip slightly flexed. There are a number of approaches to this block, and a rough guide to the position of the sciatic nerve is the midpoint of a line joining the posterior superior iliac spine to the ischial tuberosity. After eliciting paraesthesia, 10–20 ml 0.25% plain bupivacaine are injected.

Ankle block

This is carried out for reduction of fractures, toe surgery or postoperative analgesia.

The nerves supplying the ankle are the anterior tibial nerve, musculocutaneous nerve, saphenous nerve, sural nerve and posterior tibial nerve. These nerves can be blocked by a subcutaneous and intradermal weal raised circumferentially around the ankle between the medial and lateral malleolus behind the malleoli.

The total amount of local anaesthetic agent used is 20–30 ml 0.5% plain bupivacaine.

SPINAL ANALGESIA

History. The first spinal analgesic was given by Leonard Corning in New York in 1885. The first planned spinal analgesia for surgery was undertaken by August Bier in 1898, using cocaine.

Indications

- Orthopaedic surgery, hip replacements, knee replacements.
- Urological surgery, transurethral resection of prostate.
- Haemorrhoidectomy and vaginal repair.
- Obstetric anaesthesia.

Contraindications

- Blood clotting disorders.
- Local skin sepsis at the site of injection.
- A deformed back.
- Abnormality of the nervous system, for example an expanding cerebral lesion, tumour or cyst.
- Patients with an enlarged prostate coming for other surgery.

Technique

At the preanaesthetic visit, the patient is offered the option of spinal anaesthesia and if this is accepted, consent is obtained. The anaesthetic room and the equipment necessary for resuscitation is kept ready. The equipment necessary for conducting spinal analgesia comprises 22–26 gauge spinal needles with an introducer, 2 ml and 5 ml syringes, swabs, a swab-holder, antiseptic solution (chlorhexidine) and sterile towels.

The aim of the block is to enter the lumbar dural sac below the termination of the spinal cord and inject the local anaesthetic directly into the cerebrospinal fluid. Spinal analgesia can be performed in two positions: lateral and sitting.

Lateral position

The patient is placed with the back parallel to the edge of the table (which can be tilted), knees flexed onto abdomen and head flexed into chest.

The hips and shoulders are kept parallel to the table to avoid rotation of the vertebral column. After preparing the skin, and covering with the towels, the landmarks are identified. An imaginary line joining the highest points of the iliac crests indicates the approximate level of the interspace between L4 and L5. It is important not to choose an injection site any higher than the L1–L2 interspace because the spinal cord, which ends at the level of L1, could be damaged.

A skin weal is raised at the chosen level and a small incision made to prevent the core of skin being carried through into the intra- or extradural space by the spinal needle. A Sise introducer, or a 19 gauge needle, is inserted, through which the spinal needle is introduced. The needle is then slowly pushed forward at right angles to the back. It passes through the following layers:

- skin
- subcutaneous tissue
- interspinous ligament
- ligamentum flavum
- epidural space
- theca (dura mater).

When the dura mater is pierced, a click is often felt, followed by a free flow of CSF on withdrawal of the stylet. Once the CSF is flowing freely, the local anaesthetic agent is injected.

Sitting position

The patient (especially if obese or pregnant) is placed across the table with the feet resting comfortably on a stool. The patient places his or her arms on the assistant's shoulder, with the spine flexed and the chin pressed on the sternum. The procedure as described in the lateral position is carried out during the insertion of the spinal needle. This position is also helpful if perineal surgery is planned.

Local anaesthesia drug

The local anaesthetic, 1–4 ml 0.5% heavy bupivacaine (Marcain), is injected. Once the drug is injected in the CSF, the patient is placed in the required position without delay, tilting the table as necessary. For abdominal surgery, the table is levelled as soon as the analgesia reaches the umbilicus (T10), and it should finally reach the subcostal arch (T6–T8).

Other drugs that can be used are heavy cinchocaine (Nupercain), 1–2 ml; and 5% lignocaine, 0.8–1.5 ml.

Factors influencing the height of spinal analgesia are:

- the dose of drug injected: the higher the concentration and dosage, the longer its effect lasts;
- the position of the patient: if the patient is sitting, hypobaric (plain) solution tends to float and hyperbaric (heavy) solution tends to sink;
- the volume of fluid injected: the height of analgesia is directly proportional to the volume of local anaesthetic agent;
- the rate and force of injection: a slow gentle injection is necessary to get a good, effective block;
- barbotage (to mix): by withdrawal and injection of the CSF, the drug is widely distributed.

Physiology of spinal analgesia

1. *Nervous system.* At the outset of spinal analgesia, the nerve fibres are blocked in the order:
   (a) autonomic preganglionic B fibres;
   (b) temperature and pain fibres;
   (c) fibres carrying vibratory and proprioceptive impulses;
   (d) pinprick fibres;
   (e) touch fibres;
   (f) motor nerves.
During recovery, sympathetic activity returns before sensation.

2. *Respiratory system.* In general, a spinal anaesthetic will have minimal effects on the respiratory system. However, higher levels of spinal block will paralyse first the abdominal muscles and then the intercostal muscles, interfering with coughing. In an uncontrolled 'total' spinal, where the level of the block is very high, the phrenic nerves (C3, C4 and C5) may be blocked, paralysing

the diaphragm. If this happens, the patient needs to be ventilated until the block wears off.

3. *Cardiovascular system*. A fall in blood pressure, due to vasodilatation, is seen in the first 20 minutes after spinal anaesthesia. In an uncontrolled 'total' spinal, the cardiac sympathetic nerves (T2–T4) may also be blocked, contributing to the hypotension and causing bradycardia (a slow heart rate). Treatment consists of intravenous fluids, oxygen via a face mask, i.v. ephedrine 5–30 mg, atropine 0.2–0.6 mg or glycopyrronium 0.2 mg if there is bradycardia.

4. *Gastrointestinal system*. The small gut is contracted as a result of vagal influence. Nausea and vomiting can occur from hypotension, increased peristalsis or traction on the nerve endings in the viscera. Treatment consists of correcting the hypotension, reassurance and an antiemetic (metoclopramide 10 mg i.m. or i.v.).

5. *Genitourinary system*. Hypotension can lead to a decreased renal blood flow. Post-spinal retention of urine, requiring catheterization, may be seen.

6. *Body temperature*. Vasodilatation causes heat loss, and absence of sweating can lead to hyperpyrexia in hot climates.

Complications during spinal analgesia

- Nausea and vomiting
- Hiccups
- Precordial discomfort
- Hypotension
- Restlessness
- Failed spinal analgesia.

Sequelae

Headache. This may be seen in the first 72 hours postoperatively and can be very severe. Using the smallest possible needle and pencilpoint or Quincke needles decreases the risk of a headache. Classically, the headache starts in the occipital region and is made worse by sitting up or an erect posture. It is relieved by lying down.

Treatment consists of oral rehydration, avoiding strong light, aspirin and bedrest. If the headache persists, treatment is aimed at reducing the CSF leak (which is thought to be the cause):

- An epidural catheter is inserted, through which 1 L of Hartmann's solution is injected over 24 hours.
- An epidural blood patch with 10–20 ml of autologous blood is administered (the patient's own blood is injected aseptically into the epidural space).

Retention of urine. This can be treated with either carbachol 0.5–1.0 mg i.m. or catheterization.

EPIDURAL ANALGESIA (EXTRADURAL BLOCK)

History

This it was introduced by Corning in 1885 and made popular in Britain by Massey Dawkins.

Anatomy

The epidural or extradural space lies between the spinal dura mater and the vertebral canal, and has a diameter of 0.5 cm. Its boundaries are superiorly the foramen magnum, inferiorly the sacrococcygeal membrane, anteriorly the posterior longitudinal ligament and posteriorly the anterior surfaces of the laminae. The contents of the epidural space include the dural sac, spinal nerve roots, the epidural plexus of veins, spinal arteries, lymphatics and fat.

The epidural space is a potential space with a negative pressure.

Indications

- Upper abdominal operations.
- Lower abdominal operations, such as hernia repair.
- Operations on the lower limb.
- Obstetric anaesthesia and analgesia.
- Postoperative pain relief.

Contraindications

These are the same as for spinal analgesia.

Technique

The procedure is explained to the patient and informed consent is obtained. Equipment necessary for resuscitation is kept ready, and an intravenous cannula is inserted into a vein. The patient is placed in either a lateral or a sitting position (see the technique for spinal analgesia above).

The back is painted with antiseptic solution and covered by fenestrated towel (towel with a hole to expose the area of needle insertion). Because the dural sac (containing the spinal cord) is not pierced by the epidural needle, an epidural can be sited at any level. Most routine epidurals will be sited below L1.

A 16 or 18 gauge Tuohy needle is inserted at the interspace chosen. The needle passes through skin, subcutaneous tissue, the supraspinous and interspinous ligaments and ligamentum flavum, and into the epidural space.

The following signs indicate that the needle is in the epidural space:

1. sudden ease of injection of air or normal saline from a freely running syringe attached to the needle, i.e. a loss of resistance to injection;
2. deflation of Macintosh's epidural space indicator balloon;
3. 'sucking' into the open hub of the epidural needle of a carefully placed 'hanging drop' of fluid.

Equipment (Fig. 6.30). The sterile pack consists of towels, a Tuohy needle and syringes (10 ml, 20 ml, a Portex loss-of-resistance syringe, a catheter and a filter).

Local anaesthetic drug

Once the Tuohy needle is in the epidural space, a catheter is inserted through the needle and taped to the skin after removing the needle. The catheter is aspirated to check for blood (accidental cannulation of the epidural vein) or CSF (accidental spinal placement). A test dose of 3–5 ml of either 1% lignocaine or 0.25% plain bupivacaine (Marcain) is injected and, if there

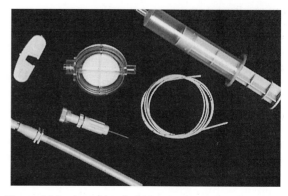

Figure 6.30 An epidural miniset showing a Tuohy needle, catheter, filter and loss of resistance syringe.

is no evidence of accidental spinal analgesia, the remaining solution is injected as follows: bupivacaine 0.25% plain 10 ml for obstetric analgesia, and 20–30 ml for abdominal operations, depending on the extent of the block required.

Site of action of local anaesthetic. When the local anaesthetic is injected in the epidural space, analgesia is brought about by direct action of the local anaesthetic on the nerve roots in the epidural space. Signs of accidental spinal analgesia are (1) a rapid onset of analgesia with the test dose, and (2) evidence of motor nerve block with the test dose.

The nerve fibres that are blocked are the anterior and posterior nerve roots, mixed spinal nerves, and the white and grey rami communicantes.

Factors influencing the spread of epidural analgesia

1. The age of the patient (the elderly require less than the young).
2. The volume of solution.
3. The speed of injection.
4. The position of the patient.

Management of the patient during epidural anaesthesia

The problems and management during epidural analgesia and anaesthesia are similar to those of spinal analgesia.

Complications

- Hypotension, which is corrected with i.v. fluids and ephedrine.
- Inadequate block, which needs to be corrected or supplemented with general anaesthesia.
- Total spinal analgesia, which is treated with IPPV, fluids and vasopressors (for example ephedrine).
- Accidental intravenous injection (causing seizures and/or ventricular fibrillation), treated by IPPV, antiseizure medication and cardiac massage.

INTRAVENOUS FLUIDS

Most patients undergoing elective operations are denied food and water for 8–12 hours preoperatively. This can result in a considerable loss of water and electrolytes. Water is lost via the kidneys, lungs and skin, and a small amount through the gastrointestinal tract. That portion of water lost from the skin and lungs is called 'insensible loss' (ranging from 800 to 1000 ml/day in a normal adult). Water is excreted as urine at the hourly rate of 1 ml/kg body weight (about 1700 ml in a 70 kg adult per day).

Routine i.v. therapy in elective operations

It is essential to give one-third to one-half again of the estimated fluid requirement during the course of a major operation in the adult, the solutions used being dextrose saline or Hartmann's solution.

Fluids and fluid requirements come in several different classes and compartments, which are useful to know when trying to work out how much and what needs replacement. These are:

- maintenance requirements
- intraoperative requirements
- blood loss
- preoperative deficits
- abnormal losses.

Maintenance fluids

These are fluid requirements to keep the body 'ticking over' when there are no extraordinary losses. The fluid used is usually dextrose saline. There are several different formulae for working out maintenance, for example:

4 ml/kg/h for the first 10 kg	40 ml
2 ml/kg/h for the next 10 kg	20 ml
1 ml/kg/h for every subsequent kg	$\underline{25\ ml}$
	= 85 ml/h
	for a 45 kg boy

It should be noted that basic fluid requirements increase by about 10% for every degree rise in body temperature above 37°C.

If the patient has been fasting from midnight without a drip and does not arrive in theatre until 3 p.m., for example, then – even before the knife hits her skin – she will be 85 ml × 15 h = 1.3 L short of fluid thereafter, for every hour of surgery.

Intraoperative fluid requirements

In general, Hartmann's solution or saline is used.

These requirements are greater than simple maintenance requirements for all but the shortest and most peripheral of operations because of:

- third spacing
- increased losses
- blood loss.

Third spacing refers to the loss of fluid from the intravascular space into the intracellular space. This tends to occur in proportion to the level of tissue trauma (handling) and usually lasts 72 hours, whereupon all the fluid reverts back to where it belongs. The fluid of choice here may be Hartmann's solution, as the loss is essentially of sodium-rich, potassium-containing fluid. If losses are substantial, colloid may be required.

In general, if the operation involves minimal tissue trauma (e.g. open reduction of the ankle), the requirements are 4 ml/kg/h of operation. If tissue trauma is moderate (e.g. open chole-cystectomy), requirements are 6 ml/kg/h of operation. For major tissue trauma (e.g. abdominal aortic aneurysm repair), the requirements are 8 ml/kg/h and above and may continue postoperatively.

Abnormal losses. These include increased loss from exposed gut (water), intraoperative loss via the respiratory tract from dry anaesthetic gases, and loss via an ileus or nasogastric tube (sodium-rich fluid ± potassium).

Blood loss. The estimated blood volume (EBV) is 70 ml/kg. The acceptable blood loss (ABL) depends upon the patient's medical condition, the preoperative haemoglobin level and the possibility of continued blood loss.

It is usually about 10% of blood volume, i.e. 7 ml/kg; up to this volume, it is possible to replace blood with either colloid 1 ml for 1 ml, or crystalloid 3 ml for 1 ml. Thus in a 50 kg woman:

$$70 \times 50 = 3.5 \text{ L EBV}$$
$$\therefore 10\% \text{ of EBV} = 350 \text{ ml}$$

Up to 350 ml, replace with either 350 ml haemacell or a similar substance, or $3 \times 350 =$ 1 L of Hartmann's solution.

Conditions associated with deficits in blood volume are shown in Box 6.5, and the physical signs of hypovolaemia are outlined in Table 6.7.

Box 6.5   Conditions associated with deficits in blood volume and ECF

Trauma	Pancreatitis
Burns	Bowel obstruction
Sepsis	Chronic systemic hypertension
Prolonged gastrointestinal losses	Chronic diuretic use

Table 6.7   Physical signs of hypovolaemia

	Loss of volume		
	5%	10%	15%
CNS	Clear	Clouded	?Stupor
Lips	Dry	Dry	Very dry
Pulse	Normal	Increased	Rapid
Respiration	Normal	Increased	Laboured
Blood pressure	Normal	Normal, postural drop	Low
Urinary output	Normal	Decreased	May be zero

The clinical indicators of the adequacy of replacement are:

- heart rate (good only in children);
- blood pressure: the definition of postural drop is >20 mmHg on standing ± a rise in heart rate of 20 beats/min;
- central venous pressure;
- urine output;
- the patient stops complaining of thirst.

Fluid therapy in the dehydrated patient. The patient's degree of dehydration is assessed preoperatively (see p. 206) and fluids given accordingly.

BLOOD: CONSTITUENTS, TRANSFUSION AND BLOOD SUBSTITUTES

The amount of blood in the human body is approximately 70 ml/kg body weight. Thus the normal human adult blood volume is 4.5–5.0 L.

The functions of blood are:

1. In transport: nutrients from the gastrointestinal tract to the cells; oxygen from the lungs to the cells; waste products from the cells to the organs of excretion; heat formed in the more active tissues to all parts of the body, thus helping in the regulation of body temperature; and hormones transported to all parts of the body.
2. In the regulation of acid–base balance.
3. In immunological reactions.

Constituents of blood

From the above functions, it can be seen that the blood is a complex fluid containing nutrients absorbed from the alimentary canal, oxygen taken up in the lungs, waste products produced by cellular activity, hormones, antibodies and other substances. It is also clear that the composition of the blood varies with place and time. The overall composition of blood is as follows:

- Plasma (a light yellow liquid): about 55% of the blood volume.
- Suspended solids, for example platelets, white cells and red blood cells.

— Three proteins forming from 6–8% of the plasma proteins are serum albumin (4.5%), serum globulin (2.0%) and fibrinogen (0.3%). They contribute to the viscosity and, to a lesser extent, the osmotic pressure of the blood. Fibrinogen plays a major role in coagulation. Of the three forms of globulin (alpha, beta and gamma), gammaglobulin is concerned with the immunization of the body against foreign cells and substances.
— Supplies for cells: glucose (0.1%), fat, amino acids and salts.
— Cellular products: enzymes, antibodies and hormones.
— Cellular waste products (nitrogenous) such as urea and uric acid.
- Gases: oxygen, carbon dioxide, nitrogen.
- Formed elements: these constitute about 45% of the blood volume. They are the red blood cells (RBCs or erythrocytes), the carriers of oxygen and carbon dioxide; the white blood cells (WBCs or leukocytes), scavengers and immunizing agents; and the platelets, essential for blood coagulation.

Indications for blood transfusion

- When a person loses considerable amounts of blood owing to haemorrhage, a transfusion is necessary to save his life. The guidelines are loss of 10% or more of blood volume in a child, and loss of 15% or more of blood volume in an adult.
- To treat anaemia or some blood deficiency.

Unfortunately, the bloods of different people are not all exactly alike, and failure to transfuse the appropriate type of blood is likely to cause the death of the recipient. Hence, it is necessary to know the physiology of blood grouping and matching before giving transfusions.

One of the reasons one person's blood may not be suitable for another person is that the recipient may be allergic to some of the proteins in the blood cells of the donor. Antibodies in the recipient's plasma will cause agglutination (clumping) and haemolysis (rupture) of the in-jected cells. This 'haemolytic blood transfusion reaction' can easily kill the patient.

Blood groups and blood typing (cross-matching)

The transfusion of blood became possible after Landsteiner described the main groups of the ABO system in 1900.

The ABO blood group system is the most important blood group system to be considered in transfusion practice because, in normal individuals, antibodies occur to any blood cell ABO marker (antigen) not present on that individual's own blood cells. For example, in people belonging to blood group A, their own red cells carry A antigen (marker) and their blood serum contains antibodies to B antigen (Table 6.8).

A blood transfusion is compatible when the recipient's blood does not contain any antibodies against the donor's blood. This usually means transfusing blood of the same type (i.e. group A blood to a group A patient). However, because AB type patients have no antibodies (Table 6.8), they can receive A, B or O blood, and because type O blood has no markers (antigens), it can be given to A, B and AB type patients.

Incompatible blood transfusions, in which the recipient's blood contains antibodies against the donor blood, will cause instant agglutination and rupture of the donor red cells – the haemolytic blood transfusion reaction. As mentioned above, this can kill the patient. All blood samples taken for cross-matching must be fully labelled and checked against the patient's identity band. Before being given to the patient, each unit of blood must be checked against the laboratory's form and the patient's identity band; careful checking should prevent an incorrect unit of blood being given to the wrong patient. Most incompatible blood transfusions occur because of mistakes made in the ward or theatre.

Table 6.8 Antigens and antibodies in the ABO group

ABO group	Red cell antigen present	Red cell antibodies present in serum
A	A	Anti-B
B	B	Anti-A
AB	A and B	No antibodies
O	No marker	Anti-A and Anti-B

Autologous transfusion

In autologous transfusion, the blood donor and recipient are the same person. The advantages of autologous transfusion are:

- the avoidance of infectious diseases associated with homologous transfusions (in which the donor and recipient are different people);
- the avoidance of immunological complications such as febrile and anaphylactoid reactions;
- the avoidance of an impaired response to bacterial infection;
- that compatible homologous blood may not be available for patients with rare blood groups so autologous blood is the only option;
- that the use of autologous transfusion is acceptable to some patients who either refuse homologous transfusion on religious grounds or fear contracting an infectious disease.

Autologous transfusion can take place in the following manner:

1. *Preoperative autologous donation.* This type of transfusion is considered in elective surgical procedures for which blood would be ordinarily cross-matched. In this procedure, the patient donates 1 unit of blood each week.

2. *Intraoperative blood salvage.* There are three techniques of intraoperative blood salvage, of which the semicontinuous flow centrifugation devices are important. These are used when large volumes of blood loss is anticipated, for example liver transplantation or total joint replacement.

3. *Isovolaemic haemodilution.* Isovolaemic haemodilution consists of elective withdrawal or surgical loss of whole blood with the simultaneous administration of a crystalloid or colloid solution to maintain the normal circulating volume. This technique is commonly used in cardiac surgery patients to decrease transfusion requirements and facilitate hypothermia.

Storage and handling of blood
(Table 6.9)

Blood for transfusion should be stored at the correct temperature of 4–6°C. The refrigerator is fitted with an automatic temperature-recording device and a battery-operated alarm system. The temperature limits must be rigidly observed in order to preserve the red cells and minimize the multiplication of chance bacterial contaminants. Food and pathological specimens must never be stored in the blood refrigerator. Blood for transfusion should not be left out of the refrigerator for more than 30 minutes before transfusion; if it is, it should be discarded. It can, however, be contained in a specially approved transport cool box, suitable for whole blood as well as packed cells, for 18 hours. Once hung, a bag of blood should be completely transfused within 5 hours or the remnants discarded. Packed red cells, unless concentrated in a sterile plastic transfer pack, must be used within 12 hours; similarly fresh frozen plasma, fibrinogen or albumin should be used within 3 hours.

Hazards of transfusion

1. *Bacterial contamination.* Even under aseptic conditions, 2% of stored blood is contaminated by Gram-negative bacteria. Hence blood should be stored at 4–6°C and discarded once out of the refrigerator for more than 30 minutes.

2. *Febrile reactions.* These are due to pyrogens, i.e. polysaccharide products of bacterial metabolism that used to be present in the blood bottles, and have decreased considerably since the use of disposable bags and transfusion sets.

3. *White cell reactions* (technically 'febrile non-haemolytic transfusion' reactions). These are *not* an 'allergy' as lay men understand the term. Such reactions occur in 1–2% of all transfusions and can be controlled with antihistamines such as chlorpheniramine (Piriton). These mild reactions are due to white cells in the donor blood and should not be confused with the severe reactions caused by ABO incompatibility.

4. *Transmission of disease.* In the past, malaria, syphilis, brucellosis and serum hepatitis were fairly common, but with testing of all donor blood, brucellosis, malaria and syphilis transmission no longer occurs. Serum hepatitis and, recently, acquired immune deficiency syndrome

Table 6.9   Blood, plasma and their products available for transfusion

Presentation	Indication	Useful points
Whole blood: blood 420 ml + acid citrate dextrose 120 ml	• Acute or chronic haemorrhage • Blood dyscrasias such as aplastic anaemia	For routine preservation, acid citrate dextrose (ACD) is the anticoagulant of choice. Blood-life expires in 21 days
Concentrated red cells	• Anaemias in which increased haemoglobin rather than blood volume is needed • Transfusion in patients with heart failure	Blood-life expires in 21 days
Freshly drawn whole blood	• Helpful in exchange transfusion in neonates • In patients with bleeding owing to thrombocytopenia	Blood-life expires in 21 days. Gives viable red blood cells and platelets
'Washed' red cells (leukocyte poor)	• In patients selected for and in post-organ transplantation • Patients with immune deficiency diseases or receiving massive irradiation • Paroxysmal nocturnal haemoglobinuria	When manual techniques are used, this form is viable for 6 hours
Fresh frozen plasma (FFP)	• After massive transfusions • To correct overdose of oral anticoagulants	Chances of serum hepatitis B are increased. Thawed FFP should be used immediately
Plasma protein fraction (PPF) concentrate	• In burns • To increase the fluid volume	Hepatitis virus is inactivated. Shelf-life is 2 years
Albumin (human albumin)	Hypoalbuminaemia	There is no risk of hepatitis. Should be used within 3 months of preparation
Cryoprecipitate	Factor VIII deficiency	Increased risk of hepatitis B. Preparation lasts for 3 months
Fibrinogen	Low fibrinogen levels following massive bleeding, defective clotting (disseminated intravascular coagulation)	Risk of hepatitis B high
Platelet concentration	• Low platelets (below 40 000/mm^3) before major surgery • Following massive transfusion • Bleeding associated with low platelet count	Platelets retain their activity for 2–3 days at 40°C
Leukocyte transfusions ('Buffy coat')	• Leukopenia (low white cell count) in patients on cytotoxics • Severe infection • Primary granulocytopenia	Cell separator used on donor blood

(AIDS) are screened for in all donor blood. However, transmission of these diseases through infected blood products still occurs, the risk being greatest in those requiring multiple donations, for example haemophiliacs.

5. *Decreased red cell survival*. Normally, the half-life of transfused cells is 32 days, but in 30% of the transfusions the red cells survive only 14–16 days.

6. *Acidity of stored blood*. Acid citrate dextrose (ACD) blood has a pH of 7.1 and becomes much more acidic (pH 6.6) the longer it is stored. Massive transfusion with stored blood can cause severe metabolic acidosis.

7. *Citrate toxicity*. Stored blood contains 120 ml ACD solution. The citrate can bind to plasma calcium in the recipient, leading to cardiac arrhythmias in patients receiving massive blood transfusions or in newborn babies. Patients with severe liver disease (who cannot metabolize citrate) are also vulnerable.

8. *Problems with cold blood*. Administration of large volumes of cold blood to anaesthetized patients or children can cause hypothermia and cardiac arrhythmias. Thus blood should be warmed, using a blood warmer, during transfusion.

9. *Haemolytic reactions*. These are due to incompatibility of blood groups and occur in 0.2–0.3% of transfusions.

10. *Potassium toxicity*. Freshly drawn and stored blood contains approximately 4–5 mEq/L potassium, which increases to 30 mEq/L by the expiry date of the unit.

Blood filters are routinely used during blood transfusion, to prevent microaggregates from the stored blood entering the patient's circulation. For massive blood transfusion in a short time, a pressure infusor is used (Fig. 6.31).

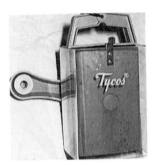

Figure 6.31   Pressure infusor.

If a severe febrile or haemolytic reaction is detected or suspected, the transfusion is stopped and the remainder of the transfused blood and the giving set returned to the blood bank, accompanied by a fresh specimen of blood from the patient. The basic scheme then followed is:

Reports of grouping and
cross-matching, and the blood bag
label, are checked
↓
Blood grouping and
cross-matching of the post-
transfusion blood from the
patient are repeated
↓
The transfusion set is cultured
for organisms
↓
The transfusion bag is
cultured for anaerobic
and aerobic organisms. The

Method of detection of a blood transfusion reaction

If a minor allergic or febrile reaction occurs during a blood transfusion, an antihistamine such as chlorpheniramine (Piriton) is given, and the transfusion continued cautiously.

Table 6.10   Plasma substitutes (volume expanders)

Presentation	Indication	Useful points
Dextran 70 Dextran 40	• Effective blood or plasma substitute • Dextran 40 (low molecular weight) prevents sludging of red cells in deep vein thrombosis	Maintain blood volume for up to 3 days Interfere with cross-matching, so blood should be taken for cross-match before giving dextran
Cross-linked gelatin (Haemaccel)	Shock due to haemorrhage, burns, etc.	Similar viscosity and osmotic pressure to that of plasma. Does not interfere with cross-matching
Hetastarch (Hespan)	Volume expander	Remains in the body for 24–36 hours. Contraindicated in bleeding disorders
Gelofusine	Volume expander	

expiry date of blood bag
is checked

↓

Urine from the patient is
examined for
haemoglobin and red cell
breakdown products.

SPECIALTIES OF ANAESTHESIA

ENT ANAESTHESIA

Most of the patients undergoing ENT surgery
are children and young adults, and a number of
operations are performed as day cases. The
airway (mouth and pharynx) is shared by both
the surgeon and the anaesthetist. The important
procedures carried out are outlined below.

Adenoidectomy and tonsillectomy

Premedication consists of trimeprazine (Vallergan)
or diazepam (see p. 146 for details). An oral
endotracheal tube is passed after inhalational or
i.v. induction. In adults, nasotracheal intubation
is preferred for tonsillectomy. Postoperative
analgesia is given and tracheal extubation carried
out with the patient slightly head down in a
lateral position.

For the management of the postoperative
bleeding tonsil, see page 210.

Nasal operations

Submucous resection, rhinoplasty, submucous
diathermy and excision of nasal polyps are the
common nasal operations.

A standard general anaesthetic employing an
oral endotracheal tube and spontaneous or controlled ventilation is employed. A throat pack
is inserted during surgery and the patient is
positioned 10° head up.

Preoperatively, the nose is prepared by the
surgeon using either cocaine or lignocaine, with
adrenaline to decrease the vascularity of the
nose.

Microlaryngoscopy

Anaesthesia is induced, and a small size (5.5 or
6.0 mm) cuffed endotracheal tube is passed;
this allows the surgeon to examine the larynx
(see Fig. 6.22 above). Either intermittent suxamethonium or atracurium is used for relaxation
of the vocal cords.

Laryngectomy

If respiratory obstruction is expected, inhalational
induction is used and intubation carried out with
a small size tube. When the larynx is dissected out,
a sterile tracheostomy tube and connections are
kept ready before the trachea is divided. The
patient's lungs are ventilated with 100% oxygen
for 2 minutes, the tracheal tube is withdrawn
into the larynx, and the tracheostomy tube is inserted by the surgeon in the divided trachea and
firmly secured. Anaesthesia is carried out through
the tracheostomy tube until the end of the surgery.

Laser surgery

Anaesthesia for laser surgery

Lasers are used to cut or coagulate tissue in
difficult-to-reach locations. A focused laser beam
can deliver approximately 2500 calories per second
to the target site. Lasers produce a relatively
'dry' or bloodless field by instantly sealing off
small blood vessels as they cut.

Hazards with the use of lasers are:

- *Atmospheric contamination*. Tissue vaporization
  by laser surgery can produce smoke, which
  can cause nausea, headache and carbon
  deposits in the lung. A smoke evacuator can
  prevent the dispersion of smoke.
- *Perforation*. Misdirected laser energy may
  perforate a viscus or a large blood vessel.
- *Embolism*. Venous gas embolism can occur,
  particularly during hysteroscopic surgery
  with Nd-YAG lasers.
- *Energy transfer to another location*. Pressing the
  laser control trigger at the wrong time can
  deliver damaging laser energy to the eyes or
  endotracheal tube.

- *Endotracheal tube fires*. With the energy delivered by laser, any hydrocarbon material, such as plastic and rubber, can burn, particularly in an oxygen-enriched atmosphere.

The methods that have been used to decrease the incidence of fire include:

- reduction of the flammability of the endotracheal tube by using red rubber tubes, foil-wrapped PVC endotracheal tubes and moistened pledgets;
- the use of Venturi ventilation through a rigid metal bronchoscope;
- using the lowest concentration of oxygen compatible with good saturations (usually between 24 and 40%);
- an intermittent apnoea technique.

The patient's eyes (non-operated) should be taped and covered with an opaque, saline-soaked knit or metal shield. Operating theatre personnel should wear safety goggles or lenses specific for the laser wavelength in use. Regular eyeglasses are sufficient but contact lenses are not.

UK regulations for laser safety

Hospitals in the UK work within the European Standards body (the ISO) and follow the British Standard European Norm (BSEN) 60825 (1992) standard governing the radiation safety of laser products. The Health & Safety at Work act needs to be referred to when setting policies and standards for the protection of staff working with lasers.

A laser is used to remove tumours or polyps from the vocal cords. Because the laser beam ignites polyvinyl chloride (PVC), either the microlaryngoscopy tubes are wrapped with protective silver foil or metal tubes are used (see Fig. 6.21 above).

Myringotomy

Children and some adults with secretory otitis media undergo examination of the ears, together with myringotomy and insertion of grommets under general anaesthesia. As these patients are treated as day-stay cases, spontaneous ventilation with a face mask or laryngeal mask is used.

Middle ear surgery

For middle ear surgery, hypotensive anaesthesia (see p. 194) is employed. A standard general anaesthesia is administered and a non-kinking oral endotracheal tube passed. The operative site should be bloodless; thus blood pressure is reduced using IPPV, halothane or isoflurane with a 10° head-up tilt. Sometimes drugs such as trimetaphan (Arfonad) or labetalol (Trandate) are employed to cause a fall in blood pressure.

DENTAL ANAESTHESIA

Dental extractions are carried out on an out-patient basis in a majority of cases; a few are admitted as inpatients. The majority of patients requiring outpatient anaesthesia are children who are either too young to cooperate with local analgesia or are mentally handicapped.

The induction of anaesthesia is inhalational in the majority of children. Halothane or sevoflurane is introduced early during induction with oxygen (30%) and nitrous oxide (70%). A mouth prop and a throat pack are inserted by the dentist once the jaw relaxes. Anaesthesia is maintained using the inhalational agent of choice in an oxygen-enriched carrier gas delivered to the patient by a nasal face mask, laryngeal mask or endotracheal tube. The anaesthetist observes the reservoir bag and makes sure that the airway is not blocked by the pack and that (if using a nasal mask) mouth breathing is avoided. At the end of the procedure, the pack is removed and the patient is transferred to the recovery room. After complete recovery, the patient is discharged.

The problems associated with dental anaesthesia are:

- *Sharing the airway*. The anaesthetist overcomes this by holding the jaw forward with the middle and ring fingers of both hands and holding the nasal mask with both thumbs.

- *A horizontal/sitting position.* A sitting-up position in the dental chair can cause hypoxia due to fainting, and in a horizontal position blood and debris can pass down the throat cavity.
- *Arrhythmias.* In approximately 25–30% of patients, transient arrhythmias such as ventricular extrasystoles are seen. Arrhythmias are especially common if halothane is used as the maintenance agent.

Intravenous induction using propofol, or etomidate or thiopentone is employed, and a nasotracheal intubation may be required in adults presenting for dental extractions who either have oral infection, which prevents the use of a local anaesthetic, or who are mentally handicapped.

Inpatient anaesthesia for the extraction of wisdom teeth or for maxillofacial surgery requires general anaesthesia with a nasotracheal tube and throat pack. Patients anaesthetized for maxillofacial surgery receive antiemetics as a routine measure.

PAEDIATRIC ANAESTHESIA

There are a number of anatomical and physiological differences between adults and children. A few major features are listed here.

The larynx is higher in children (C3–C4) than in adults. The epiglottis is floppy, and a straight laryngoscope blade elevates the epiglottis to visualize the vocal cords (C5–C6). Respiration is rapid (from about 30/min in the newborn to 16–20/min in a 2-year-old child), and the tidal volume is 7 ml/kg.

The mean heart rate ranges from 140 beats/min in the neonate to 100 beats/min in a 6-year-old. Babies do not tolerate bradycardia as cardiac output depends on heart rate. Blood pressure is around 90/60 mmHg, reaching 120/70 mmHg at around 16 years of age. Blood volume at birth is 80 ml/kg, and in a 6-year-old child 75 ml/kg. Blood transfusion is recommended if the blood loss exceeds 10% of blood volume.

The daily fluid requirements are 100 ml/kg in infants below 10 kg body weight, between 10 and 20 kg 1000 ml and 50 × (wt in kg – 10) ml/kg in a child below the age of 1 year. Maintenance fluid in children is 1/4 normal saline in 5% dextrose, intraoperative fluid losses are replaced with blood or Ringer's solution. Buretrols or Imeds are used to control infusion volumes precisely.

Neonates lose body heat rapidly from the exposed head, so the operating theatre temperature is raised to reduce this heat loss. A fall in body temperature can lead to respiratory depression, a fall in cardiac output and the prolonged action of drugs.

Children less than 18 months old are at risk of hypoglycaemia (low blood sugar) after anything but the shortest fasting period.

Anaesthetic management

The child is premedicated according to body weight (see p. 147). Anaesthesia is induced with an inhalational, i.v. or i.m. technique. Inhalational induction is carried out directly by mask or by placing the T-piece in the anaesthetist's hands near the child's face. Intravenous induction is made pain-free by the application of EMLA cream to the back of the hands 1 hour preoperatively. An Ayres T-piece is used for short periods of spontaneous ventilation with a fresh gas flow 2.5 times the minute volume of the child, i.e. tidal volume × respiratory rate × 2.5.

Jackson Rees' modification of the T-piece consists of an open-ended reservoir bag that can be used for IPPV. The fresh gas flow on the anaesthetic machine is adjusted as follows: 1000 ml + 100 ml/kg body weight per minute. A minimum gas flow of 3 L/min is required for this system.

The endotracheal tube (ETT) used for intubation should be small enough to allow a slight leak of gases during IPPV, and the size of ETT is calculated as (age in years ÷ 4) + 4.5 (see p. 286 for tube sizes). The narrowest part of the child's airway is at the cricoid ring, compared with the vocal cords in adults. A cuff on the ETT is not necessary in children below 9 years of age.

Monitoring. In addition to observation of the patient, a precordial or oesophageal stethoscope is an essential monitor. The intensity of heart sound picked up by the stethoscope varies with the stroke volume, which in itself acts as an indicator of cardiac output.

Other monitoring devices, such as temperature probes, ECG and blood pressure monitors, are used. Regular BM stix (blood sugar tests) are essential in the under-twos for all but the shortest of operations.

Drugs

The routine drugs used for adult anaesthesia are also used in children. Postoperative analgesia prescribed can range from paracetamol elixir for mild-to-moderate pain, to nerve blocks such as caudal epidural or penile block for circumcision; to ilioinguinal block for herniotomies and orchidopexy. Opiates such as papaveretum (Omnopon) or pethidine are given for severe pain.

Neonatal anaesthesia

Neonates coming for surgery are at a great disadvantage because their temperature maintenance mechanisms are immature. The incubator and operating theatre temperatures are increased during the surgical procedure, and the baby's temperature is monitored. Intubation is the rule for all but the shortest operations, and IPPV is commenced with a low concentration of an inhalational agent. Drugs are prepared in 1 or 2 ml syringes and a 22 G or 24 G cannula is inserted intravenously. A three-way tap is attached for the injection of drugs, plasma and blood.

One of the most common neonatal operations carried in district general hospitals is the repair of pyloric stenosis. The babies are 3–8 weeks old, dehydrated and metabolically alkalotic (see p. 252) due to vomiting. An i.v. infusion is commenced, dehydration and acid–base imbalance are corrected, and a nasogastric tube is passed. An i.v. induction and endotracheal intubation are carried out, and, as it is a short surgical procedure, intermittent suxamethonium or atracurium is given.

Other specific operations in the neonate are for tracheo-oesophageal fistula, diaphragmatic hernia, exomphalos, hydrocephalus and myelomeningocele.

OPHTHALMIC ANAESTHESIA

Patients presenting for eye surgery are at the extremes of age. Children present with squint and for examination under anaesthetic for congenital glaucoma. Young adults present with perforating eye injuries and diabetic complications of the eye, and the elderly present with cataracts and glaucoma.

The problems associated with ophthalmic anaesthesia are the oculocardiac reflex and maintaining intraocular pressure:

1. *Oculocardiac reflex*. Bradycardia or cardiac arrest can occur following traction on the internal rectus muscle or pressure on the eyeball. Adequate cardiac monitoring is essential. Prevention of bradyarrhythmias consists of the i.v. injection of atropine 0.3 mg or glycopyrrolate 0.2 mg.
2. *Maintaining intraocular pressure*. Ideally, the eye should be soft before the anterior chamber is opened. If the pressure is high, it is lowered by deliberate hypotension or hyperventilation using a volatile anaesthetic such as isoflurane.

Most ophthalmic procedures (e.g. for cataract, trabeculectomies) can be carried out under local anaesthesia in adults.

The joint Colleges of Ophthalmologists and Anaesthetists have recommended that an anaesthetist should be present in the theatre during local anaesthetic cases and that:

- monitoring should be carried out;
- i.v. access should be obtained;
- the equipment necessary for resuscitation should be available.

The local anaesthetic agents commonly used are:

- 2% lignocaine
- 2% lignocaine + 0.5% plain bupivacaine
- 3% prilocaine with octapressin
- 0.75% bupivacaine.

Hyaluronidase 150 IU is added to enhance the absorption of local anaesthetic.

Commonly performed blocks include:

1. *Peribulbar block*: a single-needle (medial canthus approach) and two-needle techniques have been described.

2. *Retrobulbar block*: in this technique, local anaesthetic is injected in mid orbit intraconally.

Other techniques that have been described are:

- subconjunctival (perilimbal)
- subtenon
- topical corneoconjunctival.

DAY-STAY ANAESTHESIA

Day-stay surgery has become popular because of the short waiting time for surgery and because patients can recover in their own home. A common day-stay unit consists of a separate ward using the hospital's main operating theatre complex.

Patients in the fitness grade ASA 1 or 2 undergoing operations that do not cause undue haemorrhage and severe postoperative pain are selected. A letter is sent to the patient undergoing day-stay surgery, describing what she or he should expect. It also includes the following instructions:

1. Patients should not eat or drink for 6 hours before the operation (4 hours in children).
2. Patients should be accompanied home.
3. Patients should not drink, drive or work with machinery for 24 hours after the operation.

Premedication is avoided to prevent hangover effects; young children are prescribed temazepam elixir and EMLA cream.

Surgery is mostly performed under general anaesthesia, although on some occasions regional blocks such as brachial plexus block, individual nerve blocks, intravenous regional anaesthesia, caudal block or penile block are used. Induction agents with the least hangover effects, such as propofol, methohexitone or etomidate, are used. Anaesthesia is maintained with nitrous oxide, oxygen and enflurane or isoflurane. If endotracheal intubation is required, atracurium, vecuronium or mivacurium is used. Nowadays, a number of anaesthetists use laryngeal masks to prevent sore throats.

Analgesia is provided by short-acting analgesics such as fentanyl and alfentanil. Paracetamol or diclofenac suppositories are used to decrease the incidence of postoperative pain. When the patient is fully recovered, oral analgesics, for example paracetamol, co-proxamol or co-dydramol, are prescribed. Certain patients may require analgesics such as pethidine or papaveretum for severe pain and may even need to be admitted.

Before they are discharged, all day-stay patients are seen by the anaesthetist and once again warned against driving or drinking in the following 24 hours.

THORACIC ANAESTHESIA

The common conditions requiring thoracic surgery are carcinoma of the bronchus, carcinoma of the oesophagus, metastatic disease requiring resection and certain non-malignant conditions. After preoperative assessment and investigation, patients are prepared for surgery using physiotherapy, rehydration and correction of any acid–base imbalance.

The diagnostic procedures carried out are as follows.

Bronchoscopy

This is carried out using either a fibreoptic bronchoscope or a rigid bronchoscope. Fibreoptic bronchoscopy is carried out using local anaesthetic solution, or the scope is passed via the endotracheal tube or laryngeal mask in an anaesthetized patient. Rigid bronchoscopy is carried out by the thoracic surgeons to locate bronchial tumours and for the removal of foreign bodies. The most commonly used rigid bronchoscope is the Negus.

A general anaesthetic technique is recommended. In children, deep inhalational anaesthesia with nitrous oxide/oxygen and halothane is used, the bronchoscope being passed while the child breathes spontaneously. In adults, intermittent propofol or methohexitone is used to keep the patient asleep, with suxamethonium to maintain paralysis. Ventilation is maintained using Venturi bronchoscope injectors. The Venturi jet of oxygen entrains air and produces inflation of the lungs. Expiration occurs through and round the bronchoscope.

Oesophagoscopy

Rigid oesophagoscopy is used to locate oesophageal tumours, to dilate strictures and remove foreign bodies. A general anaesthetic is given. A rapid sequence induction technique is employed because of the potential for regurgitation on induction of anaesthesia. A smaller size endotracheal tube is passed to allow the oesophagoscope to pass through the cricopharyngeal sphincter.

Mediastinoscopy

The mediastinoscope is introduced through a small incision in the suprasternal notch. It allows direct inspection and biopsy of mediastinal lesions. A general anaesthetic technique using an endotracheal tube and IPPV is employed. A large-bore i.v. cannula is sited because of the (small) risk of torrential bleeding with this procedure.

Principles of one-lung anaesthesia

In an awake, spontaneously breathing subject lying on one side, the lung nearer to the table (the dependent lung) is better perfused with blood and enjoys better ventilation. In an anaesthetized patient lying on one side, the upper lung receives better ventilation. During surgery, the upper lung is made to collapse to allow better surgical access. This leads to shunting, as the upper lung still receives blood supply but no ventilation. During lung surgery, the diseased lung is uppermost and the dependent lung receives an increased blood flow. In oesophageal surgery, in patients who may have two healthy lungs, collapsing one lung can lead to high intrapulmonary shunting. The intrapulmonary shunting can lead to a fall in arterial oxygen tension (PaO_2). A PaO_2 of 9 kPa is acceptable during one-lung anaesthesia. This is achieved by increasing the inspired oxygen concentration

and adding a positive end-expiratory pressure (PEEP) of 3–5 cmH$_2$O. PEEP improves the arterial oxygenation by increasing the functional residual capacity (FRC) of the dependent lung.

Thoracotomy

Double-lumen tubes, such as the Robertshaw, Carlen or Bronchocath (see Fig. 6.22 above), are used to provide a separate channel for the ventilation and suction of each lung. A left-sided tube is used for surgery on the right lung. The anaesthetic technique consists of the insertion of a large-bore i.v. cannula and induction with a suitable agent. If the intubation is likely to be difficult, suxamethonium is used; otherwise a large dose of non-depolarizing muscle relaxant is employed.

After the insertion of a double-lumen tube, anaesthesia is maintained with nitrous oxide, oxygen, opiates and volatile anaesthetic. The correct positioning of the tube can be checked clinically (by auscultation) or by direct examination with the fibreoptic bronchoscope.

The ECG and arterial blood pressure (non-invasive) are monitored in the majority of cases. In a few patients who are poor risk or in whom massive haemorrhage is expected, an arterial line and a CVP line are inserted. A warming blanket, blood warmer and temperature monitor are used. The patient is placed in the lateral position, with the side to be operated on uppermost. Oesophageal surgery is performed with the patient in the lateral or semi-lateral position.

Analgesia is maintained with i.v. opiates or epidural infusions, usually of local anaesthetic with an opioid. At the end of thoracotomy, a drain is placed in the pleural cavity to prevent air or fluid accumulating in the thorax in the postoperative period. The lung is reinflated before the thorax is closed and, after the closure, the drains are connected to an underwater seal.

Patients are allowed to breathe spontaneously after extubation and are given humidified 40% oxygen.

Surgical procedures carried out on the lung are described below.

Pleural abrasion. This procedure is used to treat recurrent pneumothorax or pleural effusions.

Pneumonectomy. This is carried out when a bronchial carcinoma has affected more than one lobe. The bronchus is divided and sutured. The pleural cavity is not drained, and the space eventually fills with serosanguinous fluid and fibrosis.

Bronchopleural fistula. This is a connection between the pleural cavity and the bronchial tree that may occur as a result of breakdown of a bronchial stump (e.g. following pneumonectomy), trauma or neoplasm.

The patient is dehydrated and toxic owing to the presence of infected fluid in the pleural cavity. The patient's healthy lung can be soiled by the infected fluid, so IPPV is not commenced until a double-lumen tube has been inserted and the infected area isolated. Inhalational induction is preferred.

Lobectomy. This is performed for bronchial neoplasm or bronchiectasis. A double-lumen tube is used for anaesthesia. When the lobe has been removed, the bronchus is clamped and divided and the remaining part sutured or stapled.

Other surgical procedures carried out on the thorax are:

Repair of hiatus hernia. A left-sided thoracotomy is performed. Either an ordinary endotracheal or a double-lumen tube is used.

Oesophageal myotomy. Heller's operation is carried out to treat oesophageal achalasia. This condition results in gross dilatation of the oesophagus with the collection in it of large volumes of undigested food. The anaesthetic technique consists of rapid-sequence induction following premedication with H_2 antagonists and antacids.

Surgery for carcinoma of the oesophagus. If the tumour is in the lower third, a left thoraco-abdominal incision is used. Since patients are anaemic, dehydrated and hypovolaemic, the anaesthetic technique should suit their physical condition.

NEUROSURGICAL ANAESTHESIA

In intracranial operations, the special problems involved are:

1. raised intracranial pressure
2. maintenance of the airway
3. posture such as head-up, sitting or lateral
4. the length of the operation.

Normal intracranial pressure is less than 15 mmHg; the factors that increase it are:

- pressure from outside, such as from a bony tumour;
- a space-occupying lesion, such as an abscess, neoplasm or haematoma;
- cerebral oedema;
- venous obstruction;
- arterial dilatation due to hypercarbia.

The factors that decrease the intracranial pressure are:

- head-up tilt (15–30° encourages venous drainage);
- hyperventilation (to <4 kPa);
- diuresis (mannitol or frusemide);
- CSF drainage/surgical decompression;
- dexamethasone;
- blood pressure control.

Cerebral blood flow is regulated by the following agents:

1. Arterial carbon dioxide tension: a rise in P_{CO_2} (8–11 kPa) increases cerebral blood flow (CBF) by 100%, whereas a fall in P_{CO_2} to 3.5 kPa reduces CBF to 30%.
2. Arterial blood pressure: CBF is not altered if the blood pressure is maintained at between 90 and 180 mmHg.
3. Anaesthetic agents such as nitrous oxide, halothane and ketamine increase the cerebral blood flow.

Neurological investigations such as carotid angiography and computerized axial tomography (CAT) are nowadays carried out under local analgesia. Children and uncooperative, anxious or confused adults require a general anaesthetic.

Anaesthesia

Patients are assessed preoperatively and, if there are signs of raised intracranial pressure, sedatives and narcotics are withheld. A smooth induction is carried out with thiopentone, along with a short-acting analgesic such as alfentanil to prevent fluctuations in blood pressure. The vocal cords are sprayed with 4% lignocaine, and an armoured cuffed endotracheal tube is passed. A throat pack may be inserted. IPPV with muscle relaxants, maintaining a Pco$_2$ of around 3.5 kPa, is achieved. Monitoring consists of ECG, intra-arterial blood pressure, CVP, end-tidal carbon dioxide level and use of a precordial stethoscope.

Most craniotomies are performed in the supine, brow-up position; posterior fossa surgery is carried out in the sitting position. The head is shaved under anaesthesia, with the patient in the surgical position.

Air embolism. This occurs in 2–3% of patients in the sitting position; many of the veins in the back of the neck and scalp do not collapse after they have been divided. During neurosurgery, if air enters the veins, it goes via the right side of the heart to the pulmonary artery, resulting in a mill-wheel murmur. The patient develops sudden cyanosis, hypotension and tachycardia. Treatment consists of preventing further entry of air into the circulation by compressing the neck veins, lowering the head end of the table, changing to 100% oxygen and keeping the patient on his left side so that bubbles are carried away from the pulmonary artery. The trapped air can occasionally be aspirated via the CVP or PA line.

Intracranial pressure is reduced during anaesthesia using 20% mannitol (0.2–0.5 mg/kg body weight) or frusemide 1 mg/kg.

Elective ventilation is carried out in patients who are expected to develop cerebral oedema; otherwise residual neuromuscular blockade is reversed.

Some of the specific operations carried out are described below.

Intracranial aneurysm surgery

A smooth induction and intubation are carried out. Patients are kept relatively hypertensive to encourage good brain perfusion and minimize the risk of vasospasm. If the aneurysm does burst at surgery, short periods of elective hypotension may be necessary until control of the bleeding point is gained.

Hypophysectomy

The pituitary gland is removed for tumours of the gland or for the treatment of metastatic hormone-sensitive tumours. Tracheal intubation can be difficult in patients with acromegaly, so a 'difficult intubation' set should be made available.

Anaesthesia in head injury cases

Anaesthesia may be needed in patients with head injuries, either for elevation of a depressed fracture, suturing of lacerations or compound fractures of major bones, or laparotomy. A rapid-sequence induction is carried out and a cuffed endotracheal tube passed. Necessary precautions are taken to prevent fluctuations in the intracranial pressure.

OBSTETRIC ANALGESIA AND ANAESTHESIA

In the labour ward, anaesthetists provide analgesia during labour to pregnant women and, where indicated, provide anaesthesia for procedures such as caesarean sections or the removal of retained placenta.

Analgesia

Labour is painful for a variety of reasons, such as uterine contractions and dilatation of the cervix. If the pain is abolished, both mother and fetus benefit. The methods of analgesia available during labour are:

Systemic analgesia. This is the most common method of giving analgesia, used in about 60–70%

of mothers. Pethidine is given i.m. (at dosages of 100–150 mg) 4 hourly until the second stage of labour is reached. The pain relief is not always adequate and, because pethidine and other opiates cross the placenta, babies may be born drowsy and slow to feed.

Other analgesics that have been used are pentazocine (Fortral) and meptazinol (Meptid).

Inhalational analgesia. This is used widely in the UK and, when used properly, a large proportion of women receive adequate pain relief.

Entonox is contained premixed in a cylinder containing 50% nitrous oxide in oxygen. In antenatal classes, mothers are taught to apply the face mask tightly around the face and to begin inhaling the gas as soon as a contraction is felt. The breathing should be slow and deep. When the contraction ceases, the mask can be taken off.

Epidural analgesia. This is the most effective method of pain relief during labour. Once the epidural has been carried out and the catheter inserted (see p. 175), the anaesthetist gives the first dose of 6–10 ml 0.25% plain bupivacaine (Marcain). Further top-ups are given by the midwives every 2–4 hours.

Analgesia for vaginal delivery can be effectively given using either a spinal block (see p. 173) or a caudal block. Manual removal of the placenta can be achieved effectively by using either an epidural or a spinal block.

Anaesthesia for caesarean section

The indication for caesarean section may be elective or emergency, the anaesthetic procedure being the same in each case.

The problems associated with pregnancy and anaesthesia are as follows.

Full stomach. More than half of pregnant mothers have gastric contents of more than 40 ml with a pH below 2.5 owing to delayed gastric emptying. In a number of labour wards, 30 ml of 0.3M sodium citrate is given to increase the intragastric pH to above 2.5. The gastric volume can be decreased by giving either cimetidine 200 mg i.m. or ranitidine 50 mg i.v. or i.m.

The regurgitation from the stomach and aspiration into the lungs of even small volumes of acid can cause severe and irreparable damage to the lungs.

Maternal hypotension. If the pregnant mother lies on her back, she may develop hypotension. This is due to the gravid uterus pressing on the vena cava and, in some patients, it can be severe.

Anaesthesia can be given by either a regional or a general technique.

1. Regional anaesthesia. A lumbar epidural or spinal block can be given for elective caesarean section. If the block is already present, it can be topped up for the emergency section. For an epidural block, a catheter is inserted (in a sitting position) and 10 ml 0.5% plain bupivacaine is injected; the patient is kept sitting for 12 minutes. Next, the patient is placed supine (with a wedge) and another 15 ml 0.5% plain bupivacaine is injected slowly to achieve a block up to T6. After an adequate block has been established, surgery is commenced.

2. Spinal anaesthesia using a 25G or 26G spinal needle is an effective and quicker way of obtaining anaesthesia in an emergency; 2–4 ml of hyperbaric 0.5% bupivacaine is used. The precautions are the same as those given on page 173.

Failed intubation

During emergency anaesthesia, intubation of the oesophagus instead of the trachea can lead to the death of the mother. Tracheal intubation may be especially difficult owing to:

1. a short neck;
2. large breasts obscuring the airway;
3. the inappropriate application of cricoid pressure;
4. the anaesthetist starting to intubate before the suxamethonium has begun to work;
5. anatomical abnormalities.

Factors 2–4 can easily be corrected by the anaesthetist and the assistant, whereas for anatomical problems, where the larynx cannot be visualized, a 'failed intubation drill' is carried out. The 'failed intubation drill' consists of:

- maintained cricoid pressure;
- putting the patient head down in the left lateral position;
- maintaining oxygenation with 100% oxygen, by IPPV if the effect of suxamethonium has not worn off;
- waking the patient up and sending for help.

When the senior anaesthetist arrives, the other alternatives that can be tried are:

- reintubating with a longer-bladed laryngoscope, fibreoptic laryngoscope or retrograde catheterization;
- spinal anaesthesia or epidural anaesthesia (if the catheter is in situ);
- inhalational anaesthesia.

In an emergency, when it is essential to proceed with surgery as soon as possible (e.g. fetal distress or placenta praevia), anaesthesia is maintained by the following measures:

1. Continue the application of cricoid pressure.
2. Tilt the patient head down.
3. Maintain oxygenation using 40% oxygen in nitrous oxide and add a volatile agent (halothane or isoflurane). Use bag and mask ventilation until the suxamethonium has worn off; then allow the patient to breath spontaneously, all the while maintaining cricoid pressure. It must be emphasized that this is not standard practice and should only be tried by experienced anaesthetists in an extreme emergency.

ANAESTHESIA FOR RADIOLOGY

In the UK, the radiology (X-ray) department is usually situated away from the theatre suite and is supplied with equipment that may not reflect the standard available elsewhere in the hospital. This, in association with unfamiliar environment, poor lighting or total darkness, may make the anaesthetist's task difficult. The standard anaesthetic machine check is followed (see p. 158).

Anaesthesia is required for certain diagnostic procedures such as CT or MRI scanning in the very young or the uncooperative. The patient is kept totally immobile and monitoring may be difficult as a result of inadequate lighting, a moving table or restricted access (e.g. as in whole-body CAT scanning). For CAT scanning, young children and uncooperative adults are anaesthetized. Long breathing circuits are required because of the distance between the patient and the anaesthetic machine.

Magnetic Resonance Imaging

MRI involves use of high-strength magnetic fields to provide digitalized tomographic imaging of the body. Anaesthetists and operating department personnel are sometimes involved in patient care because the quality of the image depends on the relevant part of the patient remaining immobile.

Patient monitoring and anaesthetic management are challenging because the high magnetic fields interfere with electronic monitors and the ferromagnetic components of common equipment.

Field strengths ranging from 0.15 to 2.0 tesla (T) are used with total-scanning types of up to 1.5 hours' duration.

Problems with the use of MRI.

- *Implanted objects* such as pacemakers can be inactivated or converted to an inappropriate mode.
- *Cerebral aneurysmal clips* may be detached.
- *Cosmetic tattoos* with metallic dyes can cause irritation.
- *Financial distress:* the strong magnetic field in the MRI scanner will wipe the magnetic strip on credit, bank and telephone cards.
- *Propelling of objects.* In the presence of the scanner's magnetic field, loose metal objects can become airborne, so no keys, coins or other ferromagnetic objects should be allowed into the scanning room.
- *Noise* from the MRI scanner can cause difficulty in communication, although this is less likely with more modern scanners.

- *Monitor interference.* Electron beams are affected by the static magnetic field, which distorts and displaces the image on monitors and cathode ray displays. Electrical connections to the patient act as antennae and introduce radiofrequency (RF) signals that can distort the MRI image.
- *Pulse oximetry.* These monitors are susceptible to interference from the changing magnetic field and will occasionally be deactivated for short period by RF signals. Placing the body of the pulse oximeter more than 2 m away from the magnetic field will give uninterrupted signals.
- *Blood pressure monitoring* during MRI can be accurately carried out using the oscillometric method (oscillotonometer, Dinamap, Critikon, Accutors, Datascope, etc.).
- *Anaesthesia* machines should be bolted to the walls and modified to remove ferromagnetic components. Aluminium cylinders should replace ferromagnetic ones on anaesthetic machines. Some 'MRI-compatible' ventilators are available that are pneumatically driven, fluidic-controlled and volume-cycled.
- *Respiratory gas analysis.* Oxygen analysers and capnographs should be connected to the patient with extended plastic tubing to prevent mutual interference between monitors and scanner. Plastic laryngoscopes have been made available, but the batteries in the handle can still be pulled by the magnetic field. Laryngoscopes have been modified to operate directly from a 5 V DC source connected to the MRI machine.

Problems associated with patients undergoing MRI include poor patient access and claustrophobia, because the patient table moves completely inside the scanner during imaging.

Anaesthetic techniques for MRI.

- Sedation.
- General anaesthesia with i.v. induction, and maintenance with inhalational agents.
- Total intravenous anaesthesia.

MINIMAL ACCESS SURGERY

Minimal access surgery (MAS) is continuing to grow, and with improvements in imaging and instrumentation, it will mean that the range of surgical procedures performed will continue to expand.

To obtain adequate video-assisted pictures and surgical access, the relevant body cavity is insufflated with gas to expand that cavity's potential spaces. If this gas (usually carbon dioxide or nitrogen) is inadvertently introduced into the circulation, a 'gas embolism' occurs. If the embolus is large, acute cardiovascular collapse can occur. When operating on the bladder or uterus, fluid rather than gas is used to expand the organ cavity. If very large volumes of fluid are used, absorption into the circulation may lead to fluid overload and electrolyte imbalances (sometimes called the TUR syndrome).

Gynaecological surgery

Procedures such as laparoscopy (diagnostic), laparoscopic sterilization and laparoscopy-assisted hysterectomy are all commonly carried out. These can be short procedures, and IPPV with a short-acting muscle relaxant is the preferred method of anaesthesia.

Carbon dioxide is the insufflating gas used, accidental injection of which into the blood vessels or bowel can cause complications such as gas embolism, intestinal distension, bowel perforation and pneumothorax. The carbon dioxide is absorbed across the peritoneal membranes and into the gut and circulation; during operation, the extra carbon dioxide leads to an increased ventilation requirement, and post-operatively the carbon dioxide in the gut may cause colicky abdominal pain.

Urological surgery

Patients undergoing transurethral resection (TUR) of the prostate are often elderly and can be quite frail. In order to allow visualization for TUR, sterile glycine is used. Absorption of large volumes of glycine can cause complications such as hyponatraemia, hypokalaemia, haemolysis resulting in pulmonary oedema, cardiac failure, convulsions and arrhythmias (the TUR syndrome). The volume of fluid absorbed is proportional to the size of prostate, the duration of procedure and how high the bag of glycine solution is hung above the operative site.

Intraoperative signs of fluid overload include tachycardia, hypotension and hypoxaemia. Postoperatively, the patient may present with cardiac failure, cerebral irritability and convulsions. Treatment consists of controlling the convulsions with diazepam, using diuretics to encourage a high urine output and increasing the plasma sodium concentration by the careful use of saline.

General surgery

Laparoscopic cholecystectomy, hernia repair, appendicectomy and bowel resection are some of the procedures covered by MAS.

The insufflating gas is carbon dioxide. Higher volumes are needed for upper abdominal surgery than for gynaecological surgery. The duration of pneumoperitoneum is usually prolonged. Intra-abdominal pressures of 15 mmHg can compress the venous system in the abdomen, reducing venous return to the heart and causing a fall in blood pressure. The use of the reverse Trendelenburg position (for cholecystectomy) can further aggravate this fall in blood pressure.

Physiological changes and complications with laparoscopic cholecystectomy

- Injuries to the abdominal wall vessels and gastrointestinal viscera, perforation and tears of liver and spleen following blind insertion of the trocar.
- A fall in blood pressure as a result of decreased cardiac output (see above).
- A rise in $PaCO_2$ is seen after carbon dioxide insufflation, causing increased ventilation requirements.
- Carbon dioxide embolism.

Anaesthesia

General anaesthesia with IPPV is the method of choice.

Thoracic surgery

Thoracoscopy, sympathectomy and vagotomy are the procedures carried out by the thoracic surgeon with video assistance. One-lung anaesthesia for thoracoscopic surgery is made possible through clamping of the appropriate lumen of the double-lumen tube. The non-ventilated lung will collapse spontaneously, opening up the pleural space (i.e. no gas needs to be insufflated). Because blood will continue to flow through the collapsed, non-ventilated lung, hypoxaemia can occur. Increasing the percentage of inspired oxygen or adding PEEP can prevent this (see p. 157).

HYPOTENSIVE ANAESTHESIA

Induced hypotension is defined as the deliberate reduction of blood pressure to facilitate surgery. The indications for hypotensive anaesthesia are:

- microsurgery;
- major cancer surgery where a bloodless field allows clearance of the tumour;
- to lessen blood loss in patients who object to receiving blood transfusion (e.g. Jehovah's Witnesses).

The methods of inducing hypotension are:

- hyperventilation;
- elevating the body part being operated on, for example a head-up tilt for head or neck surgery;
- higher than usual inspired concentrations of the inhalational agent;
- the use of drugs such as labetalol (Trandate), phentolamine (Rogitine), hydralazine (Apresoline), sodium nitroprusside (Nipride) and glyceryl trinitrate.

When induced hypotension is used, intra-arterial blood pressure monitoring is strongly recommended.

At the end of the surgical procedure, the blood pressure may still be low, so it is essential to keep the patient in the recovery room until the blood pressure returns to its preoperative level.

ANAESTHESIA IN PATIENTS WITH CONCURRENT DISEASE

HAEMATOLOGY

Sickle-cell anaemia and sickle-cell trait

A haemolytic anaemia that is inherited and transmitted by both sexes, this is seen in patients of West Indian or African origin and sometimes in Greeks. HbS (sickle haemoglobin) will tend to deform (sickle) and destroy the red blood cells if the patient becomes cold, acidotic, hypoxic or dehydrated. This is more common and more severe in sickle-cell anaemia than in sickle-cell trait. This is because, in sickle-cell anaemia, 90% of the haemoglobin is of S type and the patients are typed as homozygotes (SS). In sickle-cell trait, 60–70% of the patient's haemoglobin is the usual HbA and only 30–40% the abnormal HbS.

During anaesthesia, body temperature, hydration (i.v. fluids) and oxygenation is maintained. Postoperatively, oxygen therapy (35% by face mask) is continued.

Haemophilia

This is a sex-linked, recessive disorder. Females are carriers and males sufferers. It results from the deficiency of clotting factor VIII, which can lead to intra- and postoperative bleeding.

Before surgery, factor VIII is corrected using fresh frozen plasma, factor VIII concentrate or cryoprecipitate. Close cooperation with the haematologist is essential. Many haemophiliac patients have received multiple blood product transfusions during their lives, and some have been unlucky enough to become HIV- or hepatitis-positive as a result (see p. 95).

ENDOCRINE SYSTEM

Diabetes

This is a disease that affects the β-cells of the pancreas (see p. 36), altering the metabolism of fat and sugar. The resultant rise in blood sugar can eventually lead to peripheral vascular disease, retinopathy (eyes), nephropathy (kidneys) and neuropathy (nerves). Diabetics are treated either by diet, oral hypoglycaemic agents or insulin (see p. 71).

Preoperatively, if the patient is taking chlorpropamide (Diabinese), the drug is stopped the day before surgery. Other oral hypoglycaemics are stopped on the day of surgery. If the patient is on a mixture of insulins, the treatment is aimed at controlling blood sugar by using soluble insulin on a sliding scale.

If the patient is a poorly controlled diabetic, elective surgery is postponed until the blood sugar has been controlled.

Steroid therapy

The adrenocortical reserve is diminished in Addison's disease, following bilateral adrenalectomy, during steroid therapy and when a patient has received regular steroids for the past 6 months to 1 year. If such a patient is scheduled for surgery, hydrocortisone 100 g is given i.v. at the induction of anaesthesia. Steroids are continued for a variable period of time postoperatively, depending on the severity of surgery.

Carcinoid tumours

These arise from argentaffin cells of the gastro-intestinal tract. Very rarely, these tumours are malignant and produce hormones such as serotonin (5-hydroxytryptamine), histamine, and bradykinin.

Problems encountered in these patients depend on the hormone secreted, but classically include:

- skin flushing,
- episodes of tachycardia and/or hypertension,
- hypotension,
- bronchospasm,
- diarrhoea.

Preoperative preparation includes:

1. fluids;
2. H_1 (e.g. Piriton) and H_2 (e.g. ranitidine) antagonists;

3. steroids;
4. bronchodilators (e.g. aminophylline);
5. serotonin antagonists (e.g. ketanserin or cyproheptadine);
6. avoidance of indirect vasopressors;
7. vasodilator drugs immediately available.

Aprotinin (Trasylol) and steroids can be used. Central venous access and invasive blood pressure monitoring are used, as well as standard monitors.

CARDIOVASCULAR DISEASE

Anaesthesia in patients with cardiovascular disease may be hazardous.

Heart failure

These patients are at serious risk. Preoperatively, the heart failure is corrected using digitalis, diuretics and inotropes. Most anaesthesic agents make the cardiac failure worse, whereas opiates are well tolerated by the patient.

If the operation is an emergency, the patient is preoxygenated and induction agents such as etomidate or methohexitone are used. Analgesics such as alfentanil or morphine are well tolerated. The fluid balance is carefully monitored using CVP and hourly urine volume measurements (the patient must be catheterized for the latter to be accurate). These patients benefit from elective admission to the intensive care unit post operatively.

Hypertension

If the patient is an undiagnosed hypertensive, elective operation is postponed until the blood pressure is controlled. Tracheal intubation or pain can raise the blood pressure, which can be controlled using alfentanil or fentanyl during intubation and any analgesic for pain relief.

Myocardial infarction and coronary artery disease

Patients who suffer from coronary artery disease continue their heart medications as usual before surgery. Standard monitoring is applied. If the patient is very symptomatic or the surgery major, invasive blood pressure monitoring, CVP monitoring and intensive care may be necessary.

Operations within 3 months of a myocardial infarction carry a high risk of reinfarction in the perioperative (i.e. during or after surgery) period. Thoracic and upper abdominal operations carry an especially high risk.

Presence of a pacemaker

Pacemakers can be disabled or otherwise interfered with by diathermy. If diathermy must be used, it should be of the bipolar type, used in short bursts only and kept well away from the pacing system. Back-up pacing or isoprenaline should be readily available.

Heart block

This can occur due to ischaemic heart disease or previous cardiac surgery. Patients with complete heart block are usually paced (see above).

Partial heart block can proceed to complete block under general anaesthesia, so isoprenaline or temporary pacing facilities should be available in theatre.

MUSCULOSKELETAL DISEASE
Myasthenia gravis

This is a chronic disease, possibly an autoimmune reaction. Muscles all over the body are affected, which can give rise to ptosis, easy fatiguability of the muscles, weak cough, respiratory muscle weakness and dysphagia.

Myasthenia gravis is due to a reduction in the number of acetylcholine receptors at the neuromuscular junction. Its treatment consists of administration of the anticholinesterase pyridostigmine (Mestinon) and prednisolone. If a patient is scheduled for an operation, anticholinesterases are stopped on the day of surgery. If general anaesthesia is to be administered, muscle relaxants are used in very small doses, if at all. The patient is resistant to the action of suxamethonium and sensitive to all the non-depolarizing muscle relaxants. Regional techniques such as epidural or spinal blocks are suitable for surgery on the lower half of the body. The patients are transferred to intensive care for either monitoring or ventilation in the postoperative period.

Rheumatoid arthritis

This is an autoimmune disorder that occurs at any age. The difficulties arise from:

- deformity of the cervical vertebrae and temporomandibular joint, making laryngoscopy difficult;
- destruction of bone by the disease, which may make the neck unstable: extending the head at laryngoscopy can break the patient's neck;
- involvement of small joints of the larynx;
- involvement of the heart and liver;
- possible steroid therapy (see p. 195).

If a difficult intubation is anticipated, precautions are taken (p. 165) regarding management. If neck X-rays show the neck to be unstable, awake intubation, a neck collar or in-line neck traction may be necessary.

Ankylosing spondylitis

Stiffness of the cervical spine and the atlanto-occipital joint can cause difficulty during intubation.

OBESITY

Obesity is almost always due to overeating. The problems encountered in obese patients are as follows:

1. *Respiratory system*. There is decreased vital capacity and functional residual capacity, and an increase in closing volume. Some parts of the lung are underventilated, causing shunting and hypoxia. Postoperative chest complications are common.

2. *Cardiovascular system*. Hypertension, coronary artery disease and postoperative thrombosis are common. Total blood volume and cardiac work are increased.

Technically, obese patients are difficult to lift and nurse. A short, thick neck can make intubation difficult. Regional anaesthesia such as epidural and spinal, while desirable, may be impossible to perform as bony landmarks are difficult to feel.

In the postoperative period, some of these patients may not breathe adequately and may need elective ventilation in the intensive therapy unit.

RESPIRATORY SYSTEM

In patients with chest disease, defects occur in gas transport, gas mixing and blood distribution.

Bronchitis

Patients who are labelled as 'chronic bronchitics' should have preoperative physiotherapy. These patients are especially prone to coughing, straining and bronchospasm during induction. Wherever possible, regional blocks are preferred, either as the sole technique or in combination with general anaesthesia. This will allow the patient to breathe and cough adequately post-operatively without much pain. Some patients may nevertheless require ventilation in the intensive therapy unit.

Asthma

Preoperatively, patients should receive physio-therapy and their usual bronchodilators. Agents that provoke bronchospasm (e.g. thiopentone, d-tubocurarine, morphine and pethidine) are avoided. In experienced hands, i.v. induction with thiopentone is uneventful. If bronchospasm develops after induction, the patient is treated with aminophylline 5 mg/kg (approximately 250–500 mg) given slowly i.v.; hydrocortisone 100–200 mg i.v. may also be given.

RARE DISEASES THAT CAN CAUSE PROBLEMS DURING ANAESTHESIA

Condition	Difficulties
Achondroplasia	Difficult intubation
Acromegaly	Diabetes, difficult airway and intubation
Alcoholism, chronic	Resistance to anaesthetics, and delirium tremens (withdrawal crisis). Acutely intoxicated patients require lower doses of induction and maintenance agents as alcohol is a sedative. By definition, these acutely intoxicated patients will have a full stomach
Myotonus	• Characterized by the inability of skeletal muscle to relax after contracting • Can be exacerbated by cold, anticholinesterases (e.g. neostigmine) and suxamethonium • Breathing and swallowing can both be affected (respiratory failure and aspiration pneumonia) • The heart can be affected • Avoid cold and suxamethonium • Sensitive to non-depolarizing muscle blockers
Burns	• Hypovolaemia, shock • Problems with intubation (sometimes) • Hyperkalaemia following use of suxamethonium • Difficult venous access • Clotting abnormalities
Choanal atresia	Nasal obstruction in the newborn. Treated initially by oral intubation and definitively by surgery
Conn syndrome	Hypokalaemia, hypertension and oedema
Cushing's syndrome	• Hypertension, diabetes and hypokalaemia • Delicate skin
Cystic fibrosis	• Chronic lung infection. Abnormal salt loss in sweat • Bleeding tendency secondary to poor intestinal fat absorption (vitamin K, is a fat-soluble vitamin involved in blood clotting) • Atropine avoided because its effect on lung secretions can worsen the patient's chest problems (as dry phlegm is much harder to clear by coughing)
Down's syndrome (mongolism)	• Small mouth and large tongue can make intubation difficult • Heart abnormalities common • Unusually sensitive to atropine
Klippel–Feil syndrome	Difficult intubation due to congenital fusion of cervical vertebrae
Marfan's syndrome	Cataracts, high arched palate (making intubation difficult), aortic and mitral regurgitation, kyphoscoliosis
Neurofibromatosis	Difficulty in intubation due to fibromas in larynx
Pharyngeal pouch	Regurgitation of pouch contents not prevented by cricoid pressure

Porphyria | Porphyric crises (muscle weakness, pain and wildly variable blood pressure are precipitated by barbiturates, etomidate, ketamine, benzodiazepines and dehydration. 'Safe' drugs include most opioids, inhalational agents, muscle blockers and their reversing agents

Scleroderma
- Difficulty in intubation owing to restricted mouth opening, difficult veins
- Regurgitation risk
- Respiratory failure
- Renal failure

Thalassaemia | Haemolytic anaemias

COMPLICATIONS AND ACCIDENTS DURING ANAESTHESIA

Deaths associated with anaesthesia make up about 2% of overall surgical deaths, the causes being:

1. a poor preoperative medical condition;
2. failed endotracheal intubation;
3. anaphylaxis;
4. negligence or inexperience;
5. a combination of anaesthetic and surgical factors.

The complications of anaesthesia can be described as follows.

CARDIOVASCULAR SYSTEM

- Shock.
- Cardiac arrest (see p. 245).
- Cardiac dysrhythmias. The following dysrhythmias are commonly seen:
  - bradycardia: responds to glycopyrronium 0.2 mg or atropine 0.1–0.3 mg;
  - sinus tachycardia, which responds to adequate analgesia and anaesthesia and to fluid and blood replacement;
  - atrial or ventricular extrasystoles, which occur in the presence of high carbon dioxide levels. Increasing the minute ventilation and decreasing the concentration of inhalation agents will correct this;
  - supraventricular or ventricular tachycardia;
  - nodal rhythm.
- Hypertension in the recovery area, which could be due to pain, raised carbon dioxide levels, a full bladder, the patient usually being hypertensive, and emergence delirium (e.g. ketamine anaesthesia).
- Gas embolism. Gas or air can (in some special circumstances) be sucked or accidentally injected into open blood vessels or i.v. lines. If the volume of gas is large enough, cardiac arrest may occur. (See the sections on laparoscopic surgery and neurosurgery.)

RESPIRATORY SYSTEM

During anaesthesia

Obstruction.

1. Obstruction by the lips or by the tongue. The jaw is lifted forwards and upwards (see p. 246), or an oropharyngeal (Guedel) or nasopharyngeal airway is used.

2. Obstruction above the glottis. This could be due to a tooth, a foreign body, vomitus or blood. Treatment consists of suction and lifting the jaw. If suction is not available, the 'finger sweep' (see CPR) is used.

3. Obstruction at the glottis. This could be due to laryngeal spasm or foreign body impaction (e.g. teeth or vomitus); treatment is suction, or paralysis and intubation.

4. Bronchospasm. This could be due to irritant agents (enflurane, thiopentone or atracurium), an anaphylactic reaction or intrinsic asthma. The treatment of asthma consists of aminophylline 250 mg i.v. or salbutamol 2–4 µg/kg slowly i.v. In anaphylaxis, the drug of choice is i.v. adrenaline (see CPR).

5. Faulty apparatus, such as kinking of the endotracheal tube or an impacted foreign body (vomitus or sputum) in the endotracheal tube.

Coughing. Coughing occurs in patients who are not sufficiently anaesthetized by i.v. or inhalational agent and is especially likely in smokers.

Hiccup. This is due to intermittent spasm of the diaphragm, followed by a sudden closure of the glottis. It is seen during surgery around the oesophagus and around the stomach when the phrenic nerve (which supplies the diaphragm) is stimulated. It can also occur spontaneously. Treatment consists of:

- deepening the anaesthesia;
- metoclopramide (Maxolon) 5–10 mg i.v.;
- tickling the nasopharynx with a nasogastric tube.

Sweating. This is usually noticed on the face and forehead. It could be that the patient is hot, too lightly anaesthetized, in shock or underventilated. Treatment consists of deepening the anaesthesia, increasing the ventilation or treating the shock.

Complications and accidents after anaesthesia

Pneumothorax. Surgeons can accidentally open the pleura during rib resection or nephrectomy. Treatment of a pneumothorax consists of inserting a chest drain with underwater seal drainage. The most common anaesthetic cause of pneumothorax is puncture of the pleura during central venous cannulation. Very high airway pressures during ventilation may be either the cause or the result of a pneumothorax.

Hypoxaemia. All patients undergoing anaesthesia experience a fall in their functional residual capacity, a mismatch of ventilation–perfusion and shunt. These will tend to cause hypoxaemia, the severity of which depends very much on the age of the patient, the site and duration of the operation and the patient's preoperative health. The very young and the very old, those with preoperative chest problems and those having operations lasting longer than 1 hour or operations on the upper abdomen or chest will be especially at risk. Postoperative oxygen therapy is standard.

Sputum retention. Some patients may not be able to cough sputum up effectively owing to pain, sedatives or reduced movements of the diaphragm secondary to abdominal distension. This can lead to sputum retention and atelectasis (collapse) of the lung. Treatment consists in the first instance of physiotherapy. Minitracheostomy (Fig. 6.32) or intubation and ventilation may ultimately be necessary.

Acid aspiration/chemical pneumonitis (Mendelson's syndrome): The lung is normally protected from inadvertent aspiration of food or stomach contents by the intact cough or gag mechanism of the larynx. During anaesthesia and sedation, these protective mechanisms are impaired. The patient under general anaesthesia is therefore at risk of the active vomiting (a muscular and violent reflex) or regurgitation (passive and often silent) of stomach contents via the oesophagus, into the pharynx and down through the larynx into the trachea and lungs.

Stomach contents damage the lungs by several mechanisms:

1. Solids may physically obstruct the airway, trachea or bronchi.

2. The volume aspirated may be enough to cause 'drowning'.

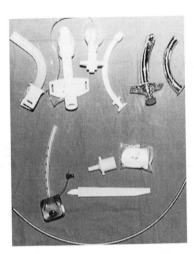

Figure 6.32 Tracheostomy tubes. Top row: plastic tracheostomy tubes with introducer and metal tracheostomy tube. Bottom row: mini tracheostomy set.

3. The acidity of the stomach contents may damage the respiratory mucosa, causing a chemical pneumonitis (especially if the pH is less than 2.5).

Evidence of aspiration:

- Tachypnoea in the spontaneously breathing patient.
- Hypoxaemia and cyanosis.
- Suspicious endotracheal aspirates.
- Soiling of the trachea evident at laryngoscopy.
- Rhonchi on auscultation.
- Abnormal chest X-ray.

Treatment consists of oxygen therapy, antibiotics, physiotherapy and intensive care.

VOMITING AND REGURGITATION

The problem of aspiration of gastric contents into the lungs is always present during induction and maintenance and immediately after anaesthesia. The risk is increased in those patients with a full stomach, abnormal gastrointestinal function, raised intra-abdominal pressure (e.g. pregnancy or laparoscopy) or impaired gastro-oesophageal sphincter function (e.g. hiatus hernia).

Prevention

Metoclopramide (Maxolon) 10 mg i.m. speeds the emptying of the stomach. Cimetidine (Tagamet) 300 mg i.v. or ranitidine (Zantac) 50 mg i.v. 1–2 hours before the induction of anaesthesia increases the pH of the gastric juice and decreases its volume. A dose of 400 mg cimetidine or 150 mg ranitidine orally has the same effect. Sodium citrate 0.3M solution 15–30 ml orally reduces the danger of aspiration. Sodium citrate is a non-particulate antacid and is therefore less likely than other antacids to cause pneumonitis if aspirated.

Management

In emergency surgery, patients either have not been fasted (i.e. they have full stomachs) or have intra-abdominal problems causing delayed gastric emptying (i.e. have full stomachs!). To decrease the risk of aspiration:

1. A large-bore nasogastric tube can be passed (effective in emptying the stomach only of liquids).
2. A stomach tube (12FG) is passed and solid food material aspirated.
3. Preoxygenation and rapid-sequence induction with cricoid pressure is carried out.
4. An endotracheal tube (cuffed in adults, uncuffed in children) is passed.

If vomiting occurs:

1. the patient is turned on one side or tilted head downwards, thus preventing the contamination of the air passages;
2. suction of the oropharyngeal region is carried out;
3. cricoid pressure is released as vomiting is active and can otherwise lead to oesophageal rupture.

If aspiration occurs:

1. suction of the trachea, followed by bronchoscopic suction and lavage, is carried out;
2. IPPV, antibiotics and bronchodilators are given in the intensive therapy unit.

NEUROLOGICAL COMPLICATIONS

Convulsions. These can be seen in patients in whom a toxic reaction occurs to ether or local anaesthetics. Treatment consists of i.v. thiopentone and oxygenation.

Hyperventilation to low levels of Pa_{CO_2} will lower the brain threshold for seizures. Therefore, while it is important to provide high levels of oxygenation, hyperventilation should be avoided.

Tremors and muscle movements. These are seen following the injection of induction agents such as methohexitone (Brietal), etomidate (Hypnomidate) and propofol (Diprivan).

Shivering. Shivering occurs after epidural, spinal and general anaesthesia. It is thought to be due to some anaesthetic effect on the hypothalamic temperature centre. It is sometimes called the 'halothane shake' although it is just as common with other anaesthetics. Pethidine 20 mg i.v. will temporarily reduce the shivering.

Delayed recovery from anaesthesia. This may be due to:

- overdose of narcotic analgesics, volatile agents or infusion of propofol;
- induced hypotension (see p. 194), hyperventilation during anaesthesia or acid–base imbalance (acidosis);
- fat embolism, air embolism and shock;
- diseases of the patient, for example hypoglycaemia, hyperglycaemia with ketosis, cerebrovascular accident (stroke) and myocardial infarction;
- overdosage of atropine (central anticholinergic syndrome). This is extremely rare and treated with physostigmine (Eserine) 1–2 mg i.v.

Peripheral nerve injuries. These injuries occur due to malposition (stretching and compression of the nerve), accidental injection of drugs directly into the nerve, use of excessive pressure in the tourniquets or leaving the tourniquet on for longer than 3 hours. Nerves can also be cut or damaged by the surgeon.

1. The brachial plexus can be stretched by (a) abduction of the arms above the head with the patient supine, (b) suspension of the arm from a bar when the patient is in the lateral position, or (c) abduction, external rotation and dorsal extension of the arm. It can be compressed against the shoulder braces that are sometimes used in the Trendelenburg position.

Stretching of the brachial plexus can be avoided by an arm board covered with pads, prevention of hyperextension and external rotation of the elbow, and padding the shoulder braces.

2. The ulnar nerve can be damaged at the elbow if the nerve is compressed against the medial epicondyle of the humerus. The elbows should always be well padded.

3. The median nerve can be damaged if i.v. injection of drugs occurs around the median nerve in the antecubital fossa.

4. The radial nerve can be damaged if the arm sags over the side of the table or is compressed against a vertical screen support.

5. The supraorbital nerve can be compressed by a metal endotracheal connector or a tight head harness.

6. The facial nerve can be damaged by firm compression between the fingers and the mandible while holding a face mask.

7. The common popliteal nerve can be damaged as a result of compression between the head of the fibula and the lithotomy pole. Damage results in foot drop. Along with ulnar nerve injury, this is the most common nerve injury in theatre.

8. The femoral nerve can be damaged by the use of a self-retaining retractor during lower abdominal surgery, or excessive angulation of the thigh when the patient is in the lithotomy position.

Other neurological complications

Postoperative headache. This occurs in 40% of all patients after general anaesthesia and in 80% of those patients who describe themselves as prone to developing headaches.

Headache is a recognized complication of dural membrane puncture (see p. 175). The dura is punctured deliberately during the performance of a spinal anaesthetic, but it can be accidentally punctured during an epidural (dural tap). The headache is classically worse on standing up and better when lying down. It is now common when large needles are used and is thought to be due to leak of CSF through the dural hole.

Extrapyramidal effect. Drugs such as phenothiazines, droperidol and metoclopramide (Maxolon) in large doses can cause involuntary movements. Treatment consists of procyclidine (Kemdarin) 10 mg i.v.

Awareness is defined as the ability of the patient to recall intraoperative events. The unparalysed patient may move during the surgery, thus warning the anaesthetist that the level of anaesthesia is too light. The paralysed patient is unable to move, and the anaesthetist must rely on the observation of clinical signs (heart rate, sweating, crying, pupil size and blood pressure) and his or her knowledge of pharmacology and dosages to estimate the level of anaesthesia. Even so, unless a volatile inhalational agent in a suitable concentration is added to the basic oxygen/nitrous oxide/opiate anaesthetic, as many as 1% of patients may be aware. The risk of awareness is highest in emergency caesarean section (no premedication and a light anaesthetic until the delivery of the baby) and trauma surgery (a light anaesthetic until the blood pressure is stable).

There are also several periods during the course of anaesthesia when the risk of awareness is high:

1. Intubation, especially rapid-sequence intubation, because the patient is not ventilated, i.e. receives no inhalational agent, until after the airway is secured with an endotracheal tube.

2. On emergence. It is probably preferable to reverse the muscle relaxant before stopping the nitrous oxide and volatile agent as there are reports of patients inadequately reversed but well aware of the closing events of their surgery.

Even if the patient is not in pain, awareness is a truly horrible experience, for which many victims require expert counselling.

POSTURE OF THE PATIENT

The problems that various positions of the patient can cause and their prevention are described below.

Supine. Pressure and stretching of the nerves of the arm can be avoided by:

- the arms being well tucked under the buttock, palm down with the wrists held by a plastic T-shaped splint;
- wrist straps firmly attached to a broad strap surrounding the table;
- neck, knees and hips being slightly flexed;
- legs being placed flat on the table and not crossed one over the other.

Prone. A pillow is placed under each shoulder and another under the pelvis to allow free breathing and to remove pressure from the abdomen. Obese patients do not tolerate this position well.

Trendelenburg. In short, fat patients steep Trendelenburg's position can cause cyanosis and dyspnoea. Prolonged head-down tilt can cause retinal detachment and cerebral oedema.

Lateral. This position makes the patient's breathing difficult, so IPPV is used.

Lithotomy. If this position is required, both legs are moved together to prevent strain on the pelvic ligaments. The knee should be outside the padded supports.

Effects of posture on various systems

Blood pressure. A head-up tilt can cause a fall in blood pressure (hypotension); this position is helpful for inducing hypotension in middle ear surgery. Other procedures that cause a fall in blood pressure are the handling and traction of the abdominal viscera, and when the table 'break' is applied for the exposure of a kidney.

Respiration. Ventilation is decreased to a large extent in the prone, jack-knife and Trendelenburg's positions, and a slight decrease occurs in the reverse Trendelenburg or lateral position.

Head and neck position. Where possible, the head should be left in a neutral position. Rotating the head to the left or right can cause stretching of the opposite side's brachial plexus (nerve injury), poor venous drainage from the head or decreased blood supply to the head (if the internal jugular vein or carotid artery is compressed).

Moving a patient. All anaesthetized patients must be moved smoothly and gently. If a canvas stretcher is not available, at least three or four members of staff should lift the patient. Moving the unconscious, anaesthetized patient is always coordinated by the person who has control of the patient's head and airway. It is necessary to ensure that no drains or i.v. lines will be left behind when the patient is moved. During recovery from anaesthesia, the patient is placed in the lateral or semi-prone position until his protective reflexes return. This helps in monitoring a free airway and prevents the aspiration of vomited material into the airway.

UROLOGICAL COMPLICATIONS

Failure to pass urine

A number of patients fail to pass adequate amounts of urine (oliguria) in the first 24 hours postoperatively. The pathological causes of oliguria are:

- prerenal – hypotension, haemorrhage and hypovolaemia;
- renal – damage to the kidneys from bacterial toxins, mismatched blood transfusion or drugs;
- postrenal – ligation of the ureter during pelvic operations (e.g. hysterectomy) and bladder neck obstruction (most often in prostatism).

Difficulty in passing urine

This occurs in about 10–15% of cases after general anaesthesia. It occurs:

- in anxious patients and those with an enlarged prostate;
- after abdominal and pelvic operations, for example haemorrhoidectomy;
- in deeply sedated patients.

Treatment consists of encouraging the patient to micturate by allowing him or her to sit up; if this fails, catheterization is carried out.

LIVER FAILURE

This can occur in the postoperative period from a number of anaesthetic and non-anaesthetic causes. Some of them are:

- drugs, including inhalational agents
- hypoxia
- blood transfusion
- hypotension
- viral hepatitis.

Patients may become sick enough to require intensive care, but there are very few curative treatments available for liver failure. The exception is jaundice as a result of gallstones, as these can be removed by surgery.

MALIGNANT HYPERPYREXIA

Malignant hyperpyrexia is a very rare inherited disease that is completely asymptomatic until triggered by anaesthetic drugs. Once triggered, the body temperature rises by 1–2°C every 5 minutes. This disease is inherited as an autosomal dominant, and is characterized by:

- cyanosis
- muscle rigidity (unrelieved by muscle relaxants)
- hyperventilation
- hypercarbia
- dysrhythmias
- acidosis
- rising body temperature
- hypertension.

Causes. Drugs such as anaesthetic agents (halothane or suxamethonium), lignocaine and tricyclic antidepressants and phenothiazines can trigger the reaction. It occurs in 1 in 100 000 adult anaesthetics and 1 in 14 000 child anaesthetics. It is associated with a mortality rate of 10–50%.

Predisposing conditions. Patients who suffer from osteogenesis imperfecta, congenital ptosis, hernias, kyphoscoliosis and cleft palate may also have inherited malignant hyperpyrexia.

Biochemical changes. Calcium is released in excess in the muscle, which in turn produces uncontrolled muscle spasm. The biochemical changes that follow lead to hypoxia, hypercarbia, hyperkalaemia, respiratory and metabolic acidosis, and disseminated intravascular coagulation.

Diagnosis. Malignant hypertension is suspected when the patient fails to relax following suxamethonium. Because the temperature is not routinely monitored during anaesthesia, cyanosis or very high ventilation requirements may be the next obvious warning sign to develop.

Management of malignant hyperpyrexia:

1. Stop the inhaled volatile agent. Do not use suxamethonium. Change the anaesthetic tubing, and do not use a circle system.
2. Hyperventilate with 100% oxygen.
3. Administer dantrolene (Dantrium) 2 mg/kg i.v., repeating the dose to a maximum of 10 mg/kg based on the Pa_{CO_2}, heart rate and body temperature.
4. Treat acidosis with sodium bicarbonate.
5. Control the body temperature (by ice, cold saline, a cooling blanket, and gastric or peritoneal lavage) until it reaches 38°C.
6. Monitor capnography and arterial blood gases, urine output, temperature and plasma potassium level.
7. Be prepared to treat hyperkalaemia and cardiac dysrhythmias.
8. The half-life of dantrolene is 4 hours, so admit the patient to the intensive therapy unit, continue monitoring and repeat the dantrolene dose as required.

Dantrolene is the only specific (curative) treatment available for malignant hyperpyrexia. All hospitals where general anaesthesia is provided must carry a stock. It is stored as a dry powder and, during treatment of an emergency, one person may need to be devoted full time to making it up.

Management for future operations. Preoperatively, oral dantrolene is given as 4 mg/kg 4 hourly. A vapourizer-free anaesthetic machine with new hoses is used. Anaesthetic agents such as thiopentone, opiates, non-depolarizing relaxants and nitrous oxide are safe. Local anaesthetics and regional techniques are also safe.

OTHER COMPLICATIONS

1. Corneal abrasions when the eyes are not taped during operations and the cornea is exposed.

2. If the operating theatre temperature falls below 21°C, the patient develops postoperative shivering and increased oxygen consumption, although postanaesthetic shivering can occur even if the theatre is warm.
3. Minor complications such as trauma to lips and backache resulting from the lithotomy position.

ANAESTHESIA FOR EMERGENCIES

Patients presenting for emergency anaesthesia are not fasted, and may have uncontrolled medical illness, uncertain diagnosis, and metabolic and cardiovascular imbalance. It is essential that they should be adequately assessed, prepared and presented for surgery. Anaesthetic management consists of preoperative assessment and preparation, intraoperative management and postoperative management.

The time available for preoperative preparation will be determined by the urgency of the surgical condition.

PREOPERATIVE ASSESSMENT AND PREPARATION

Assessment

As discussed earlier (see p. 145), a relevant past medical and drug history is taken. An enquiry is made about the patient's cardiopulmonary reserve, for example breathlessness on exertion, orthopnoea, angina and productive cough. A quick physical examination is carried out, including assessment of the airway. Laboratory investigations are reviewed and, if necessary, corrections made (e.g. hypokalaemia corrected with potassium supplements).

The major problems in emergency anaesthesia are: volaemic status, full stomach.

Volaemic status

It is essential to assess the degree of dehydration and hypovolaemia (e.g. trauma patients and patients with bowel obstruction and perforated duodenal ulcer) before the induction of anaesthesia (see p. 159).

Hypovolaemia. Blood loss (intravascular volume deficit) can be estimated from the history, measured losses, heart rate, pulse pressure, peripheral circulation, CVP pressure and urine output. Signs of severe hypovolaemia become clear (low blood pressure and tachycardia) when the blood volume is decreased by 15–20%.

Dehydration. Fluid loss (extracellular volume deficit) is difficult to assess. A rough estimation can be made, based on the time of inadequate water intake, vomiting and duration of intestinal obstruction. For convenience sake, the fluid loss can be estimated, as shown in Table 6.12. The signs and symptoms in Table 6.12 act as guidelines and, based on these, the patient is resuscitated using blood or blood substitutes for haemorrhage and normal saline (0.9%) or Hartmann's solution for dehydration.

Full stomach

The vomiting or regurgitation of gastric contents, followed by their aspiration into the tracheobronchial tree when protective laryngeal reflexes are absent, is a major disaster that can occur during general anaesthesia or when the patient is unconscious for other reasons (injury, alcohol or drugs). Vomiting occurs during light planes of anaesthesia (during induction or recovery from anaesthesia). Regurgitation is a passive process that can occur at any time and is not seen by the anaesthetist. Aspiration of gastric contents is followed by either minor chest infection or severe aspiration pneumonia.

During an elective surgical list, patients are adequately starved (for at least 6 hours), but in an emergency (e.g. ectopic pregnancy, ruptured aortic aneurysm or caesarean section) it might be essential to induce anaesthesia urgently, regardless of whether or not the stomach is empty. Moreover, the patient's surgical condition (e.g. pain following fractures, intestinal

Table 6.11   Signs of blood loss

Severity	Mild	Moderate	Severe
Percentage blood volume lost	20%	30%	40%
Approximate blood lost	1000 ml	1500 ml	Above 2000 ml
Arterial blood pressure (mmHg)	Orthostatic hypotension	Systolic below 100 mmHg	Systolic below 75 mmHg
Heart rate (beats/min)	100–110	120–140	Above 140
Urinary output (ml)	20–30	10–20	Nil
Peripheral circulation	Cold and pale	Cold and pale	Cold and clammy Peripheral cyanosis

Table 6.12   Signs and symptoms of fluid loss

Signs and symptoms of fluid loss	Amount of fluid lost (ml/70 kg body weight)	Percentage body weight lost as water
Thirst, dry tongue, decreased sweating and reduced skin elasticity	Above 2000 ml	Mild (above 4%)
Thirst, dry tongue, decreased sweating, decreased urine output, low CVP, high packed cell volume (haemoconcentration), hypotension, thready pulse, cold peripheries	Above 5000 ml	Moderate (above 7–8%)
All the above, plus coma, shock	Above 7000 ml	Severe (10–15%)

obstruction) can lead to delayed gastric emptying, and even 6 hours may not be enough time for the stomach to empty.

The factors determining the risk of gastric regurgitation are the rate of gastric emptying and the state of the lower oesophageal sphincter.

Gastric emptying

About 1–4% of the total gastric contents empty into the duodenum each minute owing to peristaltic waves. The factors that can affect gastric emptying are:

- Delayed gastric emptying:
  - Late pregnancy
  - Fear, pain, shock, anxiety
  - Sedation with opiates.
- Abnormal or absent peristalsis:
  - Peritonitis
  - Hypokalaemia or uraemia.
- Obstructed peristalsis:
  - Pyloric stenosis
  - Gastric cancer
  - Large or small bowel obstruction.

State of the lower oesophageal sphincter

The lower oesophageal sphincter (LOS) lies in the region of the cardia of the stomach; it opens during oesophageal peristalsis to allow food into the stomach. The LOS is the main barrier preventing the stomach contents flowing back into the oesophagus. 'Barrier pressure' is the difference between gastric pressure and LO pressure. Drugs such as prochlorperazine (Stemetil), anticholinesterases (neostigmine) and suxamethonium increase the barrier pressure. Drugs such as opiates, thiopentone, alcohol and atropine decrease the barrier pressure, thus increasing the tendency for gastro-oesophageal reflux.

Preparation

The preparation of a patient for emergency anaesthesia consists of resuscitation with fluids, blood and blood products (as necessary), and gastric emptying.

Gastric emptying

This is carried out by:

1. Insertion of a nasogastric tube and aspiration of gastric contents, which are liquid in nature (e.g. intestinal obstruction).

2. Insertion of a large-bore stomach tube for solid food recently eaten.

3. Neutralization of the pH of gastric contents using the non-particulate antacid 0.3M sodium citrate (30 ml). This will raise the pH of gastric contents above 2.5, and if gastric acid aspiration into the lungs does occur, the chemical damage to the lungs is less severe.

4. Decreasing the volume of gastric contents by using cimetidine (Tagamet), ranitidine (Zantac) or famotidine. Cimetidine can be given orally or i.m. (200–400 mg) and ranitidine orally (150 mg) or i.m. or i.v. (50 mg) 1–2 hours before operation.

5. The rate of gastric emptying can be increased by using metoclopramide (Maxolon) 10 mg i.m. or i.v., although this effect will be blocked by opioid drugs.

INTRAOPERATIVE MANAGEMENT

This can be discussed under the headings induction, maintenance, recovery and post-operative care. The anaesthetic machine is checked before starting anaesthesia, all drugs are drawn up into labelled syringes and the ventilator is adjusted to its proper settings. Required equipment should be checked.

Induction

As discussed earlier (see p. 145), the patient's airway is assessed for likely difficulties in performing endotracheal intubation. If the anaesthetist expects a difficult intubation, a senior anaesthetist's assistance is requested. Techniques such as awake intubation or intubation using a flexible fibreoptic laryngoscope may be necessary.

Rapid-sequence induction

This is the standard induction method for the patient at risk of aspiration (e.g. a full stomach or hiatus hernia). The patient is placed on a tipping trolley or table. The patient's head is placed in an ideal 'sniffing position' with the neck flexed on the shoulders and the head extended on the neck.

The anaesthetist is assisted by at least one skilled member of the operating theatre staff (ODP or anaesthetic nurse) to perform cricoid pressure or give an endotracheal tube, laryngoscope, etc. Before the induction of anaesthesia, heart rate and blood pressure are recorded, ECG electrodes are attached and monitoring commenced. The patient is given 100% oxygen by a face mask for 3–5 minutes before induction, and an i.v. infusion, using a large-bore cannula (14 gauge), is commenced.

The trained assistant stands on the patient's right side to apply cricoid pressure (Sellick's manoeuvre). The assistant identifies the cricoid cartilage, which lies below the thyroid cartilage. The thumb and the index finger of the right hand press the cricoid cartilage firmly backwards (posteriorly), thus compressing the oesophagus between the cricoid cartilage and the vertebral column. The cricoid cartilage forms a complete ring unlike the other cartilages of the trachea (Fig. 6.33). The patient is informed of the procedure of cricoid pressure. Some anaesthetists prefer to apply it before the i.v. injection of induction agent, while others apply it as soon as the patient loses consciousness.

With the assistant ready, the anaesthetist injects a predicted sleep dose of induction agent (e.g. thiopentone 3–5 mg/kg body weight or etomidate 0.2–0.3 mg/kg), followed rapidly by a paralysing dose of suxamethonium (1.5 mg/kg). The lungs are *not* ventilated during the short time between induction and successful intubation. As soon as the jaw relaxes, laryngoscopy and tracheal intubation are performed. Cricoid pressure is maintained by the assistant until the anaesthetist inflates the cuff, and is certain that the tube is in the trachea by auscultation of the lungs (Fig. 6.34) and that the cuff is forming an adequate seal. The cricoid pressure is released only on direct permission from the anaesthetist and not before. The endotracheal tube is then connected to the ventilator and IPPV com-

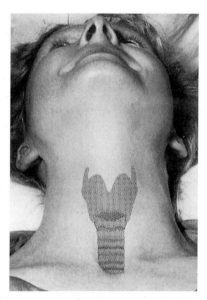

Figure 6.33 Neck region showing thyroid and cricoid cartilages. The thyroid cartilage is above and the cricoid just below.

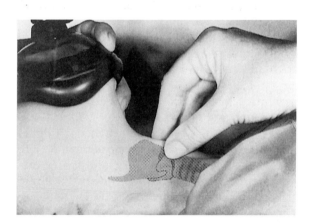

Figure 6.34 Application of cricoid pressure.

menced. The settings on the ventilator are 7–10 ml/kg body weight for tidal volume and 100 ml/kg/min for minute volume.

Awake intubation. Carried out in patients with anticipated difficulty in intubation (e.g. ankylosing spondylitis and dental abscess), the intubation can be either oral or nasal following the application of local anaesthetic to the nasal mucosa, pharynx and vocal cords (using local anaesthetic agents (see p. 165).

Fibreoptic intubation. This is carried out by an anaesthetist experienced in fibreoptic intubation, in patients for whom there is an anticipated difficulty in intubation. It should not be carried out by an inexperienced anaesthetist for the first time in an emergency. Inhalational induction is performed in patients with faciomaxillary injury or in a child with epiglottitis. Oxygen and halothane via a face mask are used for inhalational induction, and when the patient is deeply anaesthetized, endotracheal intubation is attempted. Fibreoptic intubation can also be performed in the awake patient under local anaesthesia.

Regional anaesthesia

Total i.v. regional anaesthesia (Bier's block) or brachial plexus block (interscalene or axillary approach) are used for orthopaedic procedures on the upper extremity (fracture reductions and repair of tendons).

For surgery on the lower extremity, spinal or epidural anaesthetics are employed. Spinal and epidural anaesthetics can cause profound hypotension in shocked patients or in those who have been inadequately fluid resuscitated.

Maintenance of anaesthesia

The patient is given a balanced anaesthesia consisting of Grey's triad of:

- anaesthesia
- analgesia
- muscle relaxation.

Anaesthesia. The patient is kept asleep with nitrous oxide 50–66% in oxygen and a suitable concentration of volatile inhalational agent.

Muscle relaxation. Once the patient recovers from suxamethonium, a non-depolarizing muscle relaxant such as atracurium (Tracrium) 0.45 to 0.6 mg/kg i.v. or vecuronium (Norcuron) 0.1 mg/kg is given. The longer-acting drugs are avoided in emergency surgery.

Analgesics. There are administered in small i.v. increments (e.g. fentanyl 25–200 µg, morphine 1–10 mg i.v., papaveretum 2–10 mg) until fluid and blood losses are corrected.

Monitoring

As described in an earlier section (see p. 166), all routine monitoring should be carried out. Specialist monitoring as indicated by the patient's preoperative condition or type of surgery may be necessary.

Fluid and blood therapy

Fluid balance in emergency situations is notoriously difficult to estimate. Fluid loss is corrected using Hartmann's solution; blood loss in excess of 15% blood volume in adults and 10% blood volume in children is corrected by blood transfusions. It should be remembered that these patients may be coming to theatre already having lost blood or fluid, and these losses need to be considered in addition to the intraoperative losses.

Reversal

1. At skin closure, reverse the muscle relaxant.
2. When the muscle relaxant is reversed (test with peripheral nerve stimulation) and the bandages are going on, turn off the volatile anaesthetic agent.

Pharyngoscopy is carried out to remove secretions and debris from the pharynx, and if a nasogastric tube was inserted, it is aspirated and left unspigoted.

Once respiratory activity returns and the patient is awake, he is turned onto one side (if possible), and, at the peak of inspiration, the cuff is deflated and the endotracheal tube removed. The tube is not taken out until the patient can maintain his own airway and has a gag reflex. This is because of the risk of regurgitation.

In the recovery room, the patient is given 35–40% oxygen by face mask.

POSTOPERATIVE PERIOD

Postoperatively, all patients who have undergone emergency operations are given oxygen therapy (see p. 235) and analgesics (see p. 231), and fluid therapy is written up (see p. 237). Certain patients who have undergone emergency surgery are transferred to the intensive therapy unit for elective ventilation. This includes patients with:

- extreme obesity
- prolonged period of shock
- septicaemia
- acid aspiration in the lungs
- severe lung or heart disease prior to surgery.

SPECIFIC CONDITIONS

Although the technique for emergency anaesthesia is standard, as mentioned above, certain surgical emergencies and their management are now described.

General surgery

Perforated peptic ulcer. The patient may be shocked, with a stomach likely to contain vomitable material. Before the patient arrives in the theatre, a nasogastric tube is inserted and the gastric contents emptied. Intravenous fluids are given in the form of Hartmann's solution or 0.9% normal saline.

Acute intestinal obstruction. The patient has a fluid and electrolyte imbalance, a full stomach and a distended abdomen. Intravenous fluids are given based on the degree of fluid loss (see p. 206), a nasogastric tube is passed, the stomach emptied and rapid-sequence induction employed.

Leaking/ruptured aortic aneurysm. The patient may be in shock and suffering from haematemesis (due to a leakage of the aneurysm into the duodenum). Large volumes of blood, given warmed and filtered, are needed for transfusion. The patient is anaesthetized in the operating theatre (rather than the anaesthetic room), with the surgeon scrubbed and standing by ready to operate and clamp the aorta. A rapid-sequence induction technique is used. Monitoring of arterial pressure (direct), CVP and urine output is essential.

Postoperatively, these patients are transferred to the intensive therapy unit for elective ventilation and further resuscitation.

Ear, nose and throat surgery

Post-tonsillectomy bleeding. This is an acute emergency. The patient may be in shock and is likely to have a stomach full of blood clot. Because the blood loss is not visible, estimated loss is assessed by the child's pallor, heart rate and blood pressure. An i.v. infusion is commenced. Blood is cross-matched and given when necessary.

Anaesthesia is induced with the patient on one side, head down, and the assistant applying cricoid pressure; some anaesthetists, however, prefer to have the patient lying supine. Once bleeding has been controlled, a gastric tube is passed to empty the stomach.

Gynaecology

Ectopic pregnancy. The patient may or may not be shocked. Surgery comprises ligation of the fallopian tube that is bleeding. Blood should be cross-matched, but some patients may need to go to theatre to control their bleeding before the cross-match is complete. In a life-threatening emergency, group O negative (so-called 'universal donor') blood may be given. Otherwise, fluids such as Haemaccel and Gelofusine are given to replace blood loss until the cross-matched blood is available.

Ophthalmic surgery

Perforating eye injury. Smooth anaesthesia is essential because of the danger of vitreous loss and blindness if intraocular pressure rises owing to coughing or straining. For intubation, suxamethonium is nowadays rarely used by the anaesthetist as it causes a transient rise in intraocular pressure. Vecuronium or atracurium are the muscle relaxants of choice. Intubation proceeds when the peripheral nerve stimulator indicates that muscle relaxation is complete.

FURTHER READING

Desflurane
Graham S G 1994 British Journal of Anaesthesia 72: 470–473
Weiskoff R B, Sampson D, Moore M A 1994 British Journal of Anaesthesia 72: 474–479

Laryngeal masks
Brain A I J 1991 The Intavent laryngeal mask instruction manual, 2nd edn. Intavent Intl SA, Henley-on-Thames
Maltby J R 1991 The laryngeal mask airway. Anesthesiology Review 18: 55–57
Mason D G, Bingham R M 1990 The LMA in children. Anaesthesia 45: 760–763
Pennant J H, White P F 1993 The LMA. Anesthesiology 79(1): 144–163
Tunstall M E 1989 Failed intubation in the parturient. Canadian Journal of Anaesthetics 36: 611–613 (Editorial)

Magnetic resonance imaging
Anaesthetic management for MRI 1992 Anesthesiology: 74: 121–128
Messick J M et al 1990 Anesthesia at remote locations. In: Miller R D (ed) Anesthesia. Churchill Livingstone, New York, pp 2061–2088
Rao C C et al 1988 Modification of an anesthesia machine for use during magnetic resonance imaging. Anesthesiology 68: 640

Minimal access surgery
Cunningham A J 1993 Laparoscopic cholecystectomy. Anesthetic implications. Anesthesia and Analgesia 76: 1120–1133
Hagstrom R S et al 1988 Studies in fluid absorption during transurethral prostate resection. Journal of Urology 73: 852
Holohan T V 1991 Lap cholecystectomy. Lancet 338: 801–803
Johannsen G et al 1989 The effect of general anaesthesia on the haemodynamic effects during laparoscopy with CO_2 insufflation. Acta Anaesthesiologica Scandinavica 33: 132
Rao M C 1992 Laser endoscopic sympathectomy for palmar hyperhydrosis. Lasers in Surgery and Medicine 12: 308

Anaesthesia for laser surgery
Department of Health 1984 Guidance on the safe use of lasers in medical practice. HMSO, London

Rampil I J 1992 Anaesthetic considerations for laser surgery. Anesthesia and Analgesia 74: 424–435

Ophthalmic anaesthesia
Hamilton R C 1995 Techniques of orbital regional anaesthesia. British Journal of Anaesthesia 75: 88–92
Hustead R F et al 1994 Periocular local anaesthesia: medial orbital as an alternative to superior nasal injection. Journal of Cataract and Refractive Surgery 20: 197–201
Rosen E 1993 Editorial Review: Anaesthesia for cataract surgery. European Journal of Implant and Refractive Surgery 5: 1–3

Autologous transfusion
Robertie P G, Gravlee G P 1990 Safe limits of isovolaemic hemodilution and recommendations for erythrocyte transfusion. International Anesthesiology Clinics, Vol 28: 197–204
Stehling L 1990 Autologous transfusion. International Anesthesiology Clinics 28(4): 190–194
Toy P T C Y, Strauss R G, Stehling L C 1987 Predeposited autologous blood for elective surgery: a national multicentre study. New England Journal of Medicine 316: 517–520

Anaesthesia
Aitkenhead A, Smith G 1996 Textbook of anaesthesia, 3rd edn. Churchill Livingstone, Edinburgh
Berry A J, Knos G B 1995 Anesthesiology. Williams & Wilkins, Baltimore
Davey A, Moyle J T B, Wards C S 1992 Ward's Anaesthetic Equipment, 3rd edn. W B Saunders, Philadelphia
Gaba D M 1994 Crisis management in anesthesiology. Churchill Livingstone, New York
Hall F A 1994 Minimal access surgery for nurses and technicians. Radcliffe Medical Press, Oxford
Scott D B 1989 Techniques of regional anaesthesia. Appleton & Lange, East Norwalk, CT
Mallampati S R, Gatt S P, Gugine L D 1985 A clinical sign to predict difficult tracheal intubation. A prospective study. Canadian Anaesthetic Society Journal 32: 429–434
Miller R D 1990 Anesthesia, 3rd edn. Churchill Livingstone, New York

7

Surgery

In this chapter, various incisions and suturing techniques used during surgery are listed, followed by brief descriptions of some important operations.

The patient is made optimally fit for the operation, particular attention being given to weight, nutrition, acid–base balance, anaemia, diabetes and pulmonary and cardiac disabilities.

One to one-and-a-half hours prior to surgery the patient is given a premedication (see p. 146); he is then anaesthetized (see p. 159), positioned and draped (see p. 136), and surgery is commenced.

PRINCIPLES OF SUTURING TECHNIQUE

The main types of suture (Fig. 7.1) are as follows:

1. *Simple sutures* (through-and-through). These are suitable for almost all wound closures. When applying them, it is important to invert one or both skin edges.

2. *Continuous sutures.* These are essentially similar to simple interrupted sutures, but care is taken to adjust the tension as it is very easy to make a continuous suture too tight. A continuous subcuticular suture of monofilament material gives a very neat scar.

3. *Vertical mattress sutures.* These are useful in parts of the body where the skin edges tend to invert. In this suture, the needle is passed through both skin edges twice.

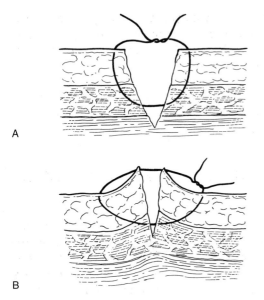

A

B

Figure 7.1 Sutures. (A) Through-and-through sutures for simple approximation. (B) Vertical mattress sutures for accurate edge-to-edge apposition.

ABDOMINAL INCISIONS

The principal abdominal incisions (Fig. 7.2) are as follows:

1. *Midline.* This is used for operations on the stomach, liver, spleen, lower bowel, uterus and rectum. The incision extends from below the xiphisternum to the umbilicus for high midline incisions, and from the umbilicus to the pubis for low midline incisions.

2. *Paramedian.* This is used to gain access to one side of the abdomen.

3. *Transverse.* This is not often used as there is a danger of damage to the nerves supplying the rectus muscle.

4. *Inguinal.* This incision is made for the repair of inguinal hernia.

5. *Pfannenstiel.* This incision is used in gynaecological operations.

6. *Subcostal.* On the right side, this incision is

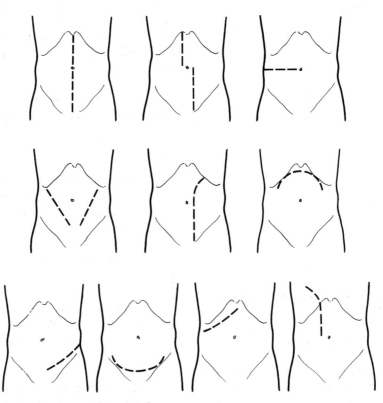

Figure 7.2 Abdominal incisions. *Top row:* midline, paramedian and transverse. *Middle row:* lumbar, hockey stick and inverted V. *Bottom row:* inguinal, Pfannenstiel, subcostal (Kocher) and abdominothoracic.

made to operate on the biliary tract, and on the left side, the stomach and spleen.

One other incision used is the Lanz incision for appendicectomy.

INSTRUMENTS

The instruments listed in Box 7.1 form the basis of a general set; they need to be arranged according to the kind of operation and the preference of the surgeon.

Box 7.1 A general set of instruments
Scalpel handles Nos 3, 4 with Nos 20 and 10 blades × 2
Dissecting forceps, toothed large (Bonney) × 2
Dissecting forceps, toothed small (Lane) × 2
Scissors, straight (Mayo) × 2
Scissors, small and large, curved on flat (Mayo)
Scissors, straight stitch
Artery forceps, straight (Moynihan) × 10
Artery forceps, curved on flat (Kelly, Dunhill) × 10
Photoclips for anchoring soiled dressing bag, diathermy leads or suction tubing, etc.
Artery forceps, straight 8 in (Spencer Wells) × 5
Probe, malleable silver
Curetting spoons, medium and large (Volkman) × 2
Sponge-holding forceps (Rampley) × 5
Sinus forceps
Needle holder, small (Kilner) × 2
Needle holder, large (Mayo) × 2
Towel clips × 5
Tissue forceps (Allis) × 5
Tissue forceps (Lane) × 5
Retractors, single hook, sharp and blunt × 2
Retractors, medium (Langenback) × 2
Retractors, large (Morris) × 2

GENERAL OPERATIONS

HEAD AND NECK SURGERY

Thyroidectomy or removal of thyroid adenoma: the partial or complete removal of the thyroid gland. The patient is placed supine with a sandbag under the shoulder blades and the neck extended.

Excision of thyroglossal duct or cyst: the removal of a congenital duct between the thyroid gland and the pharynx. The patient is placed as for thyroidectomy.

Excision of parotid tumour: the removal of a tumour in the parotid gland. The position is as for thyroid surgery.

EAR, NOSE AND THROAT SURGERY
Ear

Myringotomy. Acute otitis media is a common condition occurring in childhood, when the tympanic membrane may be perforated, releasing pus. This discharge is known as otorrhoea. Severe cases are treated by myringotomy, in which an incision is made in the tympanic membrane.

Mastoidectomy: the removal of diseased mastoid air cells. The mastoid air cells communicate with and are found posterior to the middle ear and are protected by the mastoid process of the temporal bone.

Tympanoplasty: repair of the eardrum by myringoplasty (a graft of temporal fascia).

Nose

Reduction of nasal fracture: realignment of the fractured nasal bones. If the fracture is less than 48 hours old, this is a simple 'push' under general anaesthetic.

Nasal polypectomy: the removal of the nasal polypi.

Submucous resection of the nasal septum: the removal of the deflected cartilaginous and bony parts of the nasal septum, which block the airway.

Radical antrostomy (Caldwell–Luc operation): making an opening in the antrum via the mouth, leaving a large antrostomy into the nose.

Mouth and throat

Tonsillectomy and adenoidectomy: the removal of the tonsils by either dissection or guillotine, and curetting the adenoids. The patient is placed supine with head and neck extended, and a Boyle Davis gag is used.

Direct laryngoscopy: the direct examination of the larynx with a laryngoscope.

Tracheostomy: making an opening into the trachea and inserting a tube for the purpose of maintaining an airway. The patient is placed supine with a sandbag under the shoulder blades, the neck extended and the head pushed backwards. The procedure may be performed electively or as an emergency. Permanent tracheostomies are performed during laryngectomies.

DENTAL SURGERY

Dental extraction: the removal of a tooth or root. The patient lies supine or sits with the head and neck extended.

Immobilization of a fractured mandible: the reduction of a fractured mandible, followed by immobilization, in which the upper and lower teeth are wired together.

OPHTHALMIC SURGERY

Cataract extraction: the removal of an opaque crystalline lens.

Trabeculectomy: the removal of a short length of the canal of Schlemm, allowing the two cut ends of the canal to open directly into the aqueous humour. This procedure is carried out to relieve the outflow obstruction to aqueous humour in glaucoma.

Repair of retinal detachment: sealing the retinal breaks using either cryotherapy, scleral encircling or photocoagulation.

Corneal transplants: transplanting a corneal graft from an enucleated or a cadaveric eye in the treatment of keratoconus or corneal opacities.

Enucleation: the removal of the entire eyeball because of disease or injury.

Vitrectomy: the removal of a diseased vitreous body and adhesions, and its replacement with a balanced salt solution. On some occasions, sulphur hexafluoride (SF_6) or silicone oil is injected.

BREAST SURGERY

Lumpectomy: the removal of a lump in the breast.

Simple mastectomy (Fig. 7.3): removal of the breast, leaving the chest wall muscles intact.

Excision of breast lumps. Breast lumps may be cystic or benign tumours (fibroadenomata). If a lump is detected in the breast, the initial treatment consists of aspiration with a needle and syringe. A Trucut biopsy is made for pathological identification of the lesion. In most cases, excision and biopsy of the lump and surrounding tissue are carried out. The biopsy may be sent for frozen section histology. After the pathological diagnosis, several options are available:

- wedge excision of the affected portion of the breast;
- simple mastectomy, as described above;

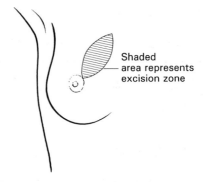

Figure 7.3 Simple mastectomy. An incision is made parallel to the border of the areola and the breast tissue excised, as shown by the shaded area.

- radical mastectomy, which consists of removing the entire breast and the pectoral muscles and lymph nodes.

THORACIC SURGERY

Bronchoscopy: the examination of the trachea and main bronchus by means of a rigid or flexible bronchoscope.

Thoracotomy: opening the chest cavity to operate on the thoracic organs. The patient is placed in the lateral position.

Lobectomy or pneumonectomy: the excision of a lobe of the lung or complete removal of the lung following thoracotomy.

Oesophagoscopy: visualizing the oesophagus. Flexible oesophagoscopy is usually under sedation; rigid oesophagoscopy requires general anaesthesia.

Oesophagectomy: the removal of a portion of the oesophagus, usually for carcinoma. The operation is carried out following thoracotomy.

Oesophagogastrectomy: the removal of part of the oesophagus and stomach, usually for a tumour of the stomach, oesophageal varices or oesophageal tumour. The operation can be carried out through a combined thoracic and abdominal incision, or separate abdominal and thoracic incisions. Some operations also require a neck incision. Patient positioning is very different for each approach and is best supervised by the surgeon.

Repair of diaphragmatic hernia (Fig. 7.4): repairing an abnormal opening in the diaphragm that allows a sliding hernia of the stomach to move into the chest. The repair is carried out via the lateral approach following thoracotomy.

CARDIAC SURGERY

This is a complex specialty requiring a team of surgeons, anaesthetists, nurses, ODPs and perfusion technicians. A number of lesions are

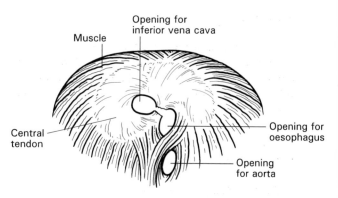

Figure 7.4 Hiatus hernia. Surgery consists of repairing the defect in the diaphragm to prevent the stomach from entering the chest.

operated on, and a brief classification of the operations is given below:

Congenital lesions

1. Patent ductus arteriosus, which requires ligation and division.
2. Coarctation of the aorta, which requires resection and end-to-end anastomosis or resection and grafting.
3. Tetralogy of Fallot, which requires repair.
4. Atrial septal defect and ventricular septal defect, which require repair.

Acquired lesions

1. Mitral stenosis, which may require either open or closed valvulotomy or valve replacement.
2. Mitral incompetence, which requires valvuloplasty or valve replacement.
3. Coronary artery disease, which requires either thromboendarterectomy, graft replacement or bypass.
4. Thoracic aortic aneurysm, which requires repair and grafting.
5. Chronic heart disease, which requires transplantation.

During the corrective procedure on the heart, the patient's circulation is maintained by temporarily bypassing the heart through a heart–lung machine. This consists of an oxygenator, arterial and venous pumps, a heat exchanger, a filter and arterial and venous cardiotomy blood reservoirs. The blood is heparinized during by-pass and cooled, and at the end of the operation the patient's own circulation is re-established in the body and the patient is separated from bypass. The residual heparin is neutralized with protamine sulphate.

ABDOMINAL SURGERY

Gastroenterostomy (Fig. 7.5): making an opening between the stomach and the jejunum. A left paramedian or midline incision is used.

Partial gastrectomy (Figs 7.6 and 7.7): resection of a part of the stomach, making an anastomosis between the remaining portion of the stomach

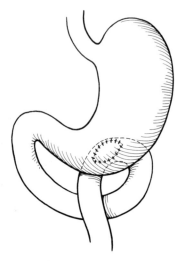

Figure 7.5 Gastrojejunostomy. A loop of the jejunum is brought nearer to the lower part of the stomach and an anastomosis made between the two.

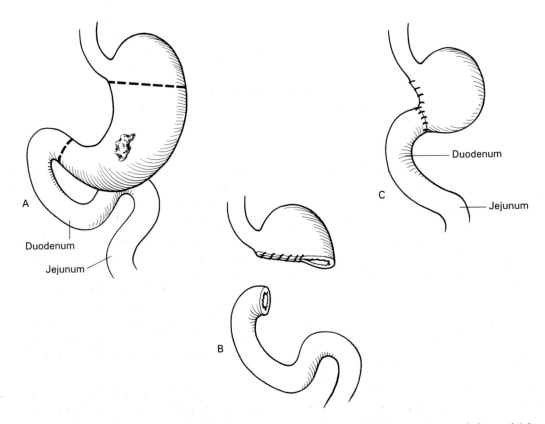

Figure 7.6 Billroth I partial gastrectomy. (A) The lines show the level of resection. (B) The gastric stump is incompletely closed. (C) The remaining opening of the gastric stump is sutured to the open end of the duodenum (gastroduodenostomy).

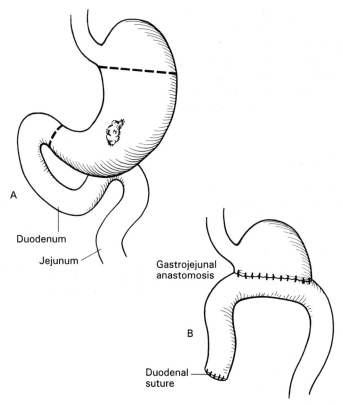

Figure 7.7 Billroth II partial gastrectomy. (A) The lines show the level of resection. (B) The duodenal stump is closed and a gastrojejunal anastomosis carried out.

and the duodenum or jejunum. It is indicated in disease of the pylorus; the distal three-quarters of the stomach is removed, along with the proximal 2–3 cm of the duodenum. The duodenal stump is closed and a gastrojejunal anastomosis performed. In Billroth I gastrectomy, the stomach is attached to the duodenum, whilst in the Billroth II operation the stomach is attached to the jejunum.

Total gastrectomy (Fig. 7.8) is performed for malignancy of the body of the stomach, the procedure resembling partial gastrectomy. It is, however, more extensive, including 2–3 cm of the lower oesophagus. A Roux-en-Y or Roux loop of 45 cm is formed when the loop of proximal jejunum is anastomosed to the oesophagus.

Vagotomy: division of the vagus nerves in association with gastrojejunostomy in the treatment of peptic ulcer.

There are three types of vagotomy:

1. truncal, in which the two main trunks of the vagus are divided as they travel alongside the oesophagus;
2. selective, in which only those fibres supplying the stomach are divided;
3. highly selective, in which the nerve fibres supplying the antrum and pylorus of the stomach are preserved and the rest divided.

Due to lack of vagal stimulation, the drainage from the pylorus of the stomach is delayed after truncal or selective vagotomy. This is treated with pyloroplasty or gastrojejunostomy.

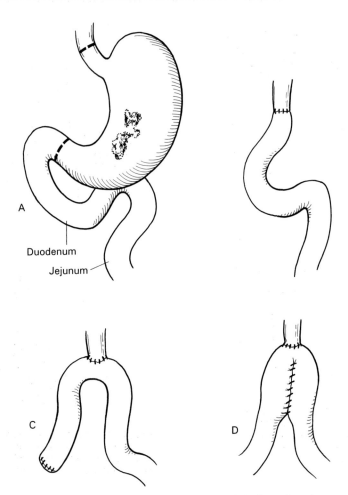

Duodenum

Jejunum

Figure 7.8 Total gastrectomy. (A) *First method:* the lines show the level of resection; (B) oesophagoduodenostomy is completed. (C) *Second method:* the duodenal stump is closed and end-to-side oesophagojejunostomy carried out; (D) side-to-side jejunostomy is completed.

Right hemicolectomy (Fig. 7.9): resection of the right half of the colon.

Appendicectomy (Fig. 7.10) is the most common emergency operation in younger patients. Through a 'grid-iron' or Lanz incision, the appendix is mobilized. Following ligation of the appendicular artery and the mesoappendix, the appendix is ligated and removed.

Volvulus. In this condition of the bowel, a loop of bowel revolves around its mesentery. The loop becomes distended and may cause com-

plete obstruction. Laparotomy consists of reducing the volvulus; bowel resection and temporary colostomy may be necessary.

Abdominoperineal resection of the rectum (Fig. 7.11): mobilizing the diseased part of the colon, which is pushed into the hollow of the pelvis for removal via the perineal route. The patient is left with a permanent colostomy.

Hartmann's procedure (Fig. 7.12): resection of a tumour that lies low in the sigmoid colon or rectum. The resection is carried out with the proximal

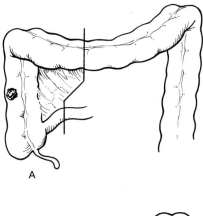

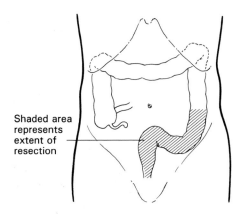

Shaded area
represents
extent of
resection

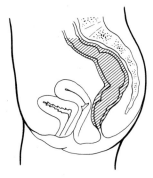

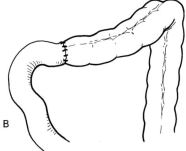

Figure 7.9 Right hemicolectomy. This is carried out for carcinoma of the colon. (A) The demarcating line shows lymph nodes in the mesentery, which are completely removed. (B) Following resection, an ileotransverse anastomosis is carried out.

Figure 7.11 Abdominoperineal resection. The extent of resection is shown by the shaded area. This operation is carried out in low anal and rectal cancer and consists of both an abdominal and a perineal resection.

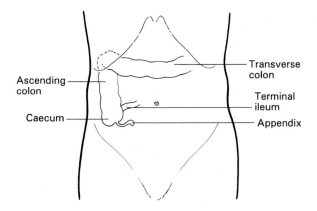

Ascending colon

Caecum

Transverse colon

Terminal ileum

Appendix

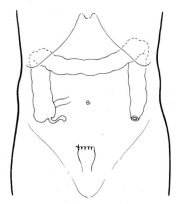

Figure 7.10 Appendicectomy. The blood supply is ligated and divided. The base of the appendix is invaginated using a purse-string suture.

Figure 7.12 Hartmann's operation is a modification of an anterior resection. The proximal end is converted into a left iliac colostomy and the lower end in the pelvic cavity is oversewn.

colon exteriorized as a descending or sigmoid colostomy. The distal stump is oversewn and left in the pelvis.

Panproctocolectomy (Fig. 7.13): removal of the whole of the colon and rectum and the formation of an ileostomy. It is carried out in the inflamed portion of the colon in patients with ulcerative colitis. If the rectum is not involved and the colitis is not extensive, a total colectomy with ileorectal anastomosis is performed.

Surgery for haemorrhoids is carried out for prolapsed piles (varicosities in the anus). The treatment consists of injecting phenol (a sclerosing agent) through a proctoscope, applying a rubber band to the neck of the pile through a proctoscope, or freezing with a cryoprobe.

Haemorrhoidectomy consists of ligating and dissecting the pile. 'Lord's procedure' (manual anal dilatation) is carried out under general anaesthetic. Four fingers are inserted to stretch the anus.

Fissurectomy: excision of a sinus or sinuses between the anal canal and the skin in the region of the anus. The patient is placed in the lithotomy or jack-knife position.

Anterior resection of the rectum: sphincter-saving resection of the rectum and part of the colon, with re-establishment of the continuity by anastomosis.

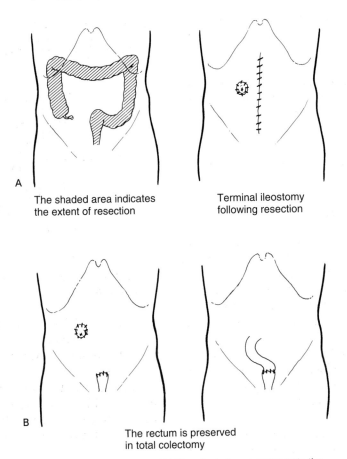

A

The shaded area indicates
the extent of resection

Terminal ileostomy
following resection

B

The rectum is preserved
in total colectomy

Figure 7.13 Protocolectomy. (A) The shaded area represents the extent of gut resection. It is carried out if the rectum needs to be excised. (B) The patient is left with a terminal ileostomy after resection.

Colostomy: establishing a temporary or permanent opening in the colon, which is brought to the surface of the abdomen.

Cholecystectomy: removal of the gallbladder. The patient lies supine with the liver bridge elevated as required.

Cholecystectomy is indicated in inflammation of the gallbladder (cholecystitis) as a result of gallstones. If a number of stones are detected, there may be a possibility of gallstones in the common bile duct. Hence an on-table cholangiogram (OTC) is carried out, in which a radio-opaque dye is injected through a small cannula in the cystic duct. This outlines the biliary tree and any stones in the track of the ducts into the duodenum.

Cholecystojejunostomy (Fig. 7.14): an anastomosis between the gallbladder and the jejunum, often with jejunojejunostomy.

Inguinal herniorrhaphy (Fig. 7.15): closing the sac that has protruded from the abdomen as either a direct hernia or an indirect hernia.

Femoral herniorrhaphy is similar to inguinal hernia, except that the sac protrudes through the femoral ring into the femoral canal.

VASCULAR SURGERY

Excision and grafting for aneurysm of the abdominal aorta: excision of a dilated portion of the abdominal aorta and insertion of a synthetic fabric prosthesis, for example Teflon or Dacron. A midline or left paramedian incision (see Fig. 7.2) is made from the xiphisternum to the pubic symphysis.

The aorta is mobilized and the aneurysm is clamped, following which an anastomosis with the prosthesis is made between the portion above the aneurysm and the common iliac arteries.

Embolectomy is a procedure carried out to remove a blood clot that has become impacted in an artery or vein and which is interfering with the circulation beyond that point. The most common site of arterial embolism is the aortic bifurcation

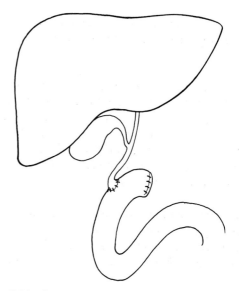

Figure 7.14 Cholecystojejunostomy: a biliary bypass operation to relieve jaundice. The shaded area represents the liver and the oval structure below it the gallbladder.

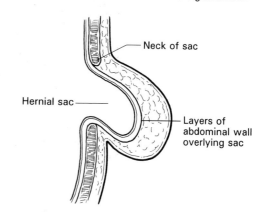

Figure 7.15 Layers of hernia encountered during inguinal herniorraphy.

at the origin of the iliac arteries. Venous embolism occurs at the junction of the inferior vena cava with the common iliac veins.

Femoropopliteal bypass graft: creating a passage for arterial blood to bypass an occluded part of the femoral artery. The patient's own saphenous vein or a Dacron graft is used.

Thromboendarterectomy: removal of an obstructing atheroma from the lumen (centre) of an artery, leaving an outer layer that is free of the disease.

The procedure is performed on major arteries such as the subclavian, vertebral and carotid arteries.

Amputations. Amputation is necessary when it is not possible to repair or save a limb because of tumour, trauma or terminal vascular disease (gangrene).

1. Syme's amputation. This type of amputation involves part of the foot being excised, leaving the heel as part of the stump.
2. Below knee. This enables a prosthesis to be fitted.
3. Gritti-Stokes. The femur is cut above the condyles and the patella is preserved.
4. Above knee is another form of amputation.

GYNAECOLOGICAL SURGERY

Dilatation of the cervix and curettage of the uterus: this is dilatation of the cervix and scraping the uterine mucosa. The patient is placed in a lithotomy position and the procedure is carried out for diagnostic purposes or following the incomplete delivery of a fetus or placenta.

Excision of a Bartholin cyst: removal of a Bartholin cyst that has formed due to blockage of the duct of one of the Bartholin glands, which lie in the labium majora on either side.

Laparoscopy: inspection of the peritoneal cavity using a laparoscope introduced through the abdominal wall. Carbon dioxide (3 L) is insufflated into the abdominal cavity to allow good visualization of the pelvic organs. Laparoscopy has multiple uses as a diagnostic procedure.

Abdominal hysterectomy: removal of the uterus through an abdominal incision. It is carried out for cancer of the uterus, persistent bleeding or uterine fibroids.

Wertheim's hysterectomy: total hysterectomy and bilateral salpingo-oophorectomy, with removal of the upper part of the vagina and lymphatic glands. It is an extensive procedure carried out for carcinoma of the cervix.

Vaginal hysterectomy: removal of the uterus through the vagina.

Lower segment caesarean section (LSCS): removal of the fetus through an incision in the abdominal wall and the uterus. LSCS is carried out for fetal distress, placenta praevia or cephalopelvic disproportion.

ORTHOPAEDICS AND TRAUMA

Fractures

Fractures occur in the following forms:

- a complete break due to trauma;
- greenstick fractures in children;
- pathological fractures due in part to pre-existing abnormal bone, for example in cancer or osteogenesis imperfecta.

Fractures may be classified as:

- *transverse*, occurring due to lateral force;
- *spiral*, occurring after a twisting force on the bone;
- *comminuted*: when bone is fragmented into three or more pieces.

If the skin over a fracture is broken, it is called an open fracture. If a fracture does not communicate with the surface, it is called a closed fracture.

The treatment of fractures consists of:

1. Reduction. Fractures may be reduced either by closed or open methods. In the closed method, the bone fragments are disimpacted and pulled into line, thus positioning the bone for healing. In the open method, the site of the fracture is opened surgically and the bone fragments are realigned and pinned or plated into position.
2. Holding the fracture. This can be done by gravity, skin traction or skeletal traction.
3. Plastering. This is carried out for the majority of fractures.

Internal fixation of a fracture is indicated when:

- a bone is prone to non-union, for example neck of femur;

- a bone is prone to malunion, for example the ankle;
- a bone is prone to pull apart, for example the olecranon.

Fixation can be achieved using a screw, Kirschner wire, K-nail, plate and screw or dynamic hip screw (DHS).

Fracture of the neck of the femur occurs mainly in elderly women after a fall. There are three types of fractures: subcapital, intertrochanteric and subtrochanteric. Subcapital fractures are classified according to the 'Garden' grading system.

Types I and II subcapital fractures are treated by inserting either Garden screws or a DHS. Type III and IV are treated by removing the head of the femur. Hemiarthroplasty is carried out using either an Austin–Moore or Thompson prosthesis.

Intertrochanteric fracture. The treatment consists of reducing the fracture under X-ray control and fixation with a DHS, a McLaughlin pin and plate or a fixed-angle screw.

Subtrochanteric fracture. These fractures are reduced on the orthopaedic table. A pin and plate (DHS) or a nail such as the Smith–Petersen nail can be used.

Arthroscopy: viewing the interior of a synovial joint, usually the knee joint, with a telescope. The most common knee injuries for which arthroscopy is required involve damage to the meniscus. Arthroscopy is performed to assess the damage and see whether repairs can be carried out through the arthroscope or whether an open menisectomy should be performed.

Decompression of the carpal tunnel. Carpal tunnel syndrome consists of compression of the median nerve between the forearm and the palm. During surgery, a tourniquet is applied and an incision made from the wrist to the palm. The flexor retinaculum is exposed and divided, thus releasing pressure on the median nerve.

NEUROSURGERY

Angiography: a serial X-ray examination of the cerebral vascular tree following the injection of a radio-opaque medium into the main artery in the neck.

Craniotomy: an incision through the scalp and underlying skull to gain access to the brain. The patient is placed supine for frontal, temporal or parietal craniotomies, and prone or in a sitting position for occipital and posterior fossa exposures.

With craniotomy, depressed fractures of the skull vault may be elevated or extradural haematomas evacuated.

Insertion of a ventriculo-atrial or ventriculo-peritoneal shunt establishes artificial CSF drainage into the heart or peritoneal cavity in cases of primary or secondary hydrocephalus.

PLASTIC SURGERY

Repair of cleft lip and palate: closing a hare-lip and bringing about the continuity of muscle necessary for modelling the underlying bone and producing a cosmetically acceptable lip. Cleft palate closure pushes the soft palate back so that it can come nearer to the posterior pharyngeal wall.

A split thickness Thiersch-type skin graft is a graft that does not include all layers of the skin but only the epidermis and the tips of the papillae of the dermis.

A full thickness Wolfe-type skin graft is a free graft that includes all the skin's layers.

Fasciectomy for Dupuytren's contracture: excision of hypertrophied palmar fascia that has caused contracture of the fingers.

UROLOGICAL SURGERY

Circumcision: partial excision of the penile foreskin.

Excision of a hydrocele: removal of a hydrocele sac in the scrotum.

Orchidectomy: removal of the testicle.

Vasectomy (Fig. 7.16): excision of part of the vas deferens.

Cystourethroscopy: examination of the interior of the urethra or urinary bladder using a cystoscope.

Prostatectomy (Fig. 7.17). There are various routes by which the prostate can be removed.

Transurethral prostatectomy is transurethral removal of the prostate gland.

Millin's retropubic prostatectomy is removal of the prostate gland through a suprapubic incision without opening the bladder.

Total cystectomy: removal of the urinary bladder and implantation of the ureters into the sigmoid colon.

Nephrectomy (Fig. 7.18): removal of the kidney. The patient is placed laterally with the kidney bridge elevated.

Nephrolithotomy, pyelolithotomy, ureterolithotomy: removal of a stone from the kidney, pelvis of the ureter, or ureter.

Renal transplantation: transplantation of a kidney from a suitable cadaver or a living related donor.

PAEDIATRIC SURGERY

Repair of hypospadias. In this condition, the urethral opening is found on the inferior surface of the penis instead of the tip. It is repaired using skin from the shaft of the penis (Dennis Browne's operation).

Orchidopexy: mobilizing the testis and placing it in the scrotum to prevent torsion of the testicle.

Herniotomy. In children, this consists of excising the hernial sac (herniotomy, compared with repair in adults).

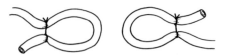

Figure 7.16 Vasectomy: the two cut ends of the vas deferens are doubly ligated with silk.

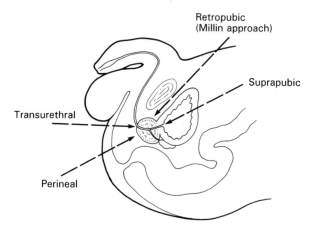

Figure 7.17 Types of prostatectomy: retropubic (Millin), transurethral, suprapubic and perineal.

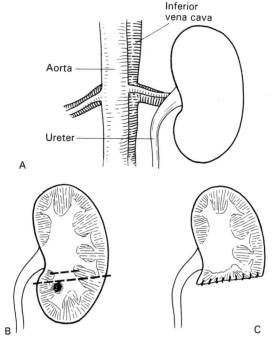

Figure 7.18 Partial nephrectomy. (A) Posterior surface of the kidney. (B) The lines indicate the level of transection of the renal calyx and renal substance. (C) Completed partial nephrectomy.

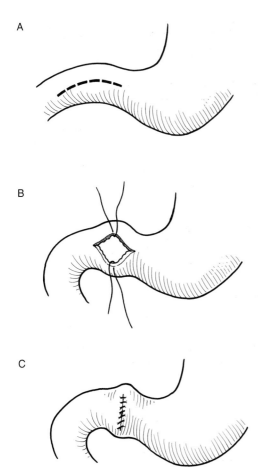

A

B

C

Figure 7.19 Pyloroplasty. (A) A longitudinal incision is made on the centre of the pylorus. (B) The edges of the incision are stretched. (C) Pyloroplasty is completed by transverse suturing.

Ramstedt's operation (Fig. 7.19): for the repair of congenital pyloric stenosis. This is carried out in neonates within the first few weeks of life. After rehydrating the baby and correcting his acid–base balance, surgery consists of cutting the hypertrophied muscles in the pyloric region of the stomach down to the submucosa. This relieves the stenosis.

8

Recovery and intensive care

RECOVERY AREA

Patients recovering from a general anaesthetic need to be monitored and nursed until they are fully awake, stable and ready to return to the ward. If these patients are not managed properly, mishaps, including death, can occur in the immediate recovery period.

Set-up of a recovery area

Recovery areas are situated in the theatre suite and supervised by members of the department of anaesthesia. They are usually managed by either a recovery sister or a charge nurse and other nursing staff. The recovery areas are open either for a 24-hour period so that the patient can remain there until the morning after the operation, or until the patient is stable enough to be discharged back to the ward, a high-dependency unit (HDU) or the intensive therapy unit (ITU) at the end of the operating session.

Equipment required in the recovery area

The patient is nursed on a trolley or a bed (if a stay of 24 hours is anticipated); both can be tilted to a head-down position quickly if the patient vomits.

Within reach of the trolley the following items should be available:

- suction apparatus and catheters;

- an oxygen supply and face masks supplying various percentages of oxygen (see p. 235);
- ECG monitors;
- Oscillotonometers/automatic blood pressure monitoring devices, for example Dinamap.

For the whole recovery area there should be the following items:

1. resuscitation equipment, including an Ambubag or rebreathing bag, face masks, laryngoscopes and endotracheal tubes;
2. a defibrillator
3. equipment for an emergency tracheostomy, including tracheostomy tubes.

Drugs in the recovery area

Each recovery area should have a cupboard for emergency drugs with facilities to stock controlled drugs. A list of the drugs that should be available in the recovery area is given in Box 8.1.

Box 8.1   Drugs available in the recovery area

General (box/boxes of):

Adrenaline: 1 in 1000 1 ml ampoules
Aminophylline: 250 mg in 10 ml
Atropine: 600 μg in 1 ml
Calcium chloride: 5% in 5 ml
Diazepam (Diazemuls): 10 mg in 2 ml
Dopamine (Intropin): 200 mg in 5 ml
Doxapram (Dopram): 50 mg in 5 ml
Ephedrine: 30 mg in 1 ml
Flumazenil: initial dose 200 μg i.v. over 15 seconds
Hydrocortisone: 100 mg in 1 ml
Isoprenaline
Labetalol (Trandate)
Lignocaine (Xylocaine): 1%, 10 ml ampoules
Metoclopramide (Maxolon): 10 mg in 2 ml
Ondansetron (Zofran): 4 mg in 2 ml or 8 mg in 4 ml
Naloxone (Narcan): 0.4 mg in 1 ml
Neostigmine (Prostigmin): 2.5 mg in 1 ml
Practolol (Eraldin)
Prochlorperazine (Stemetil): 12.5 mg in 1 ml
Propranolol (Inderal)
Sodium bicarbonate: 8.4%

Controlled drugs:

Diamorphine (Heroin)
Morphine: 10 mg in 1 ml
Pethidine: 50 mg in 1 ml
Papaveretum (Omnopon): 15 mg in 1 ml
Fentanyl

MANAGEMENT OF THE PATIENT IN THE RECOVERY AREA

At the end of the surgical procedure, the patient is wheeled into the recovery area by the anaesthetist and the recovery nurse. On arrival in the recovery area, the patient is attached to an ECG monitor, and vital signs such as pulse rate, rhythm, blood pressure, respiratory rate and colour are observed and recorded. In certain recovery areas where ECG facilities are not available, the pulse is monitored manually or by a pulse oximeter.

The following points are observed and procedures carried out carefully from the time the patient arrives in the recovery area until discharge to the ward:

1. airway maintenance
2. level of consciousness
3. postoperative analgesia
4. oxygen therapy
5. i.v. fluid therapy
6. cardiovascular problems
7. shivering
8. restlessness and excitement
9. monitoring of urinary output, drains and CVP.

AIRWAY MAINTENANCE

In the immediate postoperative period, patients are semiconscious and prone to having their airway obstructed by the tongue falling backwards and thus occluding the pharynx. The airway is maintained in these patients by either holding the lower jaw upwards and outwards, or inserting a Guedel airway into the mouth.

Positioning the patient

Patients are place in one of five positions depending on the type of surgery and level of consciousness.

1. Semi-prone. The patient lies face down with the lower arm placed behind the body, the head turned to one side and the legs flexed in the same direction as the patient's head.

2. Post-tonsillectomy. This is a position similar to the semi-prone; in addition, a pillow is placed under the chest to prevent the patient rolling forwards.
3. Lateral position. The patient lies on one side with a pillow placed behind his back (Fig. 8.1).

The above positions are used in patients who are semiconscious.

4. Supine. The patient is laid flat on his back when he is fully awake (Fig. 8.2).
5. Sitting-up. Certain obese patients do not breathe adequately if lying either on their back or on their side because their diaphragm pushes the lungs upwards, thus hindering respiratory attempts. Sitting up pushes the diaphragm downwards and allows the patient to breathe adequately.

Sometimes patients do not breathe adequately as a result of tight surgical dressings, for example after a radical mastectomy or after the application of tight dressings or plaster jackets around the head and neck.

In the immediate postoperative period, certain patients tend to vomit, so a head-down tilt of the trolley aids in drainage of the vomitus. A suction unit enables the suction of vomitus from the oropharynx using either a wide-hose suction catheter or a Yankaeur sucker.

LEVEL OF CONSCIOUSNESS

A number of patients return to the recovery area in a semiconscious state, and it is the duty of the recovery nurse to maintain the patient's airway until he is able to do so on his own.

The majority of anaesthetists prescribe oxygen therapy for all patients until consciousness has returned, and in some patients it is continued for 4–6 hours in the ward.

POSTOPERATIVE ANALGESIA

Pain according to the International Association for the Study of Pain (IASP) is defined as 'an unpleasant sensory and emotional experience

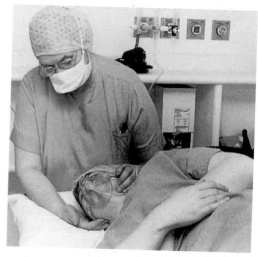

Figure 8.1   The lateral position.

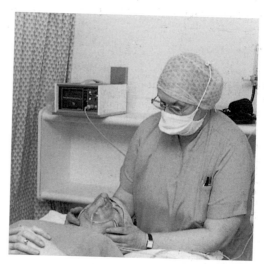

Figure 8.2   The supine position.

associated with actual or potential tissue damage, or described in terms of such damage'.

The most important reason for treating pain is humanitarian: to alleviate suffering, good analgesia reduces patient discomfort and minimizes psychological distress. Adequate pain relief has beneficial effects on several organs:

1. Pulmonary function improves and there is a decreased risk of pulmonary complications.
2. The stress response to trauma and surgery is decreased.

3. Good analgesia (e.g. epidural) improves blood flow to the lower limbs by sympathetic blockade, thus reducing the incidence of thromboembolism.

4. Pain impairs gastrointestinal function by delaying gastric emptying. When regional techniques such as epidural or spinal anaesthetics are used, normal bowel function necessary to maintain adequate nutrition returns earlier.

5. Pain in the presence of heart disease can cause unnecessary stress on the myocardium. Good analgesia (e.g. local blocks, epidurals or patient-controlled analgesia) can reduce morbidity and mortality by reducing sympathetic over-activity and catecholamine release.

6. With good postoperative analgesia, vulnerable patients such as the elderly can demonstrate normal mental function.

In 1991 a working party of the Royal College of Surgeons and College of Anaesthetists produced a report on postoperative pain. The recommendations can be summarized as follows:

- The management of pain after surgery in the UK is unsatisfactory. Evidence in the report points to several ways of improving the situation in all hospitals.
- All staff involved in the management of postoperative pain should be fully educated in this area, and traditional antiquated attitudes should be changed.
- A patient's pain should not be neglected but assessed and recorded along with other observations such as blood pressure and heart rate. It is vital that a named member of staff is responsible for a hospital policy ensuring satisfactory pain relief for all patients after surgery.
- An Acute Pain Service should be introduced into all major hospitals performing surgery in the UK.
- The introduction of new effective and safe methods for providing postoperative pain relief should be encouraged.
- The advantages of appropriate facilities in the management of postoperative pain were described.

- All major hospitals should have a high-dependency unit of sufficient size to support the needs of a modern and effective pain relief policy.
- To introduce a safe and effective policy, there is a need for properly trained staff and adequate resources.
- Research into pain relief after surgery should be encouraged.
- There is a need for powerful, safe analgesics and long-acting, non-toxic local anaesthetics.
- There are areas of doubt over the safety and efficacy of some methods of analgesia, and it is important that research into these techniques should continue.
- Monitoring of patients to detect undesirable side-effects of analgesic regimens is a major requirement.
- The development of inexpensive, easy-to-use monitors to detect the main hazards should be encouraged.
- The use of counselling and psychological methods in the management of postoperative pain should be encouraged.

The routes of administration of analgesics in the perioperative period, with their advantages and disadvantages, are described below.

Oral

This is not a practical route when treating acute pain following major surgery as the pain itself reduces gastric emptying. Postoperative vomiting will also render the oral route ineffective. However, oral analgesia is effective for minor and intermediate surgery. The drugs used include co-proxamol, co-dydramol and non-steroidal anti-inflammatory drugs (NSAIDs).

Sublingual/buccal

The advantage of these routes includes avoiding injections, although taste and nausea prevent the use of these drugs (e.g. buprenorphine).

Rectal

This route is not effective in the initial management of acute pain, but the rectal use of NSAIDs is well suited for the maintenance of analgesia. Patients should have prior warning that suppositories may be used; successful lawsuits for assault have occurred following the use of suppositories.

Transdermal

Transdermal administration of the drug fentanyl (Durogesic) gives a controlled release of analgesic. On its own, this method is not adequate for postoperative analgesia, and it may need to be topped up with small intermittent i.v. boluses. Transdermal fentanyl is used for treating the pain of malignancy.

Intranasal

A short-acting, synthetic opioid, sufentanil, has been used to produce rapid and effective analgesia.

Intramuscular

This route of administration was widely used 'as required' in the past. It is ineffective when the intensity of pain varies and there will be long periods when the patient will be in pain. The analgesia provided by intermittent i.m. injections could be improved by:

- regular and more frequent administration;
- the use of opioids with a long duration of action.

Ideally, in present-day medicine where day-stay surgery is common, a combination of i.m. analgesic, which will last into the immediate postoperative period, and rectal NSAIDs with oral analgesics is effective.

Intravenous

If given as a continuous infusion, this route is more effective than are intermittent i.m. injections. Close monitoring is required as oversedation is a possibility.

The drugs that have been commonly used for i.v. infusion are shown in Box 8.2.

Box 8.2 Postoperative analgesics for i.v. infusion	
Drug	*Infusion rate (adults)*
Morphine	1–5 mg/h
Pethidine	10–50 mg/h
Papaveretum	1–5 mg/h

The disadvantages of the continuous infusion of analgesics are:

1. Postoperative analgesic requirements vary widely with activities such as movement, physiotherapy and turning. A fixed-dose infusion is not sufficient to cater for all these situations.
2. Accumulation of the drug may occur, leading to toxicity. For example, if a patient with renal failure is given a continuous infusion of morphine, the elimination will be decreased, leading to the accumulation of active metabolites (such as morphine-6-glucuronide).
3. Respiratory and cardiovascular depression can occur with a continuous infusion.
4. Patients receiving an i.v. infusion of analgesics need to be observed frequently so that the level of infusion can be adjusted to maintain good analgesia with minimum adverse effects.

Patient-controlled analgesia

The disadvantages of i.m. or i.v. infusion have been overcome with the introduction of patient-controlled analgesia (PCA). The advantages of PCA are:

- It avoids difficulties related to inappropriate dose regimens, unpredictable drug absorption and patient variability.
- The patient is in control of his or her analgesia all the time.
- It avoids dependence upon doctors and nurses.
- The technique allows the development of a positive behaviour in patients.

PCA is used for the administration of analgesics not only by the i.v. route, but also via the epidural route. The salient features of a PCA system consist of:

1. *Drug of choice.* Morphine is the standard drug used in the UK, although pethidine and papaveretum are also used.

2. *Bolus dose.* This setting allows a bolus dose as programmed to be given as a stat dose.

3. *Lock-out interval.* A lock-out interval is set up. Once a bolus is given, the machine 'locks' and will not deliver another bolus until the lock-out time is over.

4. *Background infusion.* In the UK, a background infusion is usually not set up because of the disadvantages of continuous infusion mentioned above.

5. *4-hour dose limit.* A 4-hour dose limit can be set in order to prevent excessive analgesic being delivered to the patient.

Immediately after the surgery, analgesic requirements are high, and they need to be titrated by giving bolus doses until analgesia is established.

When the PCA device is set up, pain assessments charts are used.

The disadvantages of PCA are:

- drug errors – wrong drug, wrong concentration;
- accidental drug administration, which can occur when new syringes are connected without cross-clamping the i.v. line;
- patient factors:
  - failure to understand the PCA system;
  - intentional abuse;
  - initiation of doses by people other than the patient;
- prescribing errors:
  - incorrect demand dose
  - incorrect lock-out interval
  - high background infusion
- equipment malfunction. Syringes may empty more slowly or more quickly than programmed if the incorrect size or specification of syringe is used. Mobile telephones can reprogramme the pump computer.

The uses of PCA are:

- in postoperative pain
- as ambulatory PCA in obstetrics;
- in burns
- in terminal illness
- in major trauma.

As all opiates tend to cause postoperative nausea and vomiting (PONV), it is obligatory to prescribe antiemetics. They can be prescribed with the premedication or given intraoperatively. It is better to prevent PONV rather than have the patient suffer the side-effects of retching, increased pain, dehydration and possible admission overnight in the hospital (in the case of a day-surgery patient). Table 8.1 lists some common antiemetics and their dosages.

Epidural and intrathecal opioids

Epidural route. A catheter is introduced into the epidural (extradural) space and a local anaesthetic agent, with or without an opiate, is infused through a volumetric pump. Sites where a catheter can be inserted are the thoracic region for upper abdominal surgery and the lumbar region for lower abdominal surgery.

The dosage of various opiates which are given via epidural route are summarized in Table 8.2.

Caudal block is performed to provide pain relief in patients undergoing circumcision and haemorrhoidectomy. A dose of 0.3–0.4 ml/kg of 0.25% plain bupivacaine (Marcain) is used

Table 8.1 Common antiemetics prescribed with opiates

Drug	Dose	Route	Frequency
Premedication			
Metoclopramide (Maxolon)	10 mg	Oral/i.m./i.v.	6 hourly for i.m./i.v.
Intraoperative			
Droperidol (Droleptan)	2.5–5 mg	oral/i.v.	Once
Ondansetron (Zofran)	4 mg	i.v.	Once
Prochlorperazine (Stemetil)	12.5 mg	i.m.	6 hourly
Perphenazine (Fentazin)	5 mg	i.m.	6 hourly
Cyclizine	50 mg	i.m.	6 hourly

Table 8.2 Opiates via the extradural route

Drug	Dose	Duration
Morphine	2–5 mg	Up to 24 hours
Diamorphine (Heroin)	2.5 mg	Up to 12 hours
Fentanyl (Sublimaze)	0.1 mg	2–4 hours
Pethidine	25–50 mg	1–3 hours

The drug must be preservative free. None of the ampoules' packaging is sterile so the fentanyl ampoule must not be dropped onto the sterile trolley.

in adults, whereas 0.5–0.7 ml/kg is used in children.

Intrathecal route. Intraoperatively, a subarachnoid block is performed using 25 G or 26 G spinal needles, and preservative-free opiates (e.g. morphine, pethidine and fentanyl) are injected, the dose for morphine being 20 µg/kg body weight.

The injection of opiates via this route causes generalized analgesia lasting for 18–24 hours.

The factors influencing the action of intrathecal and epidural opioids include:

- lipid solubility
- route of administration
- elimination.

The unwanted side-effects of epidural and intrathecal opioids include:

- central: euphoria, sedation and respiratory depression;
- peripheral: itching around the face, nausea, vomiting and urinary retention.

Respiratory depression can occur as late as 24 hours following administration of the drug. Naloxone 0.4 mg i.v. in a titrated dose will reverse the respiratory depression without severing the analgesia. The dose of naloxone needs to be repeated because of its short duration of action.

Local nerve blocks

1. *Wound infiltration or wound instillation* is carried out for herniotomy, herniorrhaphy, orchidopexy, removal of breast lumps, etc. Local

anaesthetic can be instilled into drains (e.g. following mastectomy and axillary dissection) to give effective pain relief.

2. *Digital nerve block* provides postoperative analgesia following surgery on the fingers and toes.

3. *Intercostal nerve block* is occasionally carried out for pain relief in rib fractures or following open cholecystectomy.

4. *Intrapleural injection* has been used to provide analgesia for patients who have had upper abdominal surgery. Unfortunately, its side-effects, such as pneumothorax, prevent its regular usage.

5. *Femoral nerve block* is useful in analgesia for patients with a fractured neck of femur.

6. *Ankle block* is effective as a postoperative analgesic method in patients undergoing toe surgery (e.g. hallux valgus correction).

Other agents that have been used for postoperative pain include:

1. *Transcutaneous electrical nerve stimulation (TENS).* A small electric current is passed between (usually two) surface electrodes at frequencies of between 0.2 and 100 Hz. This appears to liberate endorphins (endogenous opiates), which in turn decrease the i.m. or i.v. analgesic requirement.

Acupuncture acts in the same fashion as TENS, again reducing the total analgesic requirement.

2. *Cryoanalgesia.* During certain surgical procedures (e.g. thoracotomy), intercostal nerves under direct vision are subjected to intense subzero temperatures generated by a cryoprobe (cryo = cold).

3. *Inhalational analgesia.* On some occasions, Entonox is used in the postoperative period to allow a change of dressings.

The role of ketamine as an analgesic in the postoperative period and in ITU is receiving greater attention.

OXYGEN THERAPY

In the postoperative period, a number of patients become hypoxic (suffer from lack of oxygen). The causes of hypoxia are given below.

Diffusion hypoxia

At the end of the anaesthetic procedure when the nitrous oxide is turned off, 'diffusion hypoxia' occurs. The mechanism behind 'diffusion hypoxia' is as follows.

When nitrous oxide is turned off at the end of anaesthesia, it diffuses from the blood (a high concentration of nitrous oxide) into the alveoli (a low concentration), diluting the oxygen in the alveoli. This leads to a fall in the alveolar concentration of oxygen. Administering 100% oxygen for several minutes at the end of anaesthesia will help to avoid this.

Ventilation–perfusion abnormalities

This term is used when the ventilation of the lungs does not match the blood supply to the lungs (perfusion). Oxygen delivery to the body depends upon:

- oxygen getting to those alveoli which have a blood supply;
- blood getting to the alveoli that receive oxygen.

Ventilation of lung that has no blood supply (e.g in hypotension) cannot contribute to oxygenation. The blood supply to unventilated lung (in pneumonia or collapse, for example) will not be oxygenated and will dilute the saturated blood coming from ventilated areas of the lung. Improving oxygenation depends on matching the blood supply to the ventilation.

Increased oxygen utilization

Increased metabolic activity requires increased oxygen utilization. Hypoxia will result unless extra oxygen is supplied. The most common causes of increased metabolic activity include shivering and fever. Children and pregnant women also have increased oxygen requirements.

Hypoventilation

Patients in the postoperative period may hypoventilate (decreased respiration) leading to a fall in oxygen delivery to the tissue and the retention of carbon dioxide. Some of the important postoperative conditions in which hypoventilation occurs are listed below:

- upper airway obstruction due to laryngospasm, the tongue or a foreign body;
- bronchospasm;
- intraoperative hyperventilation, which will lower the $PaCO_2$ and reduce the respiratory drive;
- respiratory depression due to opiates;
- the incomplete reversal of neuromuscular blockade, leading to muscle weakness;
- pain, which can inhibit breathing;
- obesity, causing diaphragmatic 'splinting';
- upper abdominal surgery, causing pain and reduced diaphragmatic movement;
- pneumothorax.

It is essential to administer oxygen in the postoperative period to prevent hypoxia as a result of the various causes mentioned above. If there is respiratory depression due to opiates, either naloxone (Narcan) or doxapram (Dopram) is given to reverse the depression.

'Oxygen therapy' devices (Fig. 8.3)

These are classified into:

Fixed performance devices

These devices deliver an inspired gas mixture of known composition. These are 'patient independent', which means that the oxygen concentration delivered does not change with the changing respiratory rate/rhythm of the patient.

1. Low flow systems. Anaesthetic circuits such as the Mapleson A will deliver a metered flow of oxygen and air provided the mask fits tightly on the face.

2. High airflow oxygen enrichment (HAFOE) or Venturi systems. An oxygen-driven injector entrains (traps) a fixed proportion of room air. A high flow rate (between 20 and 30 L/min) of premixed gas (oxygen + air) prevents dilution.

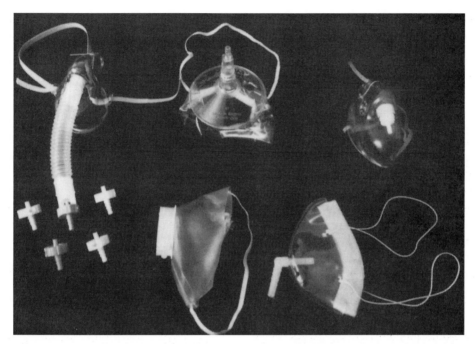

Figure 8.3 Oxygen masks. *Top row:* Venturi-type mask, Ventimask, Hudson mask. *Bottom row:* MC mask, Edinburgh mask. (From Smith J, Aitkenhead A R 1989 Textbook of anaesthesia, Churchill Livingstone, Edinburgh.)

Venturi masks. This principle should be used according to the recommendation of the manufacturers. Injectors of different sizes are used at varying oxygen flow rates to deliver set oxygen concentrations to the patient.

Variable performance devices

These devices are 'patient dependent', which means that the oxygen delivered to the patient depends on the respiration of the patient and the dead space between the face and the mask. These devices are usually sufficient for the postoperative period.

A list of masks, with the approximate oxygen concentration delivered and the flow rates that need to be set, is given in Table 8.3.

Choice of masks. An MC mask or Mapleson A circuit is used to increase oxygenation, whereas a Ventimask or Edinburgh mask is used to deliver a known oxygen concentration (e.g. to a patient with chronic obstructive airways disease).

Table 8.3 Oxygen masks

Masks	Oxygen concentration	Oxygen flow (L/min)
Mary Caterral (MC)	28–50	2
	41–70	4
	52–74	6
Hudson	24–38	2
	35–45	4
	57–61	6
	61–73	10
Harris	60	6
Edinburgh	25–29	1
	31–35	2
	33–39	3
Nasal catheter	25–29	2
	30–60	4

INTRAVENOUS FLUID THERAPY

In a large number of cases, i.v. fluid therapy is commenced in theatre. The fluids usually administered are Hartmann's solution, dextrose

4% in normal saline 0.18%, or 5% dextrose. The rate of intraoperative administration depends on the patient's weight and the type of surgery.

When the blood loss is more than 10% of blood volume in children and 15% in adults, blood transfusion is started. After checking, usually by two people, the unit of blood against the information on the patient's wristband and case notes, and the form received from the blood bank, the transfusion is commenced. In large volume transfusions, a blood filter, blood warming coil and blood warmer will help to prevent the patient receiving debris and cold blood. The transfusion of warm blood prevents the patient from becoming hypothermic.

The anaesthetist completes the fluid therapy chart before handing over the patient to the recovery nurse.

CARDIOVASCULAR PROBLEMS

Hypotension

The usual causes of hypotension are:

1. excessive premedication;
2. an overdose of general anaesthetic (e.g. a high concentration of inhalational agent delivered during anaesthesia);
3. excessive vascular absorption of the local anaesthetic (local anaesthetics depress the myocardium and cause dilatation of peripheral vessels);
4. spinal and epidural anaesthesia;
5. haemorrhage and blood loss that has not been adequately replaced;
6. motion and change of position in a vasodilated patient;
7. hypoxia, causing myocardial depression;
8. metabolic acidosis, again causing myocardial depression.

Over a period of time, the residual effects of (1), (2), (3) and (4) wear off, and when blood loss, hypoxaemia and acidosis are corrected, blood pressure returns to within normal limits. Late hypotension may be caused by vasodilatation as the patient rewarms following surgery.

Hypertension

When patients become excessively hypertensive in the postoperative period, they are at risk of a cerebrovascular accident or myocardial infarction. High blood pressure can also increase postoperative bleeding.

The important causes of postoperative hypertension are:

1. pain;
2. hypoxia and hypercarbia;
3. the excessive replacement of fluid losses;
4. following aortic grafting for abdominal aortic aneurysm;
5. a full bladder.

Adequate analgesia and oxygenation will decrease the blood pressure in conditions (1) and (2), and the use of vasodilators such as sodium nitroprusside given slowly i.v. with careful monitoring of blood pressure or chlorpromazine will treat the hypertensive response.

SHIVERING

Patients shiver in the postoperative period as a result of lowered body temperature, which in turn increases heart rate and oxygen consumption. Heat loss leading to lowered body temperature occurs:

- from breathing cold, dry gases during anaesthesia;
- when cold i.v. fluids are given;
- when the thoracic and abdominal cavities are open for prolonged periods;
- in deep planes of anaesthesia (an effect on the temperature centre in the medulla);
- in children and the elderly (because of decreased body fat insulation and increased surface area);
- due to high circulating air flows in the theatre and recovery areas.

Body temperature can be maintained by keeping the room temperature at 21°C (70°F), using closed circuits, condenser humidifiers and blood warmers, infusing warm fluids and bloods, and keeping children and the elderly warm with heated ripple mattresses, forced air warmers (the Bair hugger) and adequate wrapping (gamgee or bowel bags).

RESTLESSNESS AND EXCITEMENT

Patients may become agitated or disoriented in the postoperative period for a number of reasons, for example:

- pain;
- anxiety about recovery from the anaesthetic;
- an uncomfortable position and a full urinary bladder.

Excitement occurs as a result of:

- hypoxia following thoracic or upper abdominal operations;
- hypotension;
- the use of hyoscine, phenothiazines (chlorpromazine), barbiturates and premedicants; the use of ketamine as an anaesthetic agent, leading to postoperative hallucinations – i.e. a drug effect.

Management

This consists of relieving pain, changing the patient's uncomfortable position, emptying the bladder, oxygen therapy for hypoxia, and fluid or blood replacement to correct hypotension.

As the anaesthetic agent is eliminated, the patient gradually becomes quiet. Time and patience are important, and the patient should be comforted throughout this difficult period.

MONITORING URINARY OUTPUT, DRAINS AND CENTRAL VENOUS PRESSURE

Urinary output

In recovery areas that are open for 24 hours, it is essential to monitor urinary output as some patients develop postoperative retention of urine. In patients who have had urological surgery (prostate resection), bladder irrigation or intermittent washouts are needed to prevent clotting

of the blood, which in some cases may lead to retention of urine.

Patients who have undergone major surgical procedures (e.g. aneurysmal surgery, cardiac surgery or abdominoperineal resection of the rectum) need their bladder catheterized, and hourly monitoring of urine output using a 'urimeter' is carried out.

Wound drainage

In a number of surgical cases, the surgical wound is drained and the recovery nurse is made aware of the site of the drain or drains. When patients are positioned on trolleys or beds in the recovery area, it is essential that precautions are taken not to block or kink drains as, by observing these, it is possible to detect early haemorrhage. Following thoracic or cardiac procedures when underwater sealed drains are inserted, it is important to check that these are 'swinging' with respiration and that a large volume of blood is not being collected rapidly in the bottle. If either 'swinging' with respiration stops or larger amounts of blood start to accumulate, medical help should be sought immediately.

Central venous pressure

CVP is measured using a calibrated transducer (for blood pressure) or a manometer line. In the immediate postoperative period, CVP monitoring becomes essential for patients who have undergone major surgical procedures such as repair of an aneurysm, cardiopulmonary bypass or coronary artery bypass and valve replacements.

SPECIAL CONSIDERATIONS IN THE RECOVERY AREA

Most of the problems and management discussed above hold true for a number of surgical procedures, but the following paragraphs are relevant in the recovery of patients from specific surgical procedures.

ENT surgery

Children undergoing tonsillectomy should be nursed in the post-tonsillectomy position until they are fully awake. Bleeding post-tonsillectomy may be difficult to see as children often swallow blood rather than spit it out.

Dental and maxillofacial surgery

Patients who have a fractured jaw undergo surgical fixation followed by wiring of the jaw. The anaesthetist administers an antiemetic, for example prochlorperazine (Stemetil) or ondansetron (Zofran), intraoperatively. In the recovery area, the anaesthetist pulls the naso-tracheal tube above the vocal cords, allowing it to function as a nasopharyngeal airway. The patient is usually accompanied by wire cutters from the theatre into the recovery area. The nursing staff are informed of which wires to cut in case the patient vomits. The patient is nursed on one side with a slight head-down tilt until fully awake. The nasopharyngeal tube is then pulled out.

Ophthalmic surgery

Most patients undergoing ophthalmic surgery receive antiemetics during the intraoperative period, as vomiting, coughing and straining can increase the intraocular pressure and damage the eye. They should be nursed on one side until fully awake.

Patients who have undergone vitrectomy should be recovered according to the surgeon's recommendation.

Bronchoscopy

All patients who have received a local anaesthetic spray to their vocal cords should be observed by the recovery staff at all times as their swallowing and cough reflexes are dulled. No oral fluids should be given for at least 4 hours (or longer according to the wishes of the anaesthetist). Although patients may be fully awake after a general anaesthetic, they may still have difficulty in swallowing and speaking.

If a bronchial biopsy has been taken, there is a greater danger of haemorrhage. Control of bleeding may be difficult, so patients are usually nursed on the side from which the biopsy was taken, or in an upright, sitting position. Bronchial biopsy may occasionally cause pneumothorax, so the patient should be observed closely and a chest X-ray considered if there is unequal air entry, cyanosis or breathlessness.

Thoracic surgery

In the recovery room or HDUs all vital signs are monitored regularly. Underwater seal drains, inserted intraoperatively, should be seen to be 'swinging' (moving with respiration) and not be blocked by surgical debris or a clot. Some anaesthetists clamp the drains when moving a patient to prevent the water in the drain from entering the thorax via the tubing. Clamps should be removed at the earliest opportunity to prevent the development of tension pneumo-thorax. The drains should always be below the level of the patient's chest. Analgesia in the form of intrathecal morphine, epidural block or an infusion is prescribed.

Cardiothoracic surgery

A number of patients are transferred directly to the ITU for elective ventilation.

Paediatric surgery

Neonates who undergo surgery are quickly replaced in their incubators and returned to the special care baby unit. Larger babies are placed in their preheated cots. Some babies who are not critically ill can be recovered in the arms of the recovery staff; these babies are returned to the ward when fully awake. At all times the child's airway is maintained.

Although a fair number of anaesthetists do not prescribe analgesia for neonates, it should be prescribed based on the type of surgery the child has undergone. Analgesia in the form of pethidine, papaveretum or regional blockade can be given to older children.

Neurosurgery

Patients who undergo major neurosurgical procedures, such as posterior fossa exploration or clipping or a cerebral aneurysm, are transferred to ITU.

Vascular surgery

Patients who have had aneurysmal surgery are transferred directly to ITU. Some patients who have undergone a femoropopliteal bypass graft are sent to the HDU or ward. Before they are sent to the ward, blood loss in the drain should be measured and if necessary a blood transfusion commenced. Once the patient is stabilized, he or she can be sent back to the ward.

Vascular surgical patients usually require regular observation of the operated limbs for colour, warmth and the presence of pulses.

THE INTENSIVE THERAPY UNIT

The ITU is a specialized area in hospital where critically ill patients are given the most closely supervised level of continuous care and treatment. Compared with general wards, a larger area is allocated for each bed space. Bulky monitoring equipment occupies space, and some of this extra room is also needed for several nurses to attend to the patient at once.

Each bed area is provided with piped oxygen, air, suction and a minimum of two electric power sockets, and has sufficient space for storing drugs and carrying out physiotherapy.

Staffing in ITU

The administrative consultant in charge of the ITU is often an anaesthetist who, in addition to looking after patients, looks after the day-to-day administration of the unit.

Junior anaesthetists and nursing staff carry out a major part of patient care. The ITU junior anaesthetist liaises with other specialists and acts on the recent test results and changing physiological condition of the patient.

Design of an ITU

The ITU should be sited in close proximity to the operating department, accident and emergency department coronary care unit and labour ward. Critically ill patients are at great risk when they are moved about, so adequate precautions are taken in designing ITUs to make sure that a sufficient number of lifts, spacious corridors and doors are provided to allow easy transportation of patients and equipment.

The ITU usually has one entry and one exit point (i.e. two doors), which are attended by the receptionist or ward clerk. Through-traffic of goods or people to other hospital areas is not allowed. There are areas and rooms for reception of the patient's relatives, patient's treatment and support services.

Indications for admission to ITU

Patients who are admitted to ITU usually require life support (cardiac and respiratory) during resuscitation, diagnosis and treatment.

Other groups of patients who are admitted to the unit are those who have undergone major surgery (neurosurgery, cardiac surgery or transplants of liver or heart) or patients with organ failure (liver failure, renal failure and head injury).

Patients who are admitted to ITU are monitored continuously using highly sophisticated equipment. This monitoring is summarized in Box 8.3.

Box 8.3	Monitoring in ITU
Organ	*Monitoring*
Brain	Electroencephalogram (EEG) Cerebral function analysing monitor (CFAM) Intracranial pressure monitoring (ICP)
Cardiovascular	Electrocardiogram (ECG) Blood pressure monitoring (invasive or non-invasive) Central venous pressure (CVP) Cardiac output (transoesophageal Doppler ultrasound, Swan–Ganz catheter) Pulmonary artery pressure monitoring

Box 8.3 (*Cont'd*)	
Organ	*Monitoring*
Respiratory	Tidal volume, minute volume
	Oxygen delivery (oxygen analyser)
	Carbon dioxide production
	(carbon dioxide monitor)
	Pulse oximetry
	Arterial blood gases
Urinary	Urinary catheter
Temperature	Peripheral temperature
	Core temperature

Charts used in ITU

As patients are monitored continuously, charts are completed by the nursing staff. They show a record of physiological changes, drugs and fluids given, and laboratory results from which the medical staff can make decisions and institute treatment. Various scoring systems, such as APACHE II and III, are available to monitor the progress of critically ill patients.

A number of patients are intubated and ventilated to support their cardiovascular and respiratory systems. They tolerate the endotracheal tube and ventilator because sedatives such as midazolam (Hypnovel) and analgesics (alfentanil and morphine) are infused continuously. When the patient improves, he is gradually weaned off the ventilator.

Some patients require feeding, which is carried out using total parenteral nutrition (TPN) in patients with gastrointestinal ileus, or enteral nutrition using a nasogastric feeding tube (Clinifeed).

Predicting the outcome of critical illness

When critically ill patients are assessed for outcome after critical illness, the following patient variables are considered:

- age
- past illness
- current illness
- response to treatment
- social circumstances
- future 'quality of life'.

Outcome prediction systems are used as statistical tools only and to compare ITUs; they are not (yet) accurate enough to be applied to an individual's outcome.

Illness severity scoring systems

All ITUs have well-defined admission and treatment policies. A number of scoring systems have been developed in an attempt to quantify the relationship between disease severity and outcome.

Acute Physiology and Chronic Health Evaluation II (APACHE II). APACHE II scoring has been developed to identify prognostic groups or critically ill patients and determine the success of different forms of treatment. APACHE III has now been developed and validated, but APACHE II is still the gold standard.

The APACHE II system uses 12 physiological parameters, as shown in Box 8.4. On admission to ITU, these parameters from the critically ill patient are entered on the chart and a weighted score is assigned to each parameter. The maximum possible score is 71, although nearly all patients have scores much lower than this. A high score relates to a higher hospital mortality rate, at each 5 point increment, across a wide range of diseases.

Box 8.4   The APACHE II prognostic system
Temperature (°C)
Mean arterial pressure (mmHg)
Heart rate (bpm)
Respiratory rate
Arterial pH
Alveolar–arterial gradient (A–aDo_2) if the fractional inspired oxygen (Flo_2) is 0.5 or greater (use Pao_2 if the Flo_2 is less than 0.5)
Serum sodium level (mmol/L)
Serum potassium level (mmol/L)
Serum creatinine level (mg/100 ml)
Haematocrit (%)
White blood cell count
Glasgow Coma Scale

Therapeutic Intervention Scoring Systems (TISS). TISS assigns scores to each procedure performed on a patient in ITU, an indicator of the severity of illness and of the prognosis. The nurse/patient ratio and the staff/bed utilization are also used in TISS scoring.

A competent ITU nurse can handle up to 40–50 TISS points per day. An unacceptably high TISS score indicates that the patient needs active treatment and cannot be discharged from ITU.

TISS is a valuable administration tool for the ITU, but it cannot predict the outcome in a patient.

Sickness scoring. This is a modification of APACHE II scoring, the modifications being:

- units such as mg and mmol are converted to SI units;
- haemoglobin concentration rather than haematocrit is used;
- oxygenation is assessed using a ratio of FIO_2 and PaO_2;
- the Glasgow coma scale is modified using clinical judgment;
- the 'chronic disease' category is redefined to include conditions associated with loss of independent self-care;
- haemodynamic instability is assessed to reflect overall abnormalities rather than transient, drug-induced changes;
- daily scores are charted to assess the response to treatment.

Other predictors and scoring systems include:

1. the Simplified Acute Physiology Score;
2. Mortality Prediction Models;
3. the Injury Severity Score.

The number of patients who die in ITU used to be high because of multiorgan failure or severe septicaemia, but with advances in monitoring, organ support and antibiotics, the survival rate has improved. Patients who are admitted to ITU after cardiac surgery, neurosurgery or transplantation for postoperative observation are sent back to the ward once they have stabilized.

THE HIGH-DEPENDENCY UNIT

The HDU provides an intermediate level of care for acutely ill patients who do not require the full facilities of an ITU but need a higher intensity of medical and nursing care than can be provided in a general ward.

Patient selection

The HDU admits patients with potentially reversible acute surgical or medical conditions:

- preoperative stabilization of seriously ill emergency patients;
- postoperative care of major surgical patients (e.g. after repair of an abdominal aortic aneurysm);
- acutely ill medical or surgical patients who are not suitable for the coronary care unit (e.g. patients with diabetic ketoacidosis);
- patients with significant trauma not requiring mechanical ventilation (e.g. closed head injury with other fractures);
- patients in transition from ITU who are not yet ready to return to the general ward.

Comprehensive clinical and nursing care is provided to all the patients admitted to the HDU.

Discharge from HDU

Patients who satisfy the following criteria are discharged from the HDU:

- The original indication for admission to the HDU has been corrected.
- The optimal treatment is available on the ward.
- The condition of the patient in HDU may deteriorate and he or she need to be transferred to ITU.

TRANSPORT OF CRITICALLY ILL PATIENTS

ODPs, along with anaesthetic and recovery nurses, play a major role in the transportation of critically ill patients from ITU to theatre or other areas, such as CT scanning, MRI scanning or another ITU in a different hospital.

Safe transport of the critically ill patients involves:

- explanation to the patient (where communication is possible) or relatives of what is planned;
- stabilization of the patient optimally before transportation;

- movement of the patient in a planned, unhurried manner;
- maintaining the stability of the patient during transit, continuing all monitoring and liaising with the receiving staff.

FURTHER READING

Recovery period

Bromage P R, Camporesi E, Chestnut D 1980 Epidural narcotics for postoperative analgesia. Anaesthesia 59: 473–480

Caplan R A, Ready L B, Olson G L, Nessly M L 1986 Transdermal delivery of fentanyl for postoperative pain. Anesthesiology 65: A196

Covino R G 1988 Intrapleural analgesia. Anesthesia and Analgesia 67: 427–429

Dodson M E 1985 The management of postoperative pain. Edward Arnold, London

Modig J, Paljow L 1981 A comparison of epidural morphine and epidural bupivacaine for postoperative pain relief. Acta Anaesthesiologica Scandinavica 25: 437–441

Oh T E 1995 Intensive care manual. Butterworth, Sydney

Park G, Fulton B 1991 The management of acute pain. Oxford Medical Publications, Oxford

Shapiro G 1990 Post anaesthetic care problems. Anesthetics Clinics of North America 8: 2

Watcha M F, White P F 1992 Postoperative nausea and vomiting. Anesthesiology 77: 162–184

Intensive care

Bion J F, Aitchinson T C, Edlin S A, Ledingham I M 1988 Sickness scoring and response to treatment as predictors of outcome from critical illness. Intensive Care Medicine 14: 167–171

Braman S, Dunn S 1987 Complications of intrahospital transfer in critically ill patients. Annals of Internal Medicine 107: 469–473

Cullen D J, Civetta J M 1974 Therapeutic intervention scoring system: a method for quantitative comparison of patient care. Critical Care Medicine 2: 57–60

Gilligan J E 1985 Stabilization and transport of the critically ill. Clinics in Anaesthesiology 3: 789–810

Keene A R, Cullen D J 1983 Therapeutic Intervention Scoring System update 1983. Critical Care Medicine 11: 1–3

Knaus W A, Draper E A, Wagner D P 1985 APACHE II: a severity of disease classification system. Critical Care 13: 818–829

Merlone S, Hackel A 1995 Care of the patients during long distance transport. In: Hackel A (ed) Critical care transport. International Anesthesiology Clinics 25: 105–116

Society of Critical Care Medicine 1988 Recommendations for services and personnel for delivery of care in a critical care setting. Task force on guidelines. Critical Care Medicine 16: 809–811

Society of Critical Care Medicine 1988 Recommendations for critical care design. Task force on guidelines. Critical Care Medicine 16: 796–806

9

Cardiopulmonary resuscitation

The term 'cardiac arrest' implies a sudden interruption of cardiac output, which may be reversible with appropriate treatment. Survival from cardiac arrest is most likely when the event is witnessed, when a bystander summons help from the emergency services and starts resuscitation, when the heart arrests in ventricular fibrillation, and when defibrillation and advanced life support are initiated at an early stage. Basic life support is one link in this chain of survival.

BASIC LIFE SUPPORT

Basic life support is the emergency treatment of any condition in which the brain suddenly fails to receive enough oxygen. It involves assessment followed by action: the ABC:

- **A** is for **A**ssessment followed by **A**ction
- **B** is for **B**reathing
- **C** is for **C**irculation.

ASSESSMENT

It is essential rapidly to assess any danger to the casualty and the resuscitator from hazards such as masonry, gas, electricity, fire or traffic. Establish whether the casualty is responsive by gently shaking his or her shoulders and asking loudly, 'Are you all right?'. Be careful not to aggravate any existing injury, particularly of the cervical spine. If there is no response, shout for help or send a bystander to telephone for an ambulance (or if in hospital, the cardiac arrest team). Complete the assessment by opening the airway, checking for breathing and checking for the pulse. Loosen tight clothing around the casualty's neck and remove any obvious obstruction from the mouth; leave well-fitting dentures in place. Extend, but do not hyperextend, the neck, thus lifting the tongue off the posterior wall of the pharynx. This is best achieved by placing the hand along the casualty's upper forehead and exerting pressure to tilt the head, at the same time placing two fingertips under the point of the chin to lift it forwards. This will allow breathing to start.

Look, listen, and feel for breathing. *Look* for chest movement; *listen* close to the mouth for breath sounds; *feel* for breath sounds, and feel for air with your cheek. Look, listen and feel for 5 s before deciding that breathing is absent.

Check for a pulse. The best pulse to feel is the carotid artery, but if the neck is injured the pulse may be felt at the femoral artery. Feel for 5 s before deciding it is absent.

ACTION

Recovery position

If the casualty is unconscious but has a pulse and is breathing, place him or her in the recovery position, if necessary supporting the chin to maintain an airway. Go or telephone for help if your initial call has not been answered. If the pulse or breathing is absent, your subsequent action should again follow the ABC.

Airway

If after tilting and lifting the chin the airway still seems to be obstructed, there may be a foreign body present. First try to remove this by finger sweeps in the mouth. If this is not successful, give five firm blows between the scapulae; this may dislodge a foreign body by compressing the air that remains in the lungs, thereby producing an upward force behind the obstructing material.

If both finger sweeps and back blows fail to clear the airway, try five abdominal thrusts. In an unconscious person kneel over the casualty, make a fist of one of your hands and place it immediately below the casualty's xiphisternum. Grasp this fist with your other hand and push firmly and suddenly upwards and posteriorly. Alternate abdominal thrusts with back slaps.

BREATHING

If there is no breathing but a pulse is present, make sure that the casualty is on his or her back and give 10 breaths of expired air ventilation. Maintain the airway by tilting the head and lifting the chin. Pinch the casualty's nose closed with the fingers of your hand on the forehead. Take a deep breath, seal your lips firmly around those of the casualty and breathe out until you see the chest rising, taking about 2 s for full ventilation. The chest should rise as you blow in and fall when you take your mouth away. After 10 ventilations, if the casualty is still not breathing and help is not on its way, go and telephone for assistance. Return to the casualty, reassess the consciousness, breathing and pulse and continue ventilation as necessary, rechecking the pulse after every 10 breaths.

CIRCULATION

If the pulse is absent (cardiac arrest), it is unlikely that the casualty will recover as a result of cardiopulmonary resuscitation alone; advanced life support such as a defibrillator is urgently required. If no help has yet arrived, start chest compression.

The correct place to compress is in the centre of the lower half of the sternum. Place your middle finger on the xiphisternum and index finger on the sternum above. Slide the heel of your first hand and place it on top of the second. Press down firmly, keeping your arms straight and elbows locked. In an adult, compress about 4–5 cm, keeping the pressure firm, controlled and applied vertically. Try to spend about the same time in the compressed phase as in the released phase, and aim for a rate of 80 compressions per minute. After each 15 compressions, tilt the head, lift the chin and give two inflations. Return your hands immediately to the sternum and give 15 further compressions, continuing compression and ventilations in a ratio of 15:2.

If two trained rescuers are present, one should assume responsibility for ventilation and the other for chest compression. The compression rate should remain at 80 per minute, with a pause after each five compressions just long enough to allow a single ventilation to be given over about 2 s. Provided the casualty's airway is maintained, it is not necessary to wait for exhalation before resuming compressions.

ADVANCED CARDIAC LIFE SUPPORT

Cardiac arrest presents either as:

- ventricular fibrillation
- asystole
- electromechanical dissociation.

VENTRICULAR FIBRILLATION

Ventricular fibrillation (VF) is the most common cause of cardiac arrest in patients with ischaemic heart disease. VF is seen in up to 80–90% of patients dying suddenly outside hospital. The ECG shows a bizarre irregular waveform, random in both frequency and amplitude.

The definitive treatment of VF is the application of a defibrillatory countershock. A precordial thump may on occasions abolish the arrhythmia when applied very soon after its onset and should be considered in cases of witnessed, especially monitored, cardiac arrest.

The guidelines for defibrillation have recently been revised by the European Resuscitation Council and endorsed by the Resuscitation Council (UK). It is necessary to minimize the delay in the administration of defibrillatory shocks. The algorithm recommended for the management of VF (and pulseless ventricular tachycardia) is shown in Fig. 9.1.

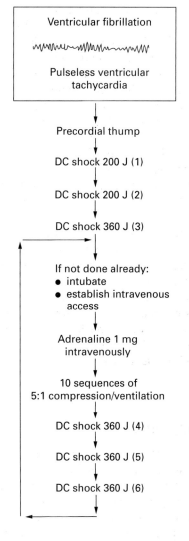

Notes:

(1) The interval between shocks 3 and 4 should not exceed 2 minutes

(2) Adrenaline should be given during each loop - i.e., every 2 to 3 minutes

(3) Continue loops for as long as defibrillation is indicated

(4) After 3 loops consider:
- an alkalising agent
- an antiarrhythmic agent

Figure 9.1 Algorithm for managing ventricular fibrillation or pulseless ventricular tachycardia.

ASYSTOLE

In asystole, ventricular standstill occurs because of the suppression of all natural or artificial cardiac pacemakers. In hospitals, 25% of cardiac arrests are due to asystole, compared with 10% outside hospital.

Asystole is diagnosed when no ventricular activity is seen on ECG. This should be confirmed by checking that the leads have not been disconnected, and that the gain and brilliance of the monitor are adequate.

The algorithm for managing asystole is given in Fig. 9.2.

ELECTROMECHANICAL DISSOCIATION

This means cardiac arrest despite normal (or near-normal) electrical excitation. Diagnosis is made from a combination of the clinical absence of cardiac output and the presence of a rhythm on the monitor. The causes of electromechanical dissociation are:

- Primary electromechanical dissociation (failure of excitation–contraction coupling):
  - myocardial infarction (inferior wall myocardial infarction);
  - β-blockers and calcium antagonists or toxins;
  - electrolyte abnormalities (hypocalcaemia and hyperkalaemia).
- Secondary electromechanical dissociation:
  - tension pneumothorax;
  - pericardial tamponade;
  - pulmonary embolus;
  - hypovolaemia.

Figure 9.3 describes the algorithm for managing electromechanical dissociation.

PROLONGED LIFE SUPPORT

Once the victim is resuscitated, he should be transferred to ITU for continued support of various organs such as brain, lungs, heart and kidneys. While in ITU, the patient is assessed for residual

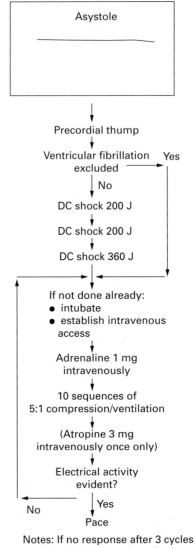

Figure 9.2 Algorithm for managing asystole.

damage, especially of the brain, following the cardiac arrest.

CARDIAC ARREST IN THE OPERATING THEATRE

If a cardiac arrest occurs in the operating theatre, the chances of a successful resuscitation are high because the precipitating causes, such as hypoxia, hypovolaemia and electrolyte imbalance, are usually reversible. Other factors that help in resuscitation are warning signs in a patient, such as cyanosis, bradycardia and hypotension, before a cardiac arrest occurs. The presence of trained staff and resuscitation equipment further contributes towards saving a patient's life.

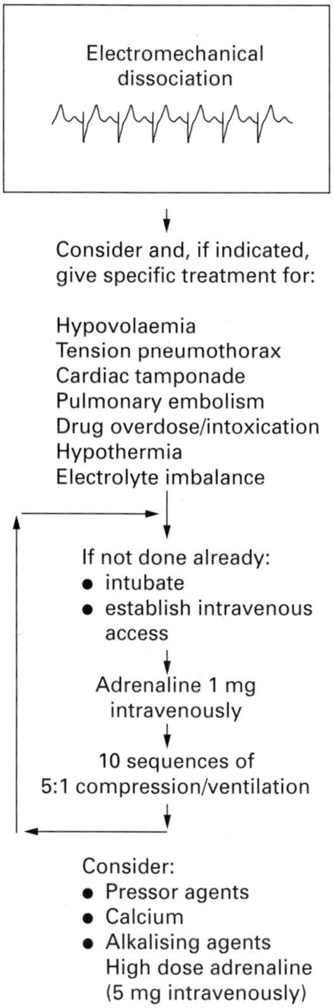

ETHICS OF RESUSCITATION

Ideally, resuscitation should be attempted only in patients whose quality of life following a successful resuscitation is likely to be good. The decision to resuscitate should depend on the wishes of the patient or of their legal representative in consultation with the doctor.

Electromechanical dissociation

Consider and, if indicated, give specific treatment for:

Hypovolaemia
Tension pneumothorax
Cardiac tamponade
Pulmonary embolism
Drug overdose/intoxication
Hypothermia
Electrolyte imbalance

If not done already:
- intubate
- establish intravenous access

Adrenaline 1 mg intravenously

10 sequences of 5:1 compression/ventilation

Consider:
- Pressor agents
- Calcium
- Alkalising agents
  High dose adrenaline
  (5 mg intravenously)

Figure 9.3 Algorithm for managing electromechanical dissociation.

FURTHER READING

Baskett P J F 1993 Resuscitation handbook, 2nd edn. Wolfe Publications, London
Colquhoun M C, Handley A J, Evans T R 1995 ABC of resuscitation, 3rd edn. British Medical Journal, London
European Resuscitation Council Advanced Life Support Working Party 1992 Guidelines for Advanced Life Support 24: 111–122
European Resuscitation Council Basic Life Support Working Group 1993 Guidelines for Basic Life Support. British Medical Journal 306: 1587–1589

10

Acid–base and electrolyte balance

Acid–base balance is a vast subject, and in this chapter an attempt will be made to simplify and correlate a few clinical situations seen in operating theatres, recovery rooms and ITUs.

The biochemistry and physiology of the lungs and kidneys are the principal basic sciences involved in acid–base balance. For the maintenance of the normal functioning of body metabolism, the composition of the cells' surroundings (extracellular) and the contents of cells (intracellular) need to be kept within certain limits. Various processes in the body, such as enzyme activity and the transport of various ions across cell membranes, are pH dependent.

WHAT IS pH?

pH describes the hydrogen ion concentration as its negative logarithm to the base 10. The normal hydrogen ion concentration is between 36 and 44 nanomols (nmol) per litre, the normal range of pH in arterial blood being 7.35–7.44. Box 10.1 shows the values of hydrogen ion concentration and their corresponding pH levels.

A member of the theatre personnel will be asked to assist the anaesthetist in obtaining an arterial blood sample and then take it to the biochemistry laboratory or the blood gas analyser machine to get the results. All blood sent for blood gas analysis must be in a preheparinized syringe. Non-heparinized samples will clot inside the delicate (and expensive) workings of the blood gas analyser. The print-out usually shows the values listed in Box 10.2.

Box 10.1 Relationship of hydrogen ion concentration to pH	
Hydrogen ions (nmol/L)	pH (units)
10	8.0
16	7.8
25	7.6
40	7.4
63	7.2
100	7.0

Box 10.2 Normal values on arterial blood gas sampling	
H+	36–44
Po_2	11–13.5 kPa
Pco_2	4.6–6.0 kPa
Standard bicarbonate	22–24 mmol/L
Actual bicarbonate	24–26 mmol/L
Base excess	–2 to +2 mmol/L

In Box 10.2, the pH is the hydrogen ion concentration as described above, Po_2 is the oxygen tension, and Pco_2 is the carbon dioxide tension.

SBC is the standard bicarbonate; this is not the actual bicarbonate of the sample but a calculated value. The bicarbonate level in the blood depends on both a renal (kidney) contribution and a respiratory (carbon dioxide) contribution. The standard bicarbonate is the bicarbonate that would be present if the patient's carbon dioxide level were normal, i.e. 5.3 kPa.

ABC is the actual bicarbonate, which is the actual bicarbonate concentration in the plasma at the patient's present body temperature and Pco_2 level.

BE is the base excess, which is defined as the amount of acid or base (in mmol/L) required to titrate the pH back to 7.40 at a temperature of 38°C with a Pco_2 of 5.3 kPa. It is a measure of the severity of the metabolic (kidney) component of an acid–base disturbance.

After interpreting the above results, it can be discovered whether the patient's acid–base imbalance (alkalosis or acidosis) is respiratory, metabolic or mixed in origin. The following definitions will further simplify the understanding of the acid–base balance:

- Acidaemia: the hydrogen ion concentration is above the normal range.
- Alkalaemia: the hydrogen ion concentration is below the normal range.
- Acidosis: a process whereby acid accumulates, and may lead to acidaemia.
- Alkalosis: a process that causes excess base and may lead to alkalaemia.

Alkalosis can be of respiratory (respiratory alkalosis) or metabolic (metabolic alkalosis) origin. Similarly, acidosis can be respiratory (respiratory acidosis) or metabolic (metabolic acidosis) in cause. In all these conditions, compensation occurs to varying degrees. Compensation involves a secondary acid–base disturbance that brings the pH changes caused by primary disturbance to within normal limits.

METABOLIC ALKALOSIS

This can occur in a patient who has been vomiting, with a consequent loss of hydrochloric acid (secreted by the stomach). Metabolic alkalosis is also seen following the ingestion of large amounts of sodium bicarbonate. Patients may present with signs of confusion as a result of a decreased cerebral blood flow and tetany due to a fall in the ionized calcium levels in the plasma. In these patients, the body compensates as far as possible by underventilating and increasing the excretion of bicarbonate in the urine.

A typical arterial blood gas picture in metabolic alkalosis is outlined in Box 10.3. The Po_2 may be high or normal.

Box 10.3 Arterial blood gas picture in metabolic alkalosis	
pH	Above 7.45
Pco_2	35–45 mmHg (4.66–5.8 kPa)
Standard bicarbonate	Above 26 mmol/L
Actual bicarbonate	Above 26 mmol/L
Base excess	above +2 mmol/L

When this metabolic alkalosis is compensated by respiratory changes (underventilation), the arterial blood gases become similar to those given in Box 10.4.

A typical arterial blood gas picture is contained in Box 10.6.

Box 10.4 Arterial blood gas picture in compensated metabolic alkalosis	
pH	7.35–7.45
P_{CO_2}	Above 45 mmHg (5.86 kPa)
Standard bicarbonate	Above 26 mmol/L
Actual bicarbonate	Above 26 mmol/L
Base excess	+2 mmol/L

Box 10.6 Arterial blood gas picture in metabolic acidosis	
pH	7.19
P_{CO_2}	33 (4.4 kPa)
Standard bicarbonate	14 mmol/L
Actual bicarbonate	13 mmol/L
Base excess	−14 mmol/L

RESPIRATORY ALKALOSIS

This occurs following hyperventilation, with a consequent fall in P_{CO_2} and a rise in pH. The effects of hypocapnia include a decreased cerebral blood flow, clouding of consciousness and a fall in blood pressure, with lowered ionized calcium and sodium levels. It prolongs the action of muscle relaxants such as gallamine and shortens the action of d-tubocurarine.

During anaesthesia, a moderate hyperventilation (P_{CO_2} of 3.0–3.5 kPa) can reduce the requirement for barbiturates and analgesia, and potentiate hypotensive anaesthesia (see p. 194).

The side-effects of hypocapnia during anaesthesia include fetal asphyxia (during caesarean section if the mother is hyperventilated), a fall in cardiac output, and cerebral changes in elderly patients due to vasoconstriction of cerebral blood vessels.

Box 10.5 shows a typical arterial blood gas picture in respiratory alkalosis.

Box 10.5 Arterial blood gas picture in respiratory alkalosis	
pH	7.5
P_{CO_2}	18 mmHg (2.4 kPa)
Standard bicarbonate	20.5 mmol/L
Actual bicarbonate	14 mmol/L
Base excess	±1 mmol/L

METABOLIC ACIDOSIS

This occurs in diabetic ketoacidosis, starvation, salicylate poisoning and acute renal failure. The clinical signs include clouding of consciousness, cold blue hands and feet, and gasping respiration.

RESPIRATORY ACIDOSIS

This occurs during the administration of anaesthesia following underventilation due to respiratory obstruction, narcotic overdose, faulty carbon dioxide absorption by the soda lime absorber and accidental administration of carbon dioxide. A rise in carbon dioxide causes an increase in cerebral blood flow and intracranial pressure, and a rise in catecholamines, which in turn cause an increase in cardiac output and contraction of the heart. Peripheral resistance is decreased. The typical arterial blood gas picture is found in Box 10.7.

Box 10.7 Arterial blood gas picture in respiratory acidosis	
pH	7.22
P_{CO_2}	80 mmHg (10.7 kPa)
Standard bicarbonate	26 mmol/L
Actual bicarbonate	31.5 mmol/L
Base excess	+2.5 mmol/L

ELECTROLYTE BALANCE

DEHYDRATION

Dehydration is defined as a reduction in the total water content of the body. There may be a pure water loss, or water and sodium may be lost together.

Causes

- Water deficiency
  - Diminished water intake.
  - Increased loss of water.

- Sodium deficiency
  - Increased sodium loss due to sweating or hyperthermia.
  - From gastrointestinal secretions due to vomiting, loss from fistulae, loss from ileostomy and jejunostomy, or gastric aspiration.
  - Urinary loss as in Addison's disease, panhypopituitarism, the diuretic phase of acute renal failure or osmotic diuresis.
  - Diarrhoea.
  - Haemorrhage.
  - The accumulation of extracellular fluid in the intestines and pleural and peritoneal cavities.
  - Decreased sodium intake due to the inability to swallow, in the postoperative period, low-sodium diets.

Symptoms and signs

- Thirst, weakness and muscle cramps.
- Oliguria (less than 400 ml/24 hours; except where cause is inappropriate high output renal disease), low blood pressure, mental confusion and hallucinations.

Investigations

- Rise in blood urea level to above 100 mg/ml.
- Plasma sodium and chloride levels increase above normal levels in pure water loss.
- Plasma sodium and chloride levels fall as sodium deficiency becomes severe in mixed water and salt loss.

Treatment

- Water deficiency
  - Give water by mouth or nasogastric tube.
  - If necessary, an i.v. infusion with 5% dextrose.
  - If water deficiency is due to diabetes insipidus, vasopressin 2–5 IU i.m. every other day.
- Sodium deficiency
  - Oral sodium chloride may be added to the diet or taken as tablets or in solution.

- Isotonic sodium chloride is given i.v., with simultaneous correction of potassium and hydrogen ion levels.
- If sodium deficiency is caused by adrenal insufficiency, hydrocortisone (25–50 mg daily) is given.

SODIUM EXCESS

This is an increase in the total amount of body sodium.

Causes

Sodium excess could be due to excessive intake or the inability to excrete sodium.

- Excess intake
  - Overtransfusion with isotonic or hypertonic sodium-containing fluids.
  - Excessive oral administration in an unconscious patient (conscious patients would complain of thirst and thus protect themselves).
- Inability to excrete sodium
  - Primary hyperaldosteronism.
  - Excessive use of corticosteroids.
  - Essential hypernatraemia.

Symptoms and signs

The symptoms and signs are usually those accompanying the disease. Hyperosmolarity (a serum sodium level above 160 mmol/L) causes cerebral symptoms such as confusion, dullness, apathy and coma.

Investigations

- Plasma sodium and chloride levels are raised (sodium up to and above 150 mmol/L)
- Potassium level is normal in essential hypernatraemia but lowered in hyperaldosteronism.
- Plasma bicarbonate is above 28 mmol/L in hyperaldosteronism.
- Urinary specific gravity is above 1020.

Treatment

- Hypernatraemia due to excess intake is treated with a sodium-free regimen together with a high water intake of 3–5 L per day.
- In essential hypernatraemia, along with a sodium-free regimen, the water intake should be restricted to 3.5 L/day.
- Primary hyperaldosteronism and Cushing's syndrome are treated with the appropriate surgical or medical therapy.

POTASSIUM DEFICIENCY

This refers to a subnormal concentration of potassium in the extracellular fluid and also in the intracellular fluid.

Causes

- Decreased intake
  - Inability to swallow.
  - Parenteral therapy without potassium supplements.
  - Special diets without potassium.
- Decreased absorption
  - Overdosage with potassium-binding ion-exchange resin (Resonium A).
- Increased urinary loss
  - Primary or secondary hyperaldosteronism.
  - Cushing's syndrome.
  - Treatment with steroids.
  - Treatment with diuretics (except spironolactone).
- Loss from the gastrointestinal tract
  - Vomiting.
  - Gastric or intestinal aspiration.
  - Fistulae or ileostomy.
  - Diarrhoea.

Symptoms and signs

- Tachycardia, extrasystoles and cardiac failure.
- The ECG shows a prolonged QT interval, a depressed ST segment and flat T waves.

- Abdominal distension and paralytic ileus.
- Weakness and hypotonia.
- Proteinuria and impaired urinary concentrating power.

Investigations

- Serum potassium level below 3.5 mmol/L.

POTASSIUM EXCESS

Potassium excess is defined as a raised concentration of potassium.

Causes

- Decreased renal excretion of potassium
  - Oliguria or anuria from any cause.
  - Use of aldosterone antagonists (e.g. spironolactone).
- Increased catabolism of endogenous proteins
  - Following trauma.
  - In untreated diabetic coma.
- Excessive intake of potassium
  - by mouth or i.v. in the presence of oliguria.

Symptoms and signs

- Mental confusion, tingling and numbness of the feet, and bradycardia.
- Irregular rhythm and heart block.
- The ECG shows peaked T waves with a potassium level of 6.5 mmol/L, followed by widening of the QRS complex, an increased PR interval, loss of the P wave, arrhythmia and cardiac arrest.

Investigations

- Serum potassium level above 5.4 mmol/L.
- If associated with renal failure, the blood urea is raised and the plasma bicarbonate is lowered.
- In adrenal failure, the plasma sodium and chloride concentrations tend to be low.

FURTHER READING

Gardner M L 1985 Medical acid–base balance: the basic principles. Baillière Tindall, London

Goldberger A 1985 A primer of water, electrolytes and acid–base syndromes. Lea & Febiger, Philadelphia, PA

11

Management of chronic pain

Chronic or intractable pain is defined as that pain which is not relieved by conventional treatment. Pain is considered to be chronic partly when it has reached a certain duration (classically 6 weeks) but especially when it has disabled the patient either physically, psychologically or socially. The intensity of pain will be influenced not only by physical factors, but also by the circumstances (environment) and by psychological and emotional factors.

PAIN MANAGEMENT SERVICES

There are three types of recognized service:

1. A single-handed practice is where an anaesthetist interested in pain relief work sees patients on a limited scale. He or she carries out simple examinations and nerve blocks.

2. A multidisciplinary service is where a number of specialists, such as a physician, surgeon, anaesthetist, neurosurgeon, psychologist, psychiatrist, physiotherapist and social worker, are involved. There is an organized outpatient clinic with adequate junior medical and nursing staff. These types of clinics are rare in the UK but are often seen in the USA.

3. The intermediate group, somewhere between the single-handed practice and multidisciplinary service, is that most often seen in the UK. This type of service is usually run by one or two consultants with an interest in pain, with outpatient facilities, arrangements for investigations, one or two inpatient beds, operating time and radio-

logical facilities to perform nerve blocks. The support staff consists of nurses specialists in pain and secretaries, with access to physiotherapists and radiologists.

The Association of Anaesthetists of Great Britain and Ireland's working party on the management of non-acute chronic pain believes and recommends the following:

- Pain management makes frequent demands on the services of physiotherapy, clinical psychology and radiology.
- Pain management should be based on an interdisciplinary rather than a multidisciplinary approach.
- Members of other disciplines that support the pain services should be experienced in dealing with this often difficult group of patients and familiar with the aims and objectives of pain management.

Referral to the pain management services

A number of referrals to pain management services are from general practitioners, orthopaedic surgeons, vascular surgeons and local hospices. To a certain extent, ophthalmologists and ENT surgeons also refer patients to the clinic.

Types of patient referred

The types of patient referred to the clinic are those suffering from:

- Vascular conditions
  - Migraine
  - Raynaud's disease
  - Claudication due to non-surgical vascular disease.
- Orthopaedic conditions
  - Backache
  - Arthritis, both osteo- and rheumatoid.
- Neurological conditions
  - Trigeminal neuralgia
  - Post-herpetic neuralgia
  - Nerve entrapment syndromes, such as scar pain and back pain
  - Pain from neuromas: stump pain

  - Central pain, for example phantom limb pain and thalamic pain
  - Pain from abnormal neural responses to trauma: dysaesthesias and hyperaesthesias.
- Pain due to carcinoma
  - Arising from the primary growth
  - Due to metastasis
  - Following treatment (e.g. radiotherapy).
- Unknown cause: atypical facial pain.

These are only a few of the wide range of conditions presenting at such a clinic.

ASSESSMENT OF PATIENTS WITH CHRONIC PAIN

All the patients referred to the pain relief clinic are assessed thoroughly, including obtaining a history and carrying out a clinical examination and investigations, and a definitive diagnosis is made, following which treatment is carried out. In some patients, in spite of lengthy investigations, no definitive cause can be found, and their pain is treated symptomatically.

A number of patients with chronic pain suffer from anxiety and depression. They are assessed by a psychologist and psychiatrist, and treatment is prescribed. Many patients fear that their pain must be a sign of cancer; physical examination and investigation can reassure both them and their doctors that this is not the case.

Chronic pain is multifactorial, and social, ethnic, religious and cultural factors all contribute to the perception of pain.

Pain measurement

Pain measurement is carried out for two reasons:

1. clinical purposes;
2. research purposes (to allow comparison of treatments).

Clinical pain measurement is carried out to determine the amount of pain related to a disease process and to assess the alleviation or worsening of the pain by treatment of an individual. Research measurement provides an insight into the nature of pain experience and allows comparison of different treatments between groups of patients.

Pain scales

The following scales are used:

- visual analogue scale
- verbal rating scale
- numerical rating scale.

The McGill pain questionnaire is a sensitive, valid and useful tool for measuring pain.

MANAGEMENT OF PATIENTS WITH CHRONIC PAIN

The management of patients with chronic pain depends on their life expectancy. Patients with a normal life expectancy suffering from chronic pain are treated differently from those who have a short life expectancy (e.g. patients with terminal cancer pain).

Patients with normal life expectancy

These patients are usually suffering from backache, post-herpetic neuralgia, Raynaud's disease or postoperative scar pain. The aim of intervention consists of a proper diagnosis and treatment. For example, a patient with backache needs to be investigated by either an orthopaedic surgeon or a neurosurgeon, and if there is a surgical cause, surgical correction should be carried out. If the patient has no surgical cause for the pain, the following line of pain management is followed:

Drugs

Patients are prescribed non-steroidal anti-inflammatory drugs (NSAIDs). For mild-to-moderate pain, acetylsalicylic acid (Aspirin), codeine or dihydrocodeine, and dextropropoxyphene (Distalgesic) are prescribed; for severe pain, buprenorphine (Temgesic), nalbuphine (Nubain) or meptazinol (Meptid) is given. Potent analgesics such as morphine and diamorphine are not prescribed as a first-line treatment, partly because of their side-effects (dizziness, nausea, constipation and risk of addiction) and partly because the opiate drugs are not particularly effective for this type of pain.

Other drugs used include carbamazepine (Tegretol), prescribed in the treatment of trigeminal neuralgia, and phenytoin (Dilantin) and sodium valproate (Epilim), prescribed for patients with post-herpetic neuralgia.

Nerve blocks

These are carried out with local anaesthetics such as 0.25–0.5% plain bupivacaine (Marcain). The blocks performed are local infiltration for scar pain and individual nerve blocks. Epidural blocks are performed for low back pain and sciatica, using 2% plain lignocaine or 0.25% plain Marcain and triamcinolone (Lederspan). The epidural blocks are performed at either the cervical, thoracic, lumbar or caudal level. Blocks are occasionally used as diagnostic tools: if blocking the nerve relieves the pain, therapy can be directed more accurately.

Alternative methods of pain relief

When the pain relief is inadequate in such patients with normal life expectancy following the use of drugs and nerve blocks, alternative lines of treatment include:

1. *Transcutaneous electrical nerve stimulation* (TENS). A small battery-operated stimulator is used to apply an electrical stimulus to the skin overlying the painful area via flexible electrodes.
2. *Acupuncture.* This treatment is based upon the principle that the insertion of needles at certain points of the body can produce analgesia. Acupuncture points are areas of low electrical resistance of the skin, and acupuncture needles are inserted to varying depths at these points. Electroacupuncture and laser acupuncture seem to have a considerable effect in the management of patients with chronic pain.
3. Hypnosis, biofeedback and operant conditioning are other alternative methods of pain relief.

A combination of drug therapy and alternative methods of pain relief can be effective.

In a multidisciplinary approach to the pain management of patients with non-malignant chronic pain, the aim should be to:

- decrease the pain;
- decrease analgesic consumption;
- improve mobility or social functioning, or decrease 'sickness behaviour';
- improve the well-being of the individual.

This is achieved by taking the patients through pain management programmes that consist of exposing the patients to various specialists, including physiotherapists, social workers, nurse specialists in pain and clinical psychologists, in a group setting. The patients discuss various factors that contribute to their pain and learn coping strategies.

Back pain is the most common pain for which patients are referred to the pain management services. Back pain occurs in about 60% of people at some time in their life, leading to sickness invalidity benefits being paid out that cost the health services approximately £480 million a year, with lost production costs totalling approximately £3.8 billion a year. Pain management programmes are ideal for such patients' rehabilitation and retraining.

Other patients who benefit from such pain management programmes include sufferers from fibromyalgia and myalgia encephalitica (ME).

Patients with short life expectancy

The aim of treatment in this group of patients is to make them pain free, and the danger of addiction to narcotic drugs and the side-effects of permanent nerve blocks do not take precedence.

The line of management consists of the following.

Drug therapy

As the aim is a pain-free patient, drugs are prescribed on a regular rather than on an 'as necessary' basis. The World Health Organization describes (and recommends) a 'pain ladder' of:

- simple analgesia
- weak opiates
- strong opiates.

In cancer or terminally ill patients, the weak opiate phase may be skipped, but the treatment programme should not go straight to opiates after diagnosis until simple analgesics (NSAIDs) have failed.

'Breakthrough' doses are also prescribed.

Subcutaneous infusions of diamorphine are set up in patients who cannot tolerate oral analgesia. Transdermal fentanyl (Durogesic) is also prescribed to alleviate patients' pain.

Nerve blocks

Before carrying out permanent blocks, temporary nerve blocks using local anaesthetic solutions are tried. This will confirm whether the block is likely to be effective. An image intensifier is essential when carrying out some blocks such as chemical sympathectomy and celiac plexus blocks. The X-ray image will confirm proper positioning of the needle before injection.

The following are some of the important nerve blocks:

- *Trigeminal nerve block.* The block of this nerve and its branches is carried out for the relief of facial pain in patients suffering from trigeminal neuralgia.
- *Intrathecal block.* This technique can be very effective, but it is rarely used as some degree of paralysis is inevitable. A hyperbaric solution of phenol in glycerine is used. If this block is performed in the sacral region, sphincter control is lost, resulting in urinary retention.
- *Autonomic blocks.* Stellate ganglion block is carried out to relieve pain of vascular origin.
- *Lumbar chemical sympathectomy* is carried out to relieve the pain of claudication and to improve blood flow to the lower limbs. It is performed using an image intensifier and 6% aqueous phenol.
- *Celiac plexus block* is carried out to relieve pain resulting from malignancy of usually the pancreas. An image intensifier and either 50% alcohol or phenol are used.

Epidural implants and opiate administration. In patients with intractable pain due to malignancy (which could be opiate sensitive or partially sensitive), epidural implantation is carried out, through which a combination of diamorphine and local anaesthetics can be infused continuously, with a facility available for the PCA mode of delivery. Other drugs that can be given through these indwelling devices include midazolam, ketamine and clonidine.

Cryoanalgesia

Cryoanalgesia is the destruction of the nerves using cold temperature probes. The probe (called a cryoprobe) consists of an insulated needle; it produces a cooling effect using nitrous oxide as the refrigerant. The probe tip can reach temperatures of up to $-80°C$, thus causing nerve destruction at the site of application.

Radiofrequency lesion

The radiofrequency lesion-maker uses a high-frequency alternating current that flows from the tip of the electrodes to the tissues. Temperatures above $45°C$ damage the nerve fibres, thus preventing the conduction of nerve impulses. This radiofrequency generator is used in the treatment of trigeminal neuralgia and in percutaneous cervical cordotomy.

Cordotomies

Anterolateral cordotomy is a procedure carried out on the anterolateral tracts of the spinal cord in which the nerve tracts are sectioned. This relieves the pain on the opposite side of the body.

Pituitary ablation

Alcohol injection into the pituitary gland is carried out in patients with severe cancer pain. This technique involves inserting a needle into the pituitary area via the transphenoidal route. After confirming the position of the needle using an image intensifier, increments of 0.1 ml absolute alcohol are injected until the desired effect is achieved.

ROLE OF OPERATING THEATRE PERSONNEL IN PAIN MANAGEMENT SERVICES

Anaesthetic nurses and the ODPs are involved in the organization of trolleys containing needles, syringes and drugs. Similarly, they are involved in the organization of nerve block sessions.

FURTHER READING

Anderson S, Bond M, Mehta M, Swerdlow M 1987 Chronic non-cancer pain. MTP Press, Lancaster
Melzack R, Wall P 1994 Pain. Churchill Livingstone, Edinburgh

Raj P 1995 Pain Medicine. C V Mosby, St Louis
Warfield C A 1991 Manual of pain management. J B Lippincott, Philadelphia, PA

12

Nursing research and statistics

NURSING RESEARCH

Nursing research has expanded considerably since the late 1980s. Nurses can utilize the findings from research and make informed decisions in the delivery of nursing care.

Nursing care can be divided into the following stages:

1. *Assessment.* This consists of the systematic collection of data from various resources, such as clients, families, patients, notes or nurses' observations.
2. *Diagnosis.* Based on the analysis of the information collected during the assessment stage, nurses can develop a nursing diagnosis.
3. *Planning.* The planning stage of the nursing process involves decision-making with regard to when and what nursing actions are needed.
4. *Intervention.* The findings of research are made use of in the intervention stage.
5. *Evaluation.* This stage evaluates the outcomes and goals achieved by the intervention stage.

Kerlinger (1973) has defined scientific research as 'the systematic, controlled, empirical and critical investigation of hypothetical propositions about the presumed relations among natural phenomena'.

METHODS OF NURSING RESEARCH

Two types of research methods are available:

1. *Qualitative research* involves the systematic collection and analysis of subjective narrative materials, with a minimum of researcher-imposed control.
2. *Quantitative research* involves the systematic collection of numerical information, often under controlled conditions, and the analysis of this information using statistical procedures.

Qualitative research emphasizes the dynamic, holistic and individual aspects of human experience. It:

- attempts to understand the entirety of a phenomenon rather than a specific concept;
- collects information without any structured format;
- has few preconceived ideas; qualitative research is principally observational and can make no causative links;
- attempts to capture the concept in its entirety;
- analyses information in an organized fashion.

Quantitative research, on the other hand, emphasizes the rules of logic and deductive reasoning. It:

- focuses on a small number of specific ideas;
- begins with preconceived ideas about how these ideas are interrelated;
- collects information in a structured format;
- analyses information using statistical procedures.

Thus, quantitative research sets out to answer a specific question about a subject. What the answer to that question might be is not 'preconceived'; i.e. quantitative research tries to establish whether there is or is not a causative link between observed phenomena.

ETHICAL CONSIDERATIONS IN RESEARCH

The protection of the rights of human subjects is a high priority amongst doctors and nurses. The ethical principles upon which the standards of ethical conduct in research are based include:

- respect for human dignity
- justice
- non-maleficence (above all, do no harm).

Respect for human dignity

This principle includes the right to self-determination, i.e. clients, subjects or patients have the right to participate – or not – in a study without prejudicing their care or being subjected to pressure. Also included is the right to full disclosure, i.e. all material or likely risks must be explained, as must the purely research nature of the project. The right to self-determination must be emphasized.

Justice

This principle includes the subjects' rights to fair treatment and to privacy.

Non-maleficence

This principle includes the clause in which the researcher should do no harm to the subject. The subject should not be exploited, either overtly or subtly. The researcher should tell the subject about potential benefits and strive to maximize these.

Research subjects' risks should be weighed against the benefits to the subjects themselves. No study is ethical if research subjects are put at risk for nebulous benefits 'to the greater good', without any possible or theoretical benefit to themselves.

INFORMED CONSENT

This means that subjects have been adequately informed regarding the research and that they are capable of comprehending the information and have the power of free choice, enabling them voluntarily to consent or decline to participate in the research, knowing the possible benefits and risks they face.

RESEARCH PROCESS

In the research process, the researcher starts at the beginning of the study (asking a question) and comes to an end-point (obtaining an answer).

The major phases of a research project are outlined below.

Phase 1: The conceptual phase

This phase involves thinking, reading, theorizing and reviewing ideas with advisors.

The four main steps in the conceptual phase are shown in Box 12.1.

Box 12.1	The conceptual phase
Step 1	Formulating and delimiting the programme
Step 2	Reviewing the related literature
Step 3	Developing a theoretical framework
Step 4	Formulating a hypothesis

Phase 2: The design and planning phase

This phase involves the investigator making a number of decisions about the methods to be used to address the research question and test the hypotheses and plan for collection of data (Box 12.2).

Box 12.2	The design and planning phase
Step 5	Selecting a research design
Step 6	Identifying the population to be studied
Step 7	Selecting measures for the research variables
Step 8	Designing the sampling plan
Step 9	Finalizing and reviewing the research plan
Step 10	Conducting the pilot study and making revisions

Phase 3: The empirical phase

This phase involves the collection of research data and the preparation of those data for analysis (Box 12.3).

Box 12.3	The empirical phase
Step 11	Collecting the data
Step 12	Preparing the data for analysis

Phase 4: The analytical phase

The data gathered in the empirical phase are subjected to various types of analysis and interpretation (Box 12.4).

Box 12.4	The analytical phase
Step 13	Communicating the findings
Step 14	Utilizing the findings

STATISTICS

Statistics is a fundamental tool for the investigative process in all biological and medical sciences. It is always essential to contact a statistician, who will assist in deciding:

- the sample size and power considerations
- questionnaires
- the choice of sample and control subjects
- the design of the study
- laboratory experiments
- displaying data
- the choice of statistical analysis.

At the planning stage, it is important to review different types of design study and consider the objectives:

- What is the major objective of the study?
- Is it clinically worthwhile?
- Are the secondary objectives stated clearly?
- Is it defined clearly?

TYPES OF STUDY

Research reports can be classified into two broad groups:

1. Longitudinal studies:
    (a) prospective studies:
        (i) deliberate interventions: randomized and non-randomized
        (ii) observational studies
    (b) retrospective studies:
        (i) deliberate intervention
        (ii) observational studies.
2. Cross-sectional studies:
    (a) disease description
    (b) diagnosis and staging: abnormal ranges and disease severity
    (c) the disease process.

Randomized trials

Randomization. In a clinical trial, the relative efficacy of treatments or interventions in human subjects is measured. In most situations, the standard treatment (control) is compared with a new treatment. Randomization is a procedure in which the assignment of a subject to a particular treatment (control or new) is determined by chance, so that outside influences or prejudices ('bias') cannot influence the trial's findings.

Parallel designs. In this type of study, one group receives the test treatment whilst another receives the standard treatment (i.e. acts as the control group).

Cross-over designs. In a cross-over design, the subject receives both the test and the control treatment in a randomized order, i.e. each subject acts as her own control.

Non-randomized trials

Historical controls. In some situations, randomization is not possible, so patients receiving the new treatment can be compared with patients of a similar age and illness severity who have received a different treatment. Because it is not possible to match patients exactly, there may be 'bias' in this type of study. Nevertheless, its findings can be very helpful.

Pretest–post-test studies. In this type of study, the relevant parameter(s) of a group of individuals are measured; the patients are then subjected to a treatment and the parameter(s) measured again. The purpose of this is to study the size of the effect of the treatment.

Cohort studies

Design. A cohort study is one in which subjects of a defined population, who have been exposed (or will be exposed) to a factor that may influence the probability of occurrence of a given disease or other outcome, can be identified. Cohort studies are observational studies, observing the progress of individuals over time.

Size of study. The required size of a cohort study depends on the size of the risk being investigated and the incidence of the particular condition under investigation. If the risk is very rare, a large number of people will need to be studied; if it is common, fewer people are required.

Problems in interpretation. Problems in interpretation arise:

- from 'bias' in choosing the study population;
- from poor study design;
- from insufficient study size;
- from misinformation from the study groups.

Post-marketing surveillance. This is a study carried out on a population of people receiving an established treatment. Post-marketing surveillance is designed to discover problems or benefits not previously identified during the treatment's trial stages. The most famous example is the relationship of thalidomide to birth defects.

Case-control studies

Design. A case-control study, which can be retrospective (historical controls) or prospective (a cohort study), starts with the identification of those with the disease of interest and a suitable control group (reference) of people without disease.

Selection of controls. The choice of an appropriate control population is important for a correct interpretation of the results, i.e. for eliminating bias.

Confounding. Confounding arises when the effects of two processes are not separated, as a result of which the effect of the treatment being studied is distorted (confounded) by other factors not controlled for in the study.

Matched study. The purpose of matching is to use efficient analytical methods to control for confounding variables that may influence results of the clinical trial. Matched pairs of patients (of similar age, gender, weight, etc.) are hopefully sufficiently similar to be able to act as controls for each other, i.e. there are no confounding variables.

Cross-sectional surveys. In this type of survey, subjects are included in the study without reference to either their exposure or their disease.

Studies of diagnostic tests

Such studies have three main uses:

- diagnosis of disease
- screening
- patient management.

Diagnosis of disease. In the process of making a diagnosis for a particular patient, a physician establishes a set of diagnostic alternatives or hypotheses.

Screening. This is the identification, among apparently healthy individuals, of those who are sufficiently at risk of a specific disorder to justify a subsequent diagnostic test or procedure, or, in certain circumstances, direct preventative action.

QUESTIONNAIRE AND FORM DESIGN

Purpose of questionnaires and forms. Forms are used to record factual information; they are used in clinical trials to follow a patient's progress and are completed by the investigator.

A questionnaire is designed to measure a person's attitude, emotional state or level of pain, and is often completed by the individual.

Types of question. There are two types of question, open and closed. In an open question, respondents are asked to reply in their own words, whilst in a closed question, the possible responses are preset, for example 'yes', 'no' or 'not sure'.

Reliability and validity. Reliability refers to whether or not the instrument or treatment will produce the same result when administered repeatedly to the same individual.

Validity means whether the instrument is actually measuring what it is supposed to measure.

Non-responders. In a questionnaire survey, some people will inevitably not respond. If the percentage of non-responders is high enough, the validity of the survey is doubtful.

METHODS OF RANDOMIZATION

Simple random. The simplest method of randomization is by tossing a coin or rolling a six-sided dice. A table of random numbers, which is computer generated, can be used.

Blocked randomization. In this type of randomization, the allocation procedure is organized in such a way that equal numbers are allocated to the assigned numbers. Thus, if there are 40 random numbers, 20 will belong to the trial group and 20 to the test group.

In multicentre trials, a randomization procedure is used for each centre to ensure balanced treatment allocation within centres.

DATA DESCRIPTION

When a set of data is collected, it is important to know their distribution. The object of data presentation, whether graphical or tabular, is to convey the essential points of a study to the reader.

Data can be:

- Numerical or quantitative. The data can be displayed as counts or values within a range, in a discrete or continuous form.
- Qualitative data:
  - Nominal data. These are simply counted but not measured.
  - Ordered categorical or ranked data. In some studies, if there are more than two categories, it is possible to order them in some way.

Displaying continuous data. The data collected can be displayed in the following ways:

- dot plots
- histograms
- box-whisker plots
- scatter plots
- survival curves.

Displaying categorical data. Categorical data can be displayed using a bar chart.

In statistics, a *population* is a theoretical concept that is used to describe an entire group. *Parameters* are quantities used to describe characteristics of such populations.

Normal distribution

The data obtained for analysis have a characteristic 'bell shape' and this is called normal distribution.

Standard error is an estimate of a parameter, which becomes more precise as the number of observations gets larger.

Standard deviation is a value around which the observations are scattered.

Confidence intervals

Confidence intervals are defined as a range of values within which most of the population (95–98%) will lie.

Use of statistics for inference

The data from various samples are collected, analysed and compared, and questions such as 'could they come from the same population?' are asked.

The concept of the null hypothesis, statistical significance, the use of statistical tests, *P* values and their relation to confidence intervals are described below.

Null hypothesis

Statistical analysis investigates the relationship between items of data, in addition to summarizing them. While conducting a study an investigator has a theory in mind, for example on the relationship between diabetes and hypertension. This theory is also known as the study hypothesis. The null hypothesis disproves rather than proves it and is usually phrased in the negative, which is the reason for its being termed 'null'.

The starting point for most statistical trials is the null hypothesis, which in general states that there is no difference between treatment A and treatment B. The trial then sets out to disprove or reject the null hypothesis.

P value

This is interpreted as the probability of obtaining the difference observed in the trial by chance alone.

A statistical 'significance test' considers the *P* value. If *P* is small (<0.05), the observed difference is very unlikely to be due to chance, i.e. there really is a difference and the null hypothesis is wrong. If the *P* value is large, the observed differences could easily be due to chance alone and the null hypothesis stands as possibly true.

Statistical inference

Hypothetical testing is a method that decides whether the data are consistent with the null hypothesis. The calculation of the *P* value is an important part of the procedure.

Hypothesis testing is summarized in three steps:

1. Choose a significance level (*P* level) of the test.
2. Conduct the study, observe the outcome and deduce the *P* value.
3. If the *P* value obtained is less than or equal to the significance level, conclude that the data are not consistent with the null hypothesis, i.e. that the null hypothesis is wrong and that there really is a difference.

   If the *P* value is greater than the significance level, the null hypothesis should not be rejected but viewed as 'not yet disproved'.

It is important to distinguish between the significance level and the *P* value. Rejecting the null hypothesis when it is in fact true, i.e. believing that there is a difference where none exists, is known as a type 1 error.

Statistical tests

There are two classes of statistical test, the parametric and the non-parametric. The Student's t-test is an example of a parametric test. For a parametric test to be valid, certain conditions should exist for the test population, principally that the population from which the test sample is drawn is normally distributed, i.e. fits a bell curve distribution.

Student's t-test

This test is used to compare the data when the sample size is small.

$$t = \frac{\text{Difference in means}}{\text{Standard error of the difference in means}}$$

There are two types of this test.

Paired t-test. This also known as the related test, or matched test, which arises when the data are paired in some natural way; for example cross-over trial or a matched case-control study.

Two-sample or unpaired t-test. The unpaired test, also known as the independent sample or unrelated test, arises when the data in the two groups are not correlated.

Non-parametric tests

Non-parametric tests make no assumption about statistical normality. The chi-squared test (χ^2) is used to assess whether an observed binomial or other distribution accords with the expected, either on the basis of knowledge of true population parameters or on theoretical grounds.

$$\chi^2 = \frac{(\text{Observation} - \text{Expectation})^2}{\text{Expectation}}$$

When calculating χ^2, the expected number in any group should not be less than five, the total number of observations should not be less than 20, and actual numbers, rather than ratios or percentages, must be used.

For values that are not continuous, alternative tests, such as the Wilcoxon signed-rank sum and Mann-Whitney U tests, are used. These tests remain the same for large or small samples but may be tedious to calculate in the large sample cases, although they are available on computer packages such as MINITAB (Minitab Inc, State College, PA, USA). These tests are also termed non-parametric or distribution-free tests.

Correlation and linear regression

Correlation and linear regression techniques are used for dealing with the relationship between two or more continuous variables.

A scatter diagram of the variables through which a trend line can be drawn shows correlation (association). The strength of the association is summarized by the correlation

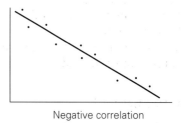

Negative correlation

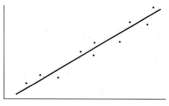

Positive correlation

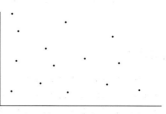

No correlation

Figure 12.1 Correlation.

coefficient, a dimensionless quantity ranging from −1 (strong negative correlation, such as jogging to heart attacks) to +1 (strong positive correlation, such as smoking and cancer). A positive correlation (Fig. 12.1) is one in which both variables increase together. A negative correlation is one in which one variable increases as the other decreases. The correlation coefficient is unaffected by the units of measurement.

In regression, we look at the dependence of one variable (the dependent variable) on another (the independent variable). The relationship is summarized by a regression equation consisting of a slope and an intercept. The slope represents the amount the dependent variable increases with each unit increase in the independent variable, and the intercept represents the value of the dependent variable when the independent variable takes the value zero.

FURTHER READING

Nursing research

Arminger B 1977 Ethics of nursing research. Profile, principles and perspective. Nursing Research 26: 330–336

Burns N, Grove S K 1987 The practice of nursing research. Conduct, critique and utilization. W B Saunders, Philadelphia

Davis A J 1989 Clinical nurses' ethical decision-making in situations of informed consent. Advances in Nursing Science 11: 63–69

Gostner S R 1974 Scientific accountability in nursing. Nursing Outlook 22: 764–768

Oiler C 1982 The phenomenological approach in nursing research. Nursing Research 31: 178–181

Robb S S 1983 Beware of the informed consent. Nursing Research 32: 132–135

Wilson H S 1989 Research in nursing: Addison-Wesley, Menlo Park, CA

Woods N F, Catanzaro M 1988 Nursing research: theory and practice. C V Mosby, St Louis

Statistics

Altman D G 1991. Practical statistics for medical research. Chapman & Hall, London

Armitage P, Berry G 1987 Statistical methods in medical research, 2nd edn. Blackwell, Oxford

Bennett A E, Ritchie K 1975 Questionnaires in medicine: a guide to their design and use. Nuffield Provincial Hospitals Trust, London

Bland J M 1987 An introduction to medical statistics. Oxford University Press, Oxford

Campbell M J, Machin D 1993. Medical statistics. A commonsense approach, 2nd edn. John Wiley & Sons, Chichester

Colton T 1974 Statistics in medicine. Little, Brown, Boston

Gardner M J, Altman D G 1989 Statistics with confidence. British Medical Association, London

Gardner M J, Gardner S B, Winter P D 1991 Confidence intervals analysis program. British Medical Association, London

McDowell J, Newell C 1987 Measuring health: a guide to rating scales and questionnaires. Oxford University Press, Oxford

13

Audit and computers

AUDIT

Audit is a peer review, described as a cycle of activity involving a systematic review of practice, the identification of problems, the development of possible solutions and the implementation of change, followed by a review.

It has been suggested that an effective system of audit consists of three elements:

1. agreed criteria for good practice;
2. methods of measuring performance against criteria;
3. mechanisms for implementing an appropriate change in practice.

Medical audit is defined as 'the systematic, critical analysis of the quality of medical care, including the procedures used for diagnosis and treatment, the use of resources, and the resulting outcome and quality of life for the patient, which should be central to any programme to enhance the overall quality of care given to the patients'.

Nursing audit

Nursing audit is defined as 'the part of the cycle of quality assurance involving the systematic and critical analysis by nurses, midwives and health visitors in conjunction with other staff, of the planning, delivery and evaluation of nursing and midwifery care, in terms of their use of resources and the outcomes for the patients, and introducing appropriate change in response to that analysis'. The objectives of nursing audit include:

- comparing the degree of quality patient care with defined criteria;
- justifying the cost incurred to human and material resources.

Audit has many similarities to research, but by critically analysing medical practices, audit aims to impose the quality of care. The differences between research and audit are outlined in Box 13.1.

Box 13.1 Differences between research and audit	
Research	*Audit*
• Randomized	• Non-randomized
• Established standards	• Compares performance and standards
• Started by researchers	• Started by service providers
• Involves comparison between treatments	• Evaluates current treatment
• Needs ethics committee approval	• Does not need ethics committee approval
• Results can be transferred to other settings	• Results are usually non-transferable to other settings
• Presents clear conclusions	• Compares performance against standards

Audit methodologies

Organizational audit

This provides a framework for the comprehensive review of services and ensures a consistency of approach to, and interpretation of, quality across the organization.

Peer review

Peer review is an activity carried out by people of the same rank, or equal to one another in status and from the same professional group.

Audit can be carried out in two dimensions, time frame and focus of evaluation. Time frame is the period in patient care during which data can be retrieved either retrospectively, prospectively or concurrently:

1. *Retrospective audit* can be carried out through patient interviews or post-discharge surveys of satisfaction. The advantages of this type of audit are the ability to review a large number of patients and/or their documents. The disadvantages of retrospective audit are that it depends on the accuracy of case records.

2. In *prospective audit*, the topic for study is selected, and cases are recorded from that point forward. This type of audit may be useful for evaluating nursing care topics that cannot be retrieved via the standard medical diagnostic coding systems.

3. *Concurrent audit* is an open audit that takes place while the patient is still receiving care. Concurrent audit reflects a quality assurance (QA) evaluation carried out whilst patient care is under way.

Criteria-based audit consists of:

- the selection of the topic for review;
- the identification of measurable criteria;
- defining/setting the standard for the aspects of care;
- compiling the audit tool and method for data collection.

Criteria-based audit allows cases to be reviewed, and those which fail to meet the standards are identified. Following discussion, changes can be defined and implemented according to the agreed plan.

Collaborative care planning is a multi-disciplinary team approach to assessing, planning, implementing and evaluating care in association with the patient during his or her stay in hospital. In this method, the quality of care is clearly defined, planned, implemented, monitored and audited.

Outcome measures include morbidity and mortality statistics, complications, readmission rates and patient satisfaction scores.

The measurement of the response to health-care intervention is of critical importance in judging advantages and disadvantages to the patients. A number of techniques are used to measure the response, including:

- pain measurement scales
- the Barthel index
- verbal feedback.

COMPUTERS

Computers play a key role in medicine, and it is essential that all the professions involved in the care of patients should have some knowledge of computing.

The budget for information technology in UK hospitals is around 0.7–0.8% of the total, compared with 1.5–2.5% in US hospitals.

Computers can be used in the areas of:

- medical equipment
- medical diagnosis
- treatment
- medical education
- medical administration
- clinical data collection.

MEDICAL EQUIPMENT

Computers form an integral part of the electronic equipment used in clinical diagnosis and treatment. An important part of clinical diagnosis is the detection and quantitation of signals from various pieces of equipment. Primary signals from medical equipment are converted into electrical impulses and presented as quantitative information. The devices that convert these signals are known as transducers (see Ch. 4). Transducers are used in the measurement of:

- biological potentials (e.g. ECG, EEG and EMG):
- temperature (e.g. thermometers, thermocouples, thermography and liquid crystals);
- pressure (e.g. Dinamap, tonometry and catheter tip transducers);
- electrochemical forces (e.g. dissolved gas and ion-specific electrodes);
- flow (e.g. electromagnetic flowmeters and ultrasound);
- displacement (e.g. ultrasound and strain gauges).

A transducer produces an electrical copy of the primary information. The computer converts the analogue signal into digital form, i.e. from a continuous wave to a list of numbers. The electrical signal is sampled at regular intervals and the findings are recorded as analogue-to-digital conversion.

Analysis of a digital signal

The signals produced by analogue-to-digital conversion can be analysed in two ways:

1. time domain analysis: a straightforward analysis of the variation of voltage over course of time;
2. frequency domain analysis: a complex analysis of the overall pattern of voltage analysis.

Computers and data from medical equipment

The actual analysis of electrical signals may vary from the simple to the highly complex. A simple analysis is counting events and dividing them by the time base in order to derive a rate. A complex approach is 'template' or pattern matching, in which the pattern may be real or theoretical, for example ST segment analysis on the ECG.

Analysis can be performed on-line or off-line. In the on-line approach, the signals are examined immediately without prior storage or transfer, whereas in the off-line approach, the signals are recorded onto a magnetic tape for subsequent analysis. The tape can be played back at a fraction of the original speed to allow time for complex mathematical analysis.

The anaesthetic machine

In the anaesthetic machine, electronics and microprocessors play an important role, such as in:

- the electronic control of gases and vapours in a pneumatic circuit;
- the servo-control of gases and vapours;
- the electronic monitoring of a conventional pneumatic anaesthetic machine;
- the servo-control of the depth of anaesthesia;
- integral physiological monitoring.

Electronic monitoring of an anaesthetic machine

The Engstrom ELSA anaesthetic machine is divided into two sections – an upper monitoring unit and a lower anaesthetic delivery unit – both of which are fully integrated. The anaesthetic delivery unit delivers gases and vapours in a controlled manner. The monitoring unit has transducers that convert the analogue signals from:

- gas supply pressures
- airway pressure
- inspired and expired breathing volumes
- fresh gas flows
- fresh gas temperatures
- vapourizer levels and temperature
- oxygen and carbon dioxide levels

into digital format, and it uses these signals for control and safety monitoring of the anaesthetic machine. Control messages and alarms are clearly displayed on the monitoring panel. The control and safety functions of the computer help to protect the patient from gas and electric supply failure, incorrect (high or low) vapour concentrations, disconnections and the delivery of hypoxic gas mixtures.

The microprocessor in an anaesthetic machine allows automatic intervention under certain alarm conditions:

- Failure of the oxygen supply automatically shuts off the nitrous oxide. Nitrous oxide is shut off within 5 s if a failure in oxygen supply is detected and the machine is opened to air (21% oxygen in air).
- It provides automatic relief of excessive airway pressure.
- Shutting off of the vapourizer occurs if the anaesthetic agent concentrations are set above a predetermined level.

All of these conditions lead to alarm sounds and a display in words showing the nature of the problem.

Servo-controlled anaesthesia

Control engineering is a subject that deals with the automatic or semi-automatic control of variables and the correction of errors in their control. It deals with closed-loop systems or servo-control loops.

In electronic servo-loops, an output or variable is measured by the transducers of the delivery and of the loop which convert it into an electrical signal. This signal is then compared at source with a reference value, and the difference between the two, or error signal, is used to adjust the controlling element until the output of the system is at the required value, at which point the error signal will be zero. The designs of servo-controlled loops are complex as they take into account delays, hysteresis, damping and stability (see Ch. 4).

Computers and the ECG

The computer facilitates automatic lead checking, baseline correction, on-line calculations, storage on magnetic data and transmission for remote processing. Computers in electrocardiography allow:

- arrhythmia monitoring
- ambulatory recording
- exercise testing
- comparison of the current reading with previous recordings.

Computer imaging

An image can be described as a matrix of small squares (pixels), each containing a shade of grey or a colour. If the pixels are small enough, they blend to form a smooth picture.

Various imaging systems use digital techniques (Box 13.2).

Box 13.2   Imaging systems using digital techniques

- Computerized axial tomography (CAT)
- Magnetic resonance imaging (MRI)
- Ultrasound
- Thermography
- Contrast and classical radiography
- Nuclear medicine

Computers can improve the basic quality of a digitized image using:

- enhancement techniques
- restoration
- noise reduction
- subtraction
- compression.

COMPUTERS AND THEIR ROLE IN TREATMENT

Computers can be used to carry out surveillance of management protocols for research, peer review and administrative purposes.

Computers in specific areas of medical treatment

Anaesthesia

Computers have a wide variety of actual or potential applications in anaesthesia, most of which concern data collection and analysis. They can also be used in servo-loop control systems (see p. 274).

Critical care

In critical care, rapid analysis of complex data, for example of cardiovascular and respiratory function, and fluid and electrolyte balance, is vital as a part of the treatment process.

Monitoring systems such as devices by Hewlett-Packard (Patient Data Management System) allow comparison between current findings and pre-determined criteria, and activate alarm systems appropriately. Some systems provide automatic intervention to correct detected abnormalities such as changing ventilator settings and adjustment of i.v. flow rates.

Orthopaedics

Computers, particularly with CAD/CAM technology, are used in:

- 3D reconstruction of skeletal structures;
- the production of plastic or wax models as templates for the preoperative review and sculpting of allografts;
- the design and manufacture of customized implants.

Reconstructive surgery

Computers have been used to generate and manipulate images from measurements obtained by encephalography and cephalometry in the planning of craniofacial surgery.

Stereotactic procedures

Liver biopsy. Computers have been able to construct a 3D image of the liver, allowing identification of vessels and intrahepatic tumours and facilitating needle puncture for biopsy or treatment.

Neurosurgery. A single point in the brain can be displayed using CT scanning and the target point chosen with a mouse-controlled cursor. The surgical point and the direction are then determined and converted into mechanical adjustments of the stereotactic operating table.

Virtual reality in surgery

Virtual reality is a human interaction in an environment simulated by a computer. This includes simulators for training in minimal access surgery (see p. 193) and 'telepresence surgery', in which the surgeon can operate on patients at separate and remote locations.

Nursing

Nursing staff use computers as a part of total clinical process. The specific nursing functions for which computer assistance is available include:

- care planning;
- the entry and communication of doctors' orders;
- physiological monitoring.

Automated data entry of vital signs and automated fluid balance calculators can considerably decrease the amount of time spent on charting and paperwork, as well as increasing chart accuracy. This helps nurses to spend more time in direct patient care.

COMPUTERS AND MEDICAL EDUCATION

Computers can provide an effective interaction between the student and the subject being studied. Interaction is the key contribution that a computer can give to education.

Computer-assisted learning

The computer can act as both a tutor and a laboratory. As a tutor, the computer gives a one-way information to the student, and using it as a laboratory the student can explore different strategies and the results of those strategies.

The types of computer programme used in education include:

- tutorial
- drill and practice
- problem-solving
- simulations
- games.

The advantages and disadvantages of computer-assisted learning (CAL) are shown in Box 13.3.

Box 13.3 Advantages and disadvantages of CAL

Advantages

- Each student works at his/her own pace
- The computer provides continuous feedback by assessing the student's performance
- The computer is always available, and no supervision is necessary
- CAL material can be altered and updated easily and quickly
- Computers can be used for interactive instruction

Disadvantages

- Cost
- Resistance by teachers and students
- Availability
- Reliability
- Awareness of what is available

Teleconferencing: distance learning

The concept of linking several people on different sites via a 'conference call' is familiar, and this technique is now used by surgeons in the operating theatre. They use video images and can communicate in real-time with the audience who may be either in an adjacent part of the building or thousands of miles away.

RETRIEVING DATA FOR RESEARCH USING COMPUTERS

Computerized databases (Box 13.4) are a convenient way of searching for information. The requirements are:

- a computer
- a modem
- an RS-232 serial port on the computer, which is linked via the public telephone to these databases.

Box 13.4 Computerized databases

- MEDLINE (MEDLARS)
- Excerpta Medica
- Commercial database services such as DIALOG and Bibliographic Retrieval Service (BRS)
- Institutional database services such as Paper Chase, AMA/GTE Telenet Medical Information Network (MINET), Medical Special Interest Group (Med SIG), Patient Data Query (PDQ) system, ADONIS, CDC Wonder

---

HEALTH HAZARDS ASSOCIATED WITH THE USE OF COMPUTERS

- Stress
- General aches and pains
- Visual problems
- Repetitive strain injury (RSI)
- Hearing impairment
- Facial dermatitis
- Cataracts, cancers and miscarriages (not proven but suspected)
- Loss of libido
- Sprains and broken limbs
- Burns.

FURTHER READING

Audit

Bowling A 1991 Measuring health. A review of quality of life measurement scales. Open University Press, Milton Keynes

Brar A 1989 An evaluation of patient care. Nursing Journal of India 80(10): 189

Department of Health 1989 Working for patients. Medical Audit – Working paper no. 6. HMSO, London

Finnegan E 1991 Collaborative care planning. A natural catalyst for change. Resource Management Support Unit, West Midlands Regional Health Unit

Hunt A, McEwan J, McKenna S 1986 Measuring health status. Croom Helm, London

Joint Centre for Education in Medicine 1992 Making medical audit effective. Joint Centre for Education in Medicine, London

King's Fund Centre 1990 Organisational audit project. King's Fund, London

Maas M, Jacox A 1977 Guidelines for nurse autonomy/patient welfare. Appleton-Century-Crofts, New York

Meisenheimer C 1985 Quality assurance. A complete guide to effective programmes. Aspen Publications, Maryland

NHS Management Executive 1991 A framework of audit for nursing services. HMSO, London

Phaneuf M 1974 The nursing audit. Appleton-Century-Crofts, New York

Shaw C 1990 Criteria based audit. British Medical Journal 300: 649

Tugwell P, Mongonelli E 1986 The clinical audit cycle. Australian Clinical Review 6: 101–105

Computers

Ball M J, Warnock-Materon A 1986 The case for using computers in the operating room. Western Journal of Medicine 145: 843–847

Bickers R G 1985 MEDLINE and beyond: the personal computer guide to retrieval and management of medical information. Year Book, Chicago

Brusco M J, Futch J 1993 Nurse staff planning under conditions of a nursing shortage. Journal of Nursing Administration 23: 58–64

Clayden G S, Wilson B 1988 Computer assisted learning in medical education. Medical Education 22: 456–467

Cobb H 1986 Computers in veterinary medical education. Veterinary Clinics in North America 16: 703–708

Cook V, McCorkel J 1987 Computer assisted instruction for medicine and nursing: sources and programs. Bulletin of Medical Librarian Association 75: 101–108

Cutting C, Grayson B 1986 Computer aided planning and evaluation of facial and orthognathic surgery. Clinical Plastic Surgery 13: 449–462

Dooling S L 1987 Designing computer simulations. Computers in Nursing 219: 224

Evans S 1985 Computer literacy in family medicine. Clinics in Primary Care 12: 403–413

Goh J C H, Ho N C 1990 Principles and applications of computer aided design and computer aided manufacturing (CAD/CAM) technology in orthopaedics. Annals of the Academy of Medicine Singapore 19: 706–712

Hashimoto D, Dohi T 1991 Developments of a computer-aided surgery system: three dimensional graphic reconstruction for treatment of liver cancer. Surgery 109: 589–596

McGovern K T 1994 Applications of virtual reality to surgery. British Medical Journal 308: 1054–1055

Prakash O 1983 Computing in anaesthesia and intensive care. Martinus Nijhoff, Boston

Siegel J H, Colman B 1986 Computers in the care of the critically ill. Urology Clinics of North America 13: 101–117

Wallingford K T, Humphreys B L 1990 Bibliographic retrieval: a survey of individual users of Medline. MD Computing 7: 166–171

Wyatt J 1991 Use and sources of medical knowledge. Lancet 338: 1368–1372

Appendix

(A) SI units (Système International d'Unités)

Base units	SI units	Symbol
There are seven base units and they are expressed in SI units as follows:		
Length	metre	m
Mass	kilogram	kg
Time	second	s
Amount of substance	mole	mol
Electric current	ampere	A
Thermodynamic temperature	kelvin	K
Luminous intensity	candela	cd
Other units are derived by multiplying or dividing the base units. For example:		
Volume	cubic metre	m^3
Force	newton	N
Pressure (force/area)	pascal	Pa

SI multiples and fractions

Multiples	SI prefix	Symbol
10	deca	da (D)
10^2	hecto	h
10^3	kilo	K
10^6	mega	M
10^9	giga	G
10^{12}	tera	T

Fractions	SI prefix	Symbol
10^{-1}	deci	d
10^{-2}	centi	c
10^{-3}	milli	m
10^{-6}	micro	μ
10^{-9}	nano	n
10^{-12}	pico	p

(B) Haematological values

(These values vary from laboratory to laboratory.)

		Normal values	SI units
Red cell count (RBC)	Male	5.5 ± 1	× 10^{12}/L
	Female	4.8 ± 1	× 10^{12}/L
Haemoglobin (Hb)	Male	15.5 ±	g/dl
	Female	2.5	(decilitre)
		14 ± 2.5	g/dl
Mean corpuscular volume (MCV)		85 ± 18	
Mean corpuscular haemoglobin (MCH)		29.5 ± 2.5	pg (picogram)
Reticulocytes (0.2–2.0%)		10–100	× 10^9/L
White cell count (WCC)		7.5 ± 3.5	× 10^9/L
Differential count			
Lymphocytes (20–45%)		1.5–4.0	× 10^9/L
Neutrophils (40–75%)		2.0–7.5	× 10^9/L
Monocytes (2–10%)		0.2–0.8	× 10^9/L
Eosinophils (1–6%)		0.04–0.4	× 10^9/L
Basophils (less than 1%)		Less than 0.1	× 10^9/L
Platelets		150–400	× 10^9/L
Erythrocyte sedimentation rate (ESR)		Male up to 5 mm in first hour	
(Westergren method)		Female up to 9 mm in first hour	

Coagulation tests

Test	Normal range	What does it test?
Bleeding time	1–7 min	Behaviour of blood vessels and platelets
Prothrombin time	10–14 s	Tests extrinsic system of clotting
Thrombin time	10–12 s	Conversion of fibrinogen to fibrin
Total fibrinogen assay	2–4 g/L	It is decreased in pregnancy and disseminated intravascular coagulation (DIC)
Fibrin degradation products (FDPs)	Absent or trace <10 mg/L	Detects fibrinolytic activity; increased in DIC
Partial thromboplastin time	35–45 s	

(C) Biochemical values

(These values vary from one laboratory to another.)

Plasma	Normal range	Units	Abnormalities
Sodium	135–145	mmol/L	Increased in sodium load and decreased in water excess
Potassium	3.5–5.5	mmol/L	High in renal failure, low in patients on diuretics
Chloride	96–106	mmol/L	High in patients with ureters implanted in colon and low in patients with pyloric stenosis
Bicarbonate	23–29	mmol/L	Low in acute/chronic renal failure and diabetic acidosis
Urea	2.5–7.0	mmol/L	High in renal failure, sodium loss, low in water load
Creatinine	60–120	μmol/L	High in acute and chronic renal failure
Osmolality	280–295	mosmol/kg	High in renal failure and diabetes insipidus

(C) Biochemical values *(cont'd)*

Serum	Normal range	Units	Abnormalities
Total protein	60–80	g/L	Low in malnutrition and nephrotic syndrome
Albumin	35–50	g/L	Low in malnutrition and nephrotic syndrome
Globulin	20–40	g/L	Increased in cirrhosis
Total calcium	2.12–2.62	mmol/L	Low in renal failure
Ionized calcium	1.14–1.30	mmol/L	Low in renal failure and during liver transplantation
Phosphate	0.8–1.4	mmol/L	Decreased in malnutrition

(D) Respiratory system

Composition of inspired and expired gases (pressure in kPa)

	Air	Alveolar	Expired
Oxygen	19.9	13–15	15–16
Nitrogen	75.0	78–79	77
Carbon dioxide	—	4–6	2.8–3.7
Water vapour	—	6.3	6.3

Arterial blood gases

	Range
pH	7.35–7.45
H^+	36–44 (nmol/L)
Oxygen (kPa)	11.9–13.2
Carbon dioxide (kPa)	4.8–6.3
Bicarbonate	
Actual	22–30 (mmol/L)
Standard	21–25 (mmol/L)
Base excess	± 2 mmol/L

Gas exchange

Measurement	Value/range	Unit	Symbol
Respiratory rate	12–20	/min	f
Minute volume	6–10	L/min	VE
Tidal volume	0.3–0.65	L/min	Vt
Alveolar minute volume	4–7	L/min	VA
Anatomical dead space	2	ml/kg	Vd
Oxygen consumption	11–13	mmol/min	nO_2
Carbon dioxide production	9–11	mmol/min	nCO_2
Respiratory quotient	0.8		

Simple lung function tests

Measurement	Range and units		Symbols
	Male	Female	
Forced expiratory volume	3.5 ± 1.5 L/s	2.5 ± 1.0 L/s	FEV
Forced vital capacity	4.5 ± 1.5 L	3.5 ± 1.0 L	FVC
Peak expiratory flow rate	550 ± 150 L/min	400 ± 100 L/min	PEFR

(The first two measurements are carried out using a spirometer, whereas PEFR is carried out using a peak flowmeter.)

(E) Cardiovascular system

Electrocardiogram

Wave	Duration (s)		What does it mean?
	Average	Range	
P wave	<0.10		Atrial contraction
PR interval	0.18	0.12–20.0	Atrial depolarization and conduction throughout AV node
QRS time	0.08	to 0.10	Ventricular depolarization
QT interval	0.40	to 0.43	Ventricular depolarization plus ventricular repolarization
T wave	<0.22		Ventricular repolarization

Normal pressures (mmHg)

	Range	Derived values in haemodynamics
Central venous pressure (CVP)	0–7	
Right atrium (RA)	1–10	5
Right ventricle (RV)		
Systolic	14–30	23
Diastolic	0–7	9
Pulmonary artery (PA)		
Systolic	15–30	25
Diastolic	5–12	9
Pulmonary artery wedge pressure (PAWP)	5–15	10
Left atrium (LA)	8	8

Derived values

		Value (in a 70 kg man)
Stroke volume (SV)	$\dfrac{\text{Cardiac output} \times 1000}{\text{Heart rate}}$	80/ml
Cardiac output (CO)	Stroke volume × heart rate	5 L/min
Cardiac index (CI)	$\dfrac{\text{Cardiac output}}{\text{Body surface area}}$	3.2 L/min/m²
Rate pressure product (RPP)	Systolic arterial pressure × heart rate	12 000

(F) Fluid composition of the body

	Male	Female
Total water content		
Between 18 and 45 years of age	60%	55%
Above 60 years of age	55%	45%

The volume of extracellular fluid (ECF) is 35% of total water content and the volume of intracellular fluid (ICF) is 65% of total water content.

Blood volumes	
Infant	75 ml/kg body weight
Child	70 ml/kg body weight
Adult female	70 ml/kg body weight
Adult male	75 ml/kg body weight

(G) Composition of commonly used i.v. fluids in theatre

Fluid	Na^+	K^+	Cl^- (all in mmol/L)	HCO_3	Others	pH	Glucose g/L
Dextrose	0	0	0	0		4.0	50
Dextrose 4% in 0.18% saline	31	0	31	0		4.5	40
Sodium chloride 0.9%	154	0	154	0		5.0	
Lactated Ringer's (Hartmann's)	131	5	112	29	Mg^{++} Ca^{++}		
Sodium bicarbonate 8.4%	1000	0	0	1000		8.0	
Haemaccel	145	5.1	145	0	Ca^{++}		
Dextran 70 in 0.9% NaCl	154	0	154	0		4–7	
Dextran 70 in 5% dextrose	0	0	0	0		3.5–7	50
HPPF	150	2	120			7.4	40

(H) Conversion from weight per unit volume to mmol/L

The formula used for this conversion is:

$$\text{Concentration in mmol/L} = \frac{10 \times \text{concentration in mg/100 ml}}{\text{Molecular weight}}$$

Example: Conversion of glucose 180 mg/100 ml to mmol/L, the molecular weight of glucose being 180:

$$\frac{10 \times 180 \text{ mg/100 ml}}{180} = 10 \text{ mmol/L}$$

Other conversions

Height: cm = inches × 2.54
  e.g. 10 in × 2.54 = 25.4 cm
Weight: kg = lb × 0.454

Volume: ml = fl oz × 28.5
Pressure: kPa = mmHg × 0.133
  e.g. 100 mmHg × 0.133 = 13.3 kPa

inches = cm × 0.39
  e.g. 10 cm × 0.39 = 3.9 in
lb = kg × 2.2
fl oz = ml × 0.035
mmHg = kPa × 7.5
  e.g. 10 kPa × 7.5 = 75 mmHg

Remember that:

1 gram (g) = 1000 milligrams (mg)
1 milligram (mg) = 1000 micrograms (μg)
1 mega unit = 1 000 000 units (1 million units).

A percentage solution means the number of parts of a drug in a hundred parts of the final solution. The abbreviation % (per cent) is used to express it. For example, a 5% solution of dextrose means:

5 parts of dextrose in 100 parts of the solution
1 part of dextrose in 20 parts of the solution
5 g dextrose in 100 ml of the solution.

On a number of occasions, theatre staff are asked to handle solutions (such as adrenaline or cocaine) that are expressed as dilutions. What do these dilutions mean?

1 in 5 solution means 20%
10 solution means 10%
1 in 40 solution means 2.5%
1 in 100 solution means 1%
1 in 1000 solution means 0.1%

Certain conversions/formulae used to calculate infusion rates

To convert drops/min to ml/h

$$\frac{\text{Number of drops per min} \times 60 \text{ min}}{\text{Drops per ml of giving set}} = \text{ml/h}$$

If a paediatric buretrol (giving set) that gives 60 drops/ml is used and 20 drops/min are to be given, the ml/h to be set up is:

$$\frac{20 \times 60}{60} = 20 \text{ ml/h}$$

To calculate the number of drops/min for i.v. infusion

$$\frac{\text{Volume (ml) to be infused} \times \text{drops/ml of giving set}}{\text{Time (min) over which volume is to be given}}$$

$$= \text{drops/min}$$

(This formula is used daily in recovery rooms and wards postoperatively.)

For example, an infusion of dextrose saline 500 ml is set up via an ordinary giving set that delivers 15 drops/min and it has to be delivered in 6 hours; thus the drops/min can be calculated as:

$$\frac{500 \times 15}{360 \text{ min}} = 20 \text{ drops/min}$$

Infusions of dopamine, dobutamine and sodium nitroprusside. On a number of occasions staff in anaesthetic or recovery rooms are asked to assist the anaesthetist in setting up infusions of dopamine, dobutamine or sodium nitroprusside.
Example:
800 mg dopamine added to 500 ml of 5% dextrose or
250 mg dobutamine added to 500 ml of 5% dextrose or
50 mg sodium nitroprusside added to 100 ml of 5% dextrose.

The following calculation gives the number of drops/min to be set up on an infusing device (e.g. an IVAC pump) for an infusion of the above-mentioned drugs prescribed in μg/kg/min.

$$\frac{\frac{\text{Drops/ml of}}{\text{giving set}} \times \frac{\text{Dosage prescribed}}{(\mu\text{g/kg/min})} \times \frac{\text{Volume of}}{\text{diluent}}}{\text{Amount of drug (}\mu\text{g used in solution)}}$$

$$= \frac{60 \times 70 \times 2 \times 500}{800\,000} = 5 \text{ drops/min}$$

where 60 is the drops/ml of the giving set; 70 is the body weight in kg; 2 is the prescribed dosage of dopamine in μg/kg/min; 500 ml is the diluent; and 800 000 μg dopamine is used to make up the solution.

Usually, wall charts are provided by respective manufacturers to give accurate dosage according to body weights.

Nowadays a number of anaesthetists are using syringe pumps to set up infusions of various drugs such as muscle relaxants (atracurium and vecuronium), propofol (Diprivan) or analgesics such as papaveretum (Omnopon) and alfentanil (Rapifen). The dilution of these agents varies with the individual anaesthetists and the types of syringe pumps used.

(I) Physical properties of anaesthetic agents

Name	Formula	BP* (°C)	SVP*	MAC* (%)	Blood gas coefficients
Cyclopropane	C_3H_6	−33	4800	9.2	0.45
Chloroform	$CHCl_3$	61	160	0.5	10
Enflurane	$CHFCl, CF_2$ CF_2H	56	175	1.68	1.9
Ether (Diethyl)	$C_2H_5OC_2H_5$	35	425	1.9	12
Halothane	$CF_3CHCLBr$	50	243	0.8	2.5
Isoflurane	$CF_3CHClCF_2H$	49	250	1.15	1.4
Nitrous oxide	N_2O	−88	—	105	0.47
Trichlorethylene	$CHClCCl_2$	87	60	0.17	9.0

* BP, boiling point (in °C); SVP, saturated vapour pressure at 20°C; MAC, minimum alveolar concentration.

(J) Endotracheal tube size

Children

The internal diameter of an endotracheal tube for a child may be calculated from the formula:

$$\frac{\text{Age (years)}}{4} + 4.5$$

For example, an 8-year-old child will require, according to the formula, a size 6.0 endotracheal tube. Ideally, it is advisable to use non-cuffed tubes below the age of 10 years. A range of tubes should be available, including tubes larger and smaller than the calculated size. The tube is correctly sized if an air leak around it is audible at about 20 cm H_2O pressure.

However, the formula does not hold below the 2–3 years age group, and also the length of the tube required for each age group varies. The length of an endotracheal tube for children in the 1–3 years age group is calculated as:

$$\frac{\text{Height in centimetres}}{5} + 12 = \quad \text{cm}$$

The tube is the correct length if it can be fixed easily to the face when the broad black ring at its tip is seen to be just below the vocal cords and if there is air entry to both lungs.

The formula is not accurate for infants below the age of 1 year, in whom head circumference (using the Liverpool chart) is used.

For simplicity, the chart below may be useful with regard to choosing the length (oral and nasal) and internal diameter of the tubes.

Adults

An adult female requires a size 8.0 mm or 8.5 mm cuffed endotracheal tube, whereas an adult male needs a size 9.0 or 9.5 mm tube.

The length required for size 8.0 or 8.5 mm is 21 cm for oral and 24 cm for nasal tubes. The length for a size 9.0 is 23 cm for oral and 25 cm for nasal tubes.

Endotracheal tube sizes for children

Age	Tube internal diameter (mm)	Length (cm) Oral	Nasal
0–3 months	3.0	10	
3–6 months	3.5	12	15
6–12 months	4.0	12	15
2 years	4.5	13	16
3 years	4.5	13	16
4 years	5.0	14	17
6 years	5.5	15	18
8 years	6.0	16	19
10 years	6.5	17	20
12 years	7.0	18	21

Where the age of the child is not known, or the child is not of a normal size for his or her age, an approximate tube size can be arrived at by using a tube of a diameter similar to that of the child's little finger.

Recommendations for standards of monitoring during anaesthesia and recovery (revised edition 1994)

(Published by the Association of Anaesthetists of Great Britain and Ireland)

The summary of the recommendations are:

• The Association of Anaesthetists of Great Britain and Ireland strongly recommend that the standard of monitoring during general anaesthesia should be uniform in all circumstances irrespective of the duration of anaesthesia or the location of administration.

• An anaesthetist must be present throughout the conduct of general anaesthetic.

• Monitoring should be commenced before induction and continued until the patient has recovered from the effects of anaesthesia.

• These recommendations also apply to the administration of local anaesthesia, regional analgesia or sedation where there is a risk of unconsciousness or cardiovascular or respiratory complications.

• The anaesthetist should check all equipment before use. Monitoring of anaesthetic machine function during the administration of anaesthesia should include an oxygen analyser with alarms.

During spontaneous ventilation, clinical observation and a capnometer should be used to detect leaks, disconnections, rebreathing and high pressure in the breathing system, measurements of airway pressure, expired volume and CO_2 concentration is strongly recommended when IPPV is employed.

• A pulse oximeter and capnometer must be available for every patient.

• It is strongly recommended that clinical observation of the patient should be supplemented by continuous monitoring devices displaying heart rate, pulse volume or arterial pressure, oxygen saturation, the electrocardiogram and expired carbon dioxide concentration.

Devices for measuring intravascular pressures, body temperature and other parameters should be used when appropriate. It is useful to have both waveform and numerical displays.

• Intermittent non-invasive arterial pressure measurement must be recorded regularly if invasive monitoring is not indicated. If neuromuscular blocking drugs are used, a means of assessing neuromuscular function should be available.

• Additional monitoring may be required in certain situations. These recommendations may be extended at any time on the judgement of the anaesthetist.

• A printed record of monitoring measurements provides a contemporaneous record during emergency situations and allows the anaesthetist to concentrate on managing the patient.

• When handing over to recovery staff, anaesthetists should issue clear instructions concerning monitoring during post-operative care.

Monitoring of oxygen saturation is strongly recommended for all patients and temperature monitoring is recommended for patients at risk of hypothermia.

• Standards of monitoring during transfer of sedated, anaesthetised or unconscious patients should be as high as during the administration of anaesthesia. All patients should have oxygen saturation, electrocardiogram and arterial pressure monitored. Other monitors may be appropriate in certain circumstances.

• For interhospital transfers, a specialist retrieval team based at the receiving hospital can have advantages.

Report of the Working Party on Pain after Surgery, September 1990

Aims and recommendations

• Improve hospital staff education and challenge traditional attitudes to postoperative pain relief
• Assess and record pain systematically, involving the patient whenever possible
• Responsibility for the management of pain relief policy after surgery in each hospital given to a named member of the staff
• Establish acute pain teams in all major hospitals
• Introduce new methods and utilise existing methods more effectively giving due regard to safety
• Audit and continuous appraisal of activity
• Establish appropriate facilities for the provision of adequate postoperative pain relief in all hospitals
• Provide properly trained staff and resources to these services
• Development of better and safer drugs to relieve pain
• Monitoring patients after surgery
• Safety and efficacy of new methods of pain relief
• Counselling and psychological methods of pain relief.

Further reading

Report of the Working Party on Pain after Surgery. Commission on the Provision of Surgical Services 1990 Royal College of Surgeons of England and College of Anaesthetists, London

Association of Anaesthetists of Great Britain and Ireland
Checklist for anaesthetic machines, a safety educational service sponsored by BOC Health Care

Check procedures should be performed at the beginning of each operating theatre session and are the responsibility of the anaesthetist. They may be performed by the anaesthetist or the anaesthetist working with an assistant. In the event of a change of anaesthetist the checked status of the anaesthetic machine must be agreed.

Oxygen analyser

1. The check procedure should start with the machine disconnected from all pipeline supplies and all vaporizers turned to 'off'. The electrical supply to the machine should be switched on.
2. Check that only cylinders which contain gases to be used are present on the machine, that they are securely seated and that they are turned off. A blanking plug should be fitted to any empty cylinder yoke.

Note: Carbon dioxide and cyclopropane cylinders should not normally be present on the machine unless specifically requested by the anaesthetist.

3. Open all flowmeter control valves.
4. Turn on the reserve oxygen cylinder and check the contents gauge. Oxygen should flow through the oxygen flowmeter. If there is another 'in use' oxygen cylinder turn off the reserve oxygen cylinder and repeat the test. Check that the oxygen flow control valve can adjust the flow over the full range of the flowmeter, and set a flow of approximately 5 litres/minute. The oxygen analyser display should approach 100%.
5. Turn on the reserve nitrous oxide cylinder and check the contents gauge. Nitrous oxide should now flow through the nitrous oxide flowmeter. If there is an 'in use' nitrous oxide cylinder turn off the reserve nitrous oxide cylinder and repeat the test. Check that the nitrous oxide flowmeter control valve can adjust the flow over the full range of the flowmeter, and set a flow of approximately 5 litres/minute.
6. Turn off the oxygen cylinder(s) and empty the oxygen from the system by operating the oxygen flush valve. The cylinder gauge(s) should return to zero. The primary audible alarm should operate while the oxygen pressure is decreasing. When the supply of oxygen fails, observe that the appropriate oxygen failure protection device (if fitted) functions correctly to prevent the delivery of a hypoxic gas mixture.
7. Connect the oxygen pipeline. This should restore the flow of oxygen and cancel the oxygen failure protection device. Perform a 'tug test' and check that the oxygen pipeline pressure gauge reads 400 kPa.
8. Turn off the nitrous oxide cylinder(s). Connect the nitrous oxide pipeline. This should restore the flow of gas through the nitrous oxide flowmeter. Perform a 'tug test' and check that the nitrous oxide pipeline pressure gauge also reads 400 kPa. Turn off the nitrous oxide flowmeter control valve.
9. If the anaesthetist has requested specifically that other cylinders be fitted, these should also be checked in a similar manner.
10. Turn off all the flowmeter control valves.
11. Operate the emergency oxygen flush valve and ensure there is no significant decrease in the pipeline supply pressure. Confirm that the oxygen analyser display approaches 100% during this test.

Vaporizers

1. Check that the vaporizer(s) for the required volatile agent(s) are fitted correctly to the anaesthetic machine, that any backbar locking mechanism is fully engaged and that the control knob(s) rotate through their full range(s). Turn off the vaporizer(s).
2. Check that the flow through any vaporizer is in the correct direction.
3. When charging each vaporizer ensure that the correct anaesthetic agent is used, and that the filling port is left tightly closed.
4. Where the anaesthetic machine is fitted with a pressure relief valve the following tests should be performed. (There may be a dangerous increase in pressure if these tests are performed in the absence of such a valve.)

- Set a suitable test flow of oxygen (6–8 litre/min), and with the vaporizer in the 'off' position, temporarily occlude the common gas outlet. There should be no leak from any of the vaporizer fitments, and the flowmeter bobbin will dip.
- Repeat this test with each vaporizer in the 'on' position. There should be no leak of liquid from the filling port.

Turn off the vaporizer(s), and the oxygen flowmeter control valve.

Breathing systems

1. Inspect the configuration of the breathing and scavenging systems to be used, and check that they function correctly. Ensure there are no leaks or obstructions in the reservoir bag or breathing system.

2. The 'push and twist' technique should be employed for connecting conical fittings.

3. Check that the adjustable pressure limiting 'expiratory' valve can be fully opened or closed.

4. Each breathing system poses separate problems. Make a visual check, and perform an occlusion test on the inner tube of the Bain type co-axial system. Check the function of the unidirectional valves on the circle system.

Ventilator

1. Check the normal operation of the ventilator and its controls.

2. Occlude the patient port and check that the pressure relief valve functions correctly.

3. Check that the disconnect alarm is present and operational.

4. Ensure that there is an alternative means to ventilate the patient's lungs in the event of ventilator malfunction.

Suction equipment

Check all components relating to the anaesthetic suction equipment and test for the rapid development of an adequate 'negative' pressure.

Leaks

The detection of small leaks is always a problem. Specific checks have been recommended. An oxygen analyser in the breathing system is a valuable safeguard against the delivery of a gas mixture which could result in hypoxia or awareness.

Self-assessment questions

The answers to these questions can be found on page 301.

ANATOMY AND PHYSIOLOGY

1. The nasal cavity is lined with which type of epithelium?
   A. cuboid
   B. simple
   C. ciliated
   D. squamous.

2. The tidal volume is the amount of air breathed per:
   A. breath
   B. minute
   C. hour
   D. second.

3. One of the following structures belongs to both the respiratory and digestive systems:
   A. oesophagus
   B. larynx
   C. pharynx
   D. bronchi.

4. The pH of gastric juice is normally:
   A. 1.6
   B. 5.6
   C. 7.4
   D. 11.0.

5. The membrane covering the abdominal organs is:
   A. pleura
   B. parietal peritoneum
   C. visceral peritoneum
   D. mesentery.

6. In the heart, the valve between the right atrium and right ventricle is known as the:
   A. bicuspid valve
   B. tricuspid valve
   C. mitral valve
   D. semilunar valve.

7. Which of the following is important in clotting?
   A. erythrocytes
   B. monocytes
   C. platelets
   D. white blood cells.

8. The celiac artery is divided into:
   A. phrenic, gastric and hepatic arteries
   B. splenic, gastric and hepatic arteries
   C. splenic, renal and hepatic arteries
   D. splenic, pancreatic and gastric arteries.

9. The normal white cell count is:
   A. 5000–10 000 cells/mm^3
   B. 1000–5000 cells/mm^3
   C. 10 000–30 000 cells/mm^3
   D. 500–1000 cells/mm^3.

10. The outer layer of an artery is called the:
    A. tunica media
    B. tunica intima
    C. tunica adventitia
    D. endothelium.

11. Which one of the following organs contains transitional epithelium?
    A. uterus
    B. bladder
    C. skin
    D. larynx.

12. The appendix is attached to the:
    A. colon
    B. caecum
    C. jejunum
    D. ileum.

13. Cerebrospinal fluid is found between the:
    A. pia mater and brain
    B. arachnoid mater and pia mater
    C. skull and dura mater
    D. dura mater and arachnoid mater.

14. Which part of the brain controls posture?
    A. thalamus
    B. cortex
    C. cerebellum
    D. hypothalamus.

15. Stimulation of the parasympathetic system causes:
    A. dilatation of the pupil
    B. increased heart rate
    C. decreased salivation
    D. constriction of the bronchi.

16. The second cranial nerve is the:
    A. oculomotor
    B. optic
    C. facial
    D. auditory.

17. The medulla oblongata is part of the:
    A. cerebellum
    B. cerebrum
    C. brainstem
    D. spinal cord.

18. Body temperature is controlled by the:
    A. pineal gland
    B. hypothalamus
    C. pituitary
    D. cerebrum.

19. The islets of Langerhans are found in the:
    A. spinal cord
    B. spleen
    C. pancreas
    D. kidney.

20. the loop of Henle is found in the:
    A. pancreas
    B. kidney
    C. ovaries
    D. uterus.

PHARMACOLOGY

1. A drug used for muscle relaxation is:
    A. buprenorphine (Temgesic)
    B. prilocaine (Citanest)
    C. cinchocaine (Nupercaine)
    D. atracurium (Tracrium).

2. Which one of the following drugs is used to treat acute bronchospasm?
    A. aminophylline
    B. sodium cromoglycate (Intal)
    C. digoxin
    D. frusemide (Lasix).

3. An i.v. injection of atropine causes:
    A. hypertension
    B. salivation
    C. tachycardia
    D. nausea.

4. Which one of the following drugs is a diuretic?
    A. adrenaline
    B. digoxin
    C. frusemide
    D. ranitidine.

5. Insulin is not given orally because:
    A. the blood flow through the stomach is insufficient
    B. it is irritant to the stomach mucosa
    C. it may cause peptic ulcer
    D. the gastric juice inactivates or destroys the insulin.

6. Which one of the following is not an antibiotic?
    A. chloromycetin
    B. gentamicin
    C. prednisolone
    D. penicillin.

7. Which one of the following is not used as a premedicant?
    A. lorazepam
    B. papaveretum
    C. vecuronium
    D. atropine.

8. Adrenaline is mixed with a local anaesthetic agent to:
    A. increase the heart rate
    B. decrease the blood pressure
    C. increase the rate of absorption of local anaesthetic from the site
    D. decrease the rate of absorption of local anaesthetic from the site.

9. Suxamethonium is supplied in ampoules of:
    A. 100 mg in 2 ml
    B. 100 mg in 5 ml
    C. 100 µg in 2 ml
    D. 25 mg in 2 ml.

10. Diprivan (propofol) is supplied in 20 ml ampoules containing 200 mg. What dose, in ml, should be given to a 70 kg patient if the dose is 2 mg per kg?
    A. 10 ml   C. 16 ml
    B. 14 ml   D. 18 ml.

11. One of the relaxants mentioned below is safe in patients with renal failure:
    A. alcuronium
    B. atracurium
    C. pancuronium
    D. gallamine.

12. Which one of the following drugs is a specific antidote for morphine?
    A. doxapram
    B. nikethamide
    C. naloxone
    D. neostigmine.

13. The last sensation to leave and the first to come back during general anaesthesia is:
    A. touch
    B. pain
    C. smell
    D. hearing.

14. Atropine causes:
    A. dry secretions
    B. constriction of the pupil
    C. dilatation of the pupil
    D. bradycardia.

15. Which one of the following is not an anaesthetic agent?
    A. carbon dioxide
    B. halothane
    C. cyclopropane
    D. methoxyflurane.

MICROBIOLOGY

1. Penicillin was discovered by:
   A. Koch
   B. Pasteur
   C. Fleming
   D. Penn.

2. Diplococci are found:
   A. in pairs
   B. in clusters
   C. in chains
   D. singly.

3. The organism *Pseudomonas pyocyanea* is often found to be resistant to:
   A. chlorhexidine
   B. proflavine
   C. glutaraldehyde
   D. iodine.

4. Which of the following bacteria forms spores?
   A. *Clostridium tetani*
   B. *Pseudomonas aeruginosa*
   C. Pneumococci
   D. Meningococci.

5. Gas gangrene is caused by:
   A. *Staphylococcus aureus*
   B. *Streptococcus viridans*
   C. *Clostridium welchii*
   D. *Proteus vulgaris.*

6. Aerobic bacteria multiply in the presence of:
   A. carbon dioxide
   B. oxygen
   C. hydrogen peroxide
   D. hydrogen.

7. Which of the following organisms does not cause food poisoning?
   A. Staphylococcus
   B. Salmonella
   C. Neisseria
   D. Clostridium.

8. Streptococci are usually seen in stained smears (Gram staining) as:
   A. clusters
   B. chains
   C. arranged in straight rows
   D. single organisms.

9. Urinary tract infection can be caused by:
   A. Klebsiella
   B. *Treponema pallidum*
   C. Staphylococcus
   D. Pseudomonas.

10. The organism that commonly causes tonsillitis in children is:
    A. adenovirus
    B. haemolytic Streptococcus
    C. *Candida albicans*
    D. *Staphylococcus aureus.*

11. The process time for a high-vacuum autoclave is:
    A. 20 minutes   C. 10 minutes
    B. 3 minutes   D. 30 minutes.

12. Browne's tubes are used for:
    A. lumbar puncture
    B. blood sampling
    C. testing autoclaves
    D. abdominal paracentesis.

13. The most reliable test of sterility following high-vacuum temperature autoclaving is:
    A. Thermistor   C. Bowie-Dick test
    B. spore test   D. Browne's tubes.

14. In the high-vacuum, high-pressure autoclave, the temperature probe is found in the:
    A. door
    B. jacket
    C. steam inlet
    D. drain.

15. The temperature in an autoclave is accurately measured by:
    A. a bimetallic strip
    B. a clinical thermometer
    C. temperature-sensitive tape
    D. a thermistor.

16. Microorganisms can be destroyed at:
    A. 4°C for 24 hours
    B. −20°C for 24 hours
    C. 160°C for 1 hour
    D. 40°C for 10 minutes.

17. Disinfection is:
    A. sterilization with chemicals
    B. destruction of vegetative forms of bacteria
    C. destruction of bacterial spores
    D. the same as sterilization.

18. Stewart's medium is used as a transport medium for:
    A. biochemistry
    B. bacteriology
    C. blood cross-matching
    D. histology.

19. Which one of the following organisms is used for testing an autoclave?
    A. *Bacillus steartothermophilus*
    B. *Clostridium perfringens*
    C. *Bacillus anthracis*
    D. *Bacillus subtilis.*

20. Which of the following is not a micro-organism?
    A. virus
    B. protozoa
    C. fomite
    D. bacteria.

PHYSICS AND ELECTRONICS

1. The joule is a unit of:
    A. energy
    B. temperature
    C. power
    D. resistance.

2. Temperature is normally measured in medical practice in one of the following units:
    A. kelvin
    B. kilogram
    C. centigrade
    D. celsius.

3. An ion consists of:
    A. a neutron
    B. an element
    C. an atom or molecule carrying an electrical charge
    D. a mixture of elements.

4. An atom of hydrogen contains:
    A. one electron and one proton
    B. one electron and one neutron
    C. one neutron and one proton
    D. two electrons and two protons.

5. Mass and weight are:
    A. different in that the latter varies with gravity
    B. always proportional to each other
    C. identical
    D. different in that mass varies with gravity.

6. Boyle's law applies to which one of the following?
    A. the relationship between the pressure and volume of a gas
    B. the temperature of a gas
    C. the pressure within an autoclave
    D. the difference between a gas and a vapour.

7. One of the following components allows the passage of alternating current but not direct current:
    A. inductor   C. capacitor
    B. resistor   D. solenoid.

8. **Latent heat is:**
   A. produced by the sun
   B. necessary for boiling
   C. the extra heat necessary to change a physical state
   D. necessary to increase pressure.

9. **Water boils at 100°C due to:**
   A. decreased pressure
   B. atmospheric pressure
   C. the type of container it is in
   D. increased pressure.

10. **Static electricity can be reduced by:**
    A. wearing dark clothes
    B. having humid surroundings
    C. wearing nylon clothes
    D. wearing rubber boots.

11. **The colour of the neutral wire in a 13 amp plug is:**
    A. black
    B. blue
    C. green and yellow
    D. brown.

12. **Ohm's law relates to:**
    A. voltage produced by a cell
    B. current flowing through a resistor
    C. light produced by a laser
    D. the number of ions in 100 ml of a solution.

13. **Before handling faulty mains-operated equipment, it is essential that the:**
    A. equipment is earthed
    B. fuse be removed
    C. mains should be switched off
    D. plug be removed from the mains.

14. **Radioactive isotopes emitting gamma rays should be stored in:**
    A. water
    B. a glass bottle
    C. a lead container
    D. a thick plastic container.

15. **The term ferrous metal means it:**
    A. is magnetic
    B. contains iron
    C. rusts easily
    D. conducts electricity.

16. **Low-dose radiation is hazardous to the:**
    A. nervous system
    B. skin
    C. respiratory system
    D. reproductive system.

17. **Ionization is produced by:**
    A. sound waves
    B. X-rays
    C. alpha particles
    D. neutrons.

18. **A device that converts electrical energy into mechanical energy is a:**
    A. transformer
    B. motor
    C. dynamo
    D. rectifier.

19. **Mains electrical frequency is:**
    A. 120 Hz
    B. 50 Hz
    C. 240 Hz
    D. 100 Hz.

20. **Diathermy is not recommended in:**
    A. a child
    B. an adult with a pacemaker fitted
    C. an adult with hyperthermia
    D. an elderly patient.

PATIENT CARE AND THEATRE TECHNIQUE

1. **It is essential to remove make-up and nail varnish preoperatively because it:**
   A. may obscure physical signs
   B. can react with anaesthetic agents
   C. can cause skin irritation following anaesthesia
   D. can cause cross-infection.

2. If a patient arrives in theatre with his dentures still in, the theatre personnel should:
   A. consult the anaesthetist
   B. leave them in his mouth
   C. place the dentures in a labelled pot and return them to the ward
   D. wrap them in paper and place them under the pillow.

3. Which of the following is the most suitable for wiping the scrub trolley during preparation?
   A. Dettol
   B. detergent hypochlorite
   C. Cidex
   D. Hibitane in spirit.

4. The site and side of operation in a small child should be marked:
   A. by the ward sister
   B. just before the premedication is given
   C. in the presence of the parent or guardian
   D. just before leaving for theatre.

5. False teeth should be removed prior to surgery to prevent:
   A. their breakdown
   B. biting on the endotracheal tube
   C. airway obstruction
   D. delay in anaesthetizing the patient.

6. Approved theatre footwear must be:
   A. fully insulated
   B. padded with paper
   C. fully conducting for electricity
   D. designed to conduct electrostatic charges.

7. If the surgeon wishes to open the posterior aspect of the skull, the patient may be positioned:
   A. prone
   B. supine
   C. with the neck extended
   D. in the lithotomy position.

8. For haemorrhoidectomy, the patient is placed in the following position:
   A. prone
   B. lithotomy

   C. supine
   D. left lateral.

9. In which of the following positions is a patient's respiratory function embarrassed?
   A. Trendelenburg
   B. supine
   C. left lateral
   D. reverse Trendelenburg.

10. In an unconscious patient, lifting only one leg into the lithotomy position at a time may lead to:
    A. sciatic nerve palsy
    B. pelvic damage
    C. damage of the sacroiliac joint
    D. arthritis of the hip joint.

11. Wrist drop is caused by damage to the:
    A. radial nerve
    B. median nerve
    C. ulnar nerve
    D. femoral nerve.

12. Continuous pressure on the calf muscles can lead to:
    A. bruising of the skin
    B. venous thrombosis
    C. ulcers
    D. varicose veins.

13. Which of the following is used during an abdominoperineal resection operation?
    A. perineal post
    B. lithotomy poles
    C. Lloyd-Davis poles
    D. sandbag under the loins.

14. The maximum safe abduction of an arm on a board is:
    A. 45 degrees
    B. 90 degrees
    C. 135 degrees
    D. 180 degrees.

15. After tonsillectomy, the patient should be recovered in which position:
    A. supine
    B. supine with a pillow
    C. left lateral
    D. prone.

16. The relative humidity in the operating theatre should be:
    A. 20%
    B. 50%
    C. 40%
    D. 80%.

17. A hygrometer is used to measure the level of:
    A. hydrogen in atmospheric air
    B. mercury in a tube
    C. humidity in the operating room
    D. urine in the bladder.

18. The earth or indifferent electrode on a diathermy machine:
    A. makes a wide area of contact with the patient
    B. prevents electrical interference with ECG monitors
    C. is connected to the patient by a point contact
    D. is isolated from patient contact.

19. Radiofrequency current is used in diathermy to:
    A. prevent muscle stimulation
    B. avoid burns
    C. prevent electrical interference
    D. prevent the build-up of static electricity.

20. The air ventilation systems in theatres should be:
    A. hot air
    B. water cooled
    C. positive pressure
    D. negative pressure.

ANAESTHESIA

1. Which of the following is not a laryngoscope blade?
   A. Negus
   B. Magill
   C. Shadwell
   D. Macintosh.

2. The size in millimetres (mm) marked on an endotracheal tube is to:
   A. maintain a patient's airway during an operation
   B. maintain an airtight seal with the trachea
   C. prevent the regurgitation of stomach contents
   D. prevent accidental misplacement of the tube.

3. The Macintosh laryngoscope:
   A. has a straight blade
   B. is suitable only in neonates
   C. is designed so that its tip lies in the front of the epiglottis when used
   D. is especially designed for a left-handed operator.

4. Which of the following drugs is an anticholinesterase?
   A. hyoscine
   B. sodium nitroprusside
   C. neostigmine
   D. glycopyrrolate.

5. Muscle fasciculations indicate that one of the following drugs has been used:
   A. atracurium   C. neostigmine
   B. suxamethonium   D. thiopentone.

6. To make a 2.5% solution of thiopentone, the following are mixed together:
   A. 250 mg thiopentone in 25 ml water
   B. 500 mg thiopentone in 20 ml water
   C. 1 g thiopentone in 25 ml water
   D. 250 mg thiopentone in 40 ml water.

7. Which of the following is not a muscle relaxant?
   A. atracurium   C. physostigmine
   B. vecuronium   D. suxamethonium.

8. The main reasons for humidifying inspired gases is to:
   A. keep bronchial secretions moist
   B. prevent explosions
   C. maintain the patient's fluid balance
   D. prevent cross-infection.

9. Which of the following ventilators is a pressure generator?
   A. Bennett
   B. Servo
   C. Manley
   D. Nuffield.

10. Which one of the following drugs causes respiratory depression?
   A. doxapram
   B. morphine
   C. atropine
   D. neostigmine.

SURGERY

1. Dennis Browne's operation is for:
   A. urethral obstruction
   B. epispadias
   C. hypospadias
   D. ectopia vesicae.

2. Orchidopexy is an operation for:
   A. acute infection of the testis
   B. acute pain in the testicle
   C. an undescended testis
   D. removing a malignant tumour from the testis.

3. A Pfannenstiel incision:
   A. involves dividing the external oblique muscle
   B. is mainly used for gynaecological operations
   C. is a vertical midline incision
   D. is a good incision by which to approach the liver.

4. A Kocher's incision is used for:
   A. cholecystectomy
   B. drainage of an appendicular abscess
   C. vagotomy and pyloroplasty
   D. gynaecological operations.

5. Which of the following is undertaken to demonstrate stones in the gallbladder?
   A. cystogram
   B. cholecystectomy

C. cholangiogram
D. cystometrogram.

6. A collection of blood in a tissue is an:
   A. epistaxis
   B. haematoma
   C. haemothorax
   D. haematemesis.

7. In the operations of vagotomy and pyloroplasty, the reason for doing a vagotomy is to:
   A. reduce acid secretion in the stomach
   B. prevent pain sensation reaching the brain
   C. improve the digestion of fats
   D. improve emptying of the stomach.

8. An abdominoperineal resection:
   A. is indicated in Crohn's disease
   B. requires a permanent colostomy
   C. requires a temporary colostomy
   D. requires a permanent ileostomy.

9. During a cholecystectomy, an on-table cholangiogram (OTC) is taken to demonstrate the:
   A. Hartmann's pouch
   B. common bile duct
   C. gallbladder
   D. cystic duct.

10. Haemorrhoids are:
   A. benign tumours of the rectum
   B. painful ulcers around the anus
   C. varicose veins around the anal canal
   D. a form of skin warts.

11. Achalasia of the cardia is a condition of the:
   A. bile ducts
   B. rectum
   C. heart
   D. oesophagus.

12. A Caldwell-Luc operation is performed to:
   A. drain a pelvic abscess
   B. open the maxillary sinus
   C. remove a foreign body from the nose
   D. repair the pelvic floor.

13. Ramstedt's operation is performed for:
    A. small bowel volvulus
    B. pyloric stenosis
    C. duodenal atresia
    D. intussusception.

14. In pyelolithotomy, a stone is removed from the:
    A. renal pelvis
    B. ureter
    C. kidney substance
    D. gallbladder.

15. A simple mastectomy involves the removal of the:
    A. whole breast and lymph nodes
    B. breast lump only
    C. whole breast but no lymph nodes
    D. whole breast, lymph nodes and underlying muscle.

RECOVERY AND INTENSIVE CARE

1. All of the following equipment is required in the recovery area except a:
    A. defibrillator
    B. suction unit
    C. diathermy machine
    D. ECG.

2. Following tonsillectomy, the patient is nursed in the:
    A. prone position
    B. supine position
    C. lateral position
    D. sitting position.

3. All of the following are routine postoperative analgesics except:
    A. alfentanil
    B. papaveretum
    C. pethidine
    D. nerve blocks.

4. All of the following are side-effects of intrathecal morphine except:
    A. pruritus
    B. urinary retention
    C. delayed respiratory depression
    D. hallucinations.

5. The commonly used local anaesthetic agent is:
    A. bupivacaine   C. cinchocaine
    B. lignocaine   D. prilocaine.

6. All of the following are common causes of postoperative hypoxia except:
    A. hypoventilation
    B. hyperventilation
    C. bronchospasm
    D. diffusion hypoxia.

7. The common cause of postoperative hypertension is:
    A. pain
    B. hypovolaemia
    C. residual effect of anaesthetic agent
    D. faulty monitoring equipment.

8. In the recovery area, all of the following agents can be used as antiemetics except:
    A. hyoscine
    B. metoclopramide
    C. prochlorperazine
    D. perphenazine.

9. All of the following are causes of postoperative excitement except:
    A. pain
    B. preoperative anxiety
    C. preoperative depression
    D. a full bladder.

10. All of the following are important causes of postoperative hypotension except:
    A. excessive premedication
    B. a residual effect of anaesthetic agent
    C. following spinal analgesia
    D. full urinary bladder.

CARDIOPULMONARY RESUSCITATION AND ACID–BASE BALANCE

1. Which one of the following is not a characteristic of cardiac arrest?
   A. pinpoint pupils
   B. a death-like appearance
   C. absent pulses
   D. pallor or cyanosis.

2. The normal Po_2 of arterial blood is:
   A. 95 mmHg
   B. 40 mmHg
   C. 46 mmHg
   D. 110 mmHg.

3. When two operators are available during cardiopulmonary resuscitation (CPR), the ratio of mouth-to-mouth ventilation to cardiac massage in an adult is:
   A. 2:15
   B. 1:5
   C. 1:10
   D. 1:15.

4. In the terminology of blood gases, SBC stands for:
   A. actual bicarbonate
   B. standard bicarbonate
   C. base excess
   D. base deficit.

5. Hyperventilation causes:
   A. respiratory acidosis
   B. respiratory alkalosis
   C. metabolic alkalosis
   D. metabolic acidosis.

6. Metabolic acidosis is seen in all these conditions except:
   A. diabetes
   B. salicylate poisoning
   C. hyperventilation
   D. hypoxia.

7. In ITU, junior anaesthetists carry out all duties except:
   A. liaising with senior medical staff and nursing staff
   B. liaising with other specialties
   C. taking major decisions
   D. acting on recent test results.

8. In cardiopulmonary resuscitation (CPR), adrenaline is given in:
   A. systole
   B. ventricular fibrillation
   C. ventricular tachycardia
   D. electromechanical dissociation.

9. With regard to defibrillation in cardiac arrest, which one of the following is not true?
   A. commonly used shock is delivered using an AC current
   B. current strength starts at 100 J
   C. the maximum strength that can be used is 5 J/kg in the adult
   D. the maximum strength which can be used is 2 J/kg in a child.

10. Which one of the following drugs is not used in cardiac arrest?
    A. adrenaline
    B. sodium bicarbonate
    C. calcium
    D. ranitidine.

Answers to self-assessment questions

Anatomy and physiology

1. C	6. B	11. B	16. B
2. A	7. C	12. B	17. C
3. C	8. B	13. B	18. B
4. A	9. A	14. C	19. C
5. C	10. C	15. D	20. B

Pharmacology

1. D	5. D	9. A	13. D
2. A	6. C	10. B	14. A, C
3. C	7. C	11. B	15. A
4. C	8. D	12. C	

Microbiology

1. C	6. B	11. B	16. C
2. B	7. C	12. C	17. C
3. B	8. A	13. C	18. B
4. A	9. A	14. A	19. A
5. C	10. B	15. A	20. C

Physics and electronics

1. A	6. A	11. B	16. B
2. C	7. C	12. B	17. C
3. C	8. C	13. C	18. A
4. A	9. B	14. D	19. B
5. A	10. D	15. B	20. B

Patient care and theatre technique

1. A	6. D	11. A	16. B
2. A	7. A	12. B	17. C
3. C	8. B	13. C	18. A
4. C	9. A	14. B	19. B
5. C	10. C	15. C	20. C

Anaesthesia

1. A	4. C	7. C	10. B
2. D	5. B	8. A	
3. C	6. B	9. C	

Surgery

1. C	5. C	9. B	13. B
2. C	6. B	10. C	14. A
3. B	7. D	11. D	15. B
4. A	8. B	12. B	

Recovery area and intensive care

1. C	4. D	7. A	10. D
2. C	5. A	8. A	
3. A	6. B	9. C	

Cardiopulmonary resuscitation and acid–base balance

1. A	4. B	7. C	10. D
2. A	5. B	8. A	
3. B	6. C	9. A	

Glossary

Abdomen   The largest cavity in the body, lying below the thorax and separated from it by the diaphragm.

Abdominoperineal   Relating to the abdomen and perineum. This term is used in the surgical removal of rectal cancer.

Abduct   To move away from the median line of the body; the opposite of adduct.

Ablation   Excision or removal.

Abrasion   Superficial injury to the skin or mucous membrane.

Abscess   A localized collection of pus caused by bacteria.

Acebutolol   A beta-adrenergic blocking drug used in the control of hypertension, angina pectoris and dysrhythmias.

Acetylcholine   A chemical substance (also called a neuro-transmitter) that is released by nerves at the neuro-muscular junction, resulting in the passage of a nerve impulse.

Actrapid   Neutral insulin.

Adenocarcinoma   A malignant tumour of glandular tissue, for example breast.

Adenoidectomy   Removal of adenoid tissue from the naso-pharynx.

Adenotonsillectomy   Removal of the adenoids and tonsils.

Adhesion   Following inflammation, abnormal union of two parts by fibrous tissue.

Adiposity   Excessive accumulation of fat in the body.

Adrenalectomy   Removal of the adrenal gland.

Afebrile   Without fever.

Agglutination   The clumping of red blood cells in the presence of specific immune antibodies called agglutinins.

Allograft   When a part of one person is transplanted into another person.

Amethocaine   A synthetic local anaesthetic.

Anaesthesia   Reversible loss of sensation

Anaphylaxis   When a body is presented with a foreign protein, it becomes hypersensitive and, following a second exposure, an acute reaction can result.

Aneurysm   Local dilatation of a blood vessel, usually an artery.

Antacid   An agent, for example sodium citrate, that neutralizes acidity.

Anticholinesterase   A drug that counteracts the effects of the enzyme that normally destroys acetylcholine. Neostigmine is a drug with this property.

Anticoagulant   An agent, for example heparin, that prevents clotting of the blood.

Antiemetic An agent that prevents nausea and vomiting, for example metoclopramide (Maxolon) or prochlorperazine (Stemetil).

Antihistamine An agent, for example chlorpheniramine (Piriton), that blocks the effect of histamine.

Antrostomy In ENT surgery, an artificial opening made from the nasal cavity to the antrum of the maxillary sinus to facilitate the drainage of pus.

Arteriogram A film showing arteries after the injection of an opaque substance in the X-ray department.

Arthroplasty Creation of an artificial joint.

Arthroscopy The procedure by which the inside of a joint is visualized.

Ascites Secreted fluid in the abdominal cavity. It is always abnormal.

Autoclave An apparatus used to sterilize equipment.

Avascular Bloodless.

Bifurcation Division into two branches.

Bleeding time Time required for the spontaneous stoppage of bleeding from a skin puncture (normally 1–7 minutes).

Boyle's law At standard temperature, the volume of a given mass of gas is inversely proportional to the pressure upon it.

Bronchodilator A drug, for example aminophylline, that dilates the bronchi (singular bronchus).

Bronchospasm Sudden contraction of the bronchial tubes in the presence of irritants.

Buerger's disease Disease of the peripheral blood vessels. More common in smokers.

Bursa A fibrous sac lined with synovial membrane. Bursae are present between skin and bone, and muscle and muscle.

Caecostomy Surgical procedure in which the caecum is exposed on the abdominal wall.

Caecum The beginning of the colon; it is attached to the appendix.

Carcinoid syndrome Caused by a tumour that secretes serotonin. The patient presents with asthma, bronchospasm and diarrhoea.

Cardiomegaly Enlargement of the heart.

Cardiopulmonary Related to the heart and lungs. The term cardiopulmonary bypass is used in heart surgery.

Cardioversion The use of electrical countershock to restore the heart rhythm to normal.

Cataract An opacity of the crystalline lens or its capsule in the eye.

Catgut Ligature suture of varying thickness prepared from sheep's intestines.

Chemotherapy Chemical agents used to arrest the progress of disease, for example leukaemia.

Cholangiogram A film showing the hepatic, cystic and bile ducts.

Cholecystectomy Surgical removal of the gallbladder.

Cholecystolithiasis The presence of gallstones in the gallbladder.

Choledocholithotomy Surgical removal of a stone from the common bile duct.

Cholinergic Parasympathetic nerves that liberate acetylcholine.

Cholinesterase An enzyme that breaks down acetylcholine into choline and acetic acid.

Claudication Pain caused by poor blood supply to the limbs. It may present at rest or only when the patient is walking.

Colectomy Removal of part or the whole of the colon.

Colonoscopy The use of a fibreoptic instrument (colonoscope) to view the inside of the colon.

Colporrhaphy Surgical repair of the vaginal wall. Anterior colporrhaphy repairs a cystocele and posterior colporrhaphy a rectocele.

Contracture Shortening of a muscle.

Coronary arteries An artery or arteries supplying blood to the heart.

Cryoanalgesia Pain relief achieved using a cryosurgical probe, a probe cooled to a very low temperature.

Cryosurgery Instead of a knife, an intense, controlled cold is used to destroy diseased tissue.

Cystectomy The partial or complete removal of the urinary bladder.

Cystodiathermy Application of diathermy to the urinary bladder.

Cystometrogram A record of pressure changes in the urinary bladder.

Cystostomy A fistulous opening between the urinary bladder and the abdominal wall.

Cystotomy An incision into the urinary bladder.

Dacryocystorhinostomy An operation in which the lacrimal sac in the eye is drained into the nose.

Dextrocardia Transposition of the heart to the right side of the thorax.

Dupuytren's contracture Contracture of the palmar fascia, which bends one or more fingers.

Dysphagia Difficulty in swallowing.

ECG Electrocardiogram.

Eclampsia A complication of pregnancy, resulting in fits, hypertension and coma.

Ectopic pregnancy Pregnancy outside the uterus, the fallopian tube being the most common site. The tube ruptures and bleeds between the 6th and 8th week of pregnancy; this is a surgical emergency.

Edentulous Without teeth.

Electrocochleography Recording of movement of the fluid in the internal ear.

Embolectomy Surgical removal of an embolus.

Emetic An agent that produces vomiting.

Endarterectomy Surgical removal of an atheromatous plug from an artery.

Endoscope An instrument used to visualize body cavities.

Epiglottitis Inflammation of the epiglottis.

Episiotomy An incision made in the perineum during the birth of a child to allow delivery.

Epispadias A congenital opening on the upper surface of the penis.

Epistaxis Bleeding from the nose.

Esmarch's bandage A rubber bandage that is rolled onto an arm or leg to produce a bloodless operative field.

Ethmoidectomy Surgical removal of bone (ethmoid) from the lateral wall of the nose.

Evisceration Removal of internal organs.

Extrapleural Outside the pleura.

Extraperitoneal Outside the peritoneum.

Fibroid A tumour of fibrous and muscular tissue found in the uterus.

Fibrosarcoma A malignant tumour.

Fissure A split or cut, for example an anal fissure.

Fistula An abnormal communication between two body cavities or surfaces, for example in a colostomy between the colon and the abdominal wall.

Gallie's operation Use of fascia from the thigh in the permanent repair of a hernia.

Gastroenterostomy An anastomosis between the stomach and small intestine.

Gastropexy Surgical fixation of a displaced stomach.

Haemangioma An abnormal blood vessel in any part of the body.

Haematuria Blood in the urine.

Haemodialysis A technique by which waste products are removed and essential constituents replaced in the blood.

Hemicolectomy Removal of half of the colon.

Hydronephrosis Following obstruction, urine fills up the kidney, causing its distension.

Hyperkalaemia High levels of potassium in the serum.

Hyperpituitarism Increased activity of the anterior pituitary gland, causing acromegaly or gigantism.

Hyperthermia High body temperature.

Hypertrophy Increase in the size of, for example, tissue or muscles.

Iatrogenic A complication caused by the treatment of another primary condition.

Infarction Death of tissue.

Intra-arterial Within an artery.

Intrathecal In the subarachnoid space.

Intravascular Within the blood vessels (artery or vein).

Ion A charged atom.

Jejunostomy An opening (fistula) made between the jejunum and the anterior abdominal wall for feeding purposes.

Keller's operation An operation to correct the deformity of the proximal portion of the proximal phalanx.

Keratectomy Removal of a part of the cornea.

Keratoplasty Replacing unhealthy corneal tissue with a graft.

Küntscher nail A nail used for the fixation of fractured long bones, for example the femur.

Labile Unstable.

Lacrimation Crying (as a physical rather than an emotional sign).

Laminectomy Removal of part of a degenerated disc between two vertebrae and vertebral laminae to expose the spinal cord.

Laparoscopy Insertion of an instrument (laparoscope) to visualize the abdominal contents and perform such operations as sterilization.

Laparotomy Incision of the abdominal wall to expose the contents. Its use implies that the diagnosis or operation to be performed is not fully certain.

Laryngoscope An instrument used to visualize the larynx.

Lateral Away from the midline or on the side.

Ligate To tie a blood vessel.

Lipoma A benign tumour containing fatty tissue.

Lithotrite An instrument used to crush stones in the urinary bladder.

Lugol's solution An aqueous solution containing potassium iodide and iodine. It is used in the preoperative preparation of patients undergoing thyroid surgery.

Lymphadenopathy A disease of the lymph nodes.

Lymphosarcoma A malignant tumour of lymphatic tissue.

McBurney's point A point one-third of the way between the anterior superior iliac spine and the umbilicus. This point develops maximum tenderness in acute appendicitis.

Macroglossia An abnormally large tongue.

Mammography An X-ray examination of the breast after the injection of an opaque agent.

Mastectomy Surgical removal of the breast.

Meconium A greenish-black discharge from the bowel of a newborn baby.

Medial Near to the middle.

Meibomian glands Sebaceous glands that lie in the grooves on the inner surface of the eyelids, their ducts opening on the free margins of the lids.

Melaena Black, tar-like stools as a result of gastrointestinal bleeding or iron therapy.

Multilobular Possessing many lobes.

Mydriasis Abnormal dilatation of the pupil of the eye.

Myringoplasty An operation to close a defect in the tympanic membrane of the ear using a graft (e.g. of temporal fascia).

Myringotomy An incision into the tympanic membrane (ear drum) to drain pus from the middle ear.

Necrosis Local death of tissue.

Nephrolithotomy Removal of a kidney stone.

Neuromuscular Related to nerve and muscle.

Neurotoxic Poisonous to nervous tissue.

Nuclear magnetic resonance (NMR) A non-invasive imaging technique.

Oedema Excess fluid in the tissues.

Oesophagectomy Excision of part or whole of the oesophagus.

Oncology The study of cancer.

Orthopnoea Breathlessness on lying flat.

Orthostatic Caused by an upright position.

Osteotome An instrument used for cutting bone.

Papilloedema Oedema of the optic disc in the eye, indicating raised intracranial pressure.

Para-aortic Near the aorta.

Paramedian Near the middle.

Paraphimosis The prepuce (foreskin) of the penis is retracted behind the glans; the tightness of this ring interferes with the blood flow in the glans.

Parasympathetic A part of the autonomic nervous system arising mostly from the cranial and sacral regions of the spinal cord.

Parathyroidectomy Excision of one or more parathyroid glands.

Paravertebral Near the spine.

Parenteral Not via the gastrointestinal tract.

Patellectomy Excision of the patella.

Percutaneous Through the skin.

Peritoneum The serous membrane that lines the abdominal and pelvic contents.

Phaeochromocytoma A tumour of the adrenal medulla or the sympathetic chain. It secretes adrenaline and nor-adrenaline, causing episodes of severe hypertension.

Pharyngectomy Surgical removal of the pharynx.

Polya operation Partial gastrectomy.

Polycystic Consisting of a number of cysts (especially the kidney and ovary).

Pott's fracture A fracture dislocation of the ankle.

Proctocolectomy Surgical removal of the colon and rectum.

Prolapse Falling of an organ or structure, for example prolapse of the uterus or an intervertebral disc.

Prophylaxis Prevention.

Prosthesis An artificial replacement for a missing part, for example a knee.

Pyelolithotomy An operation for the removal of a stone from the renal pelvis.

Quadriplegia Paralysis of all four limbs.

Quinsy Acute inflammation of the tonsil with abscess formation.

Radiograph An X-ray picture that is developed.

Radiologist One who specializes in X-ray diagnosis.

Radiology The study of the diagnosis of disease using X-rays.

Radiotherapist One who specializes in the treatment of disease with X-rays.

Ranula A cystic swelling below the tongue.

Rectocele Prolapse of the rectum and its herniation into the posterior vaginal wall.

Referred pain Pain occurring at a distance from its source; for example, the pain from angina pectoris can be felt in the left upper limb.

Renin A enzyme released into the blood from the kidney in response to sodium loss.

Rennin A milk-curdling enzyme present in the gastric juice of infants.

Reticulocyte A young circulating red blood cell with traces of its nucleus.

Retrobulbar Referring to the back of the eyeball.

Retrocaecal Behind the caecum, for example a retrocaecal appendix.

Retrograde Going backwards.

Rhinology A study of disease affecting the nose.

Rhinoplasty Plastic surgery of the nose.

Rhizotomy Surgical division of a root, usually the posterior root of a nerve.

Salpingectomy Surgical removal of a fallopian tube.

Salpingo-oophorectomy Surgical removal of a fallopian tube and ovary.

Salpingostomy An operation performed to restore tubal patency.

Sarcoma A malignant growth of connective tissue, muscle or bone.

Sclerotherapy The injection of sclerosing agents (e.g. phenol) for the treatment of varicose veins.

Septicaemia The presence and multiplication of living bacteria in the bloodstream.

Shirodkar's operation An operation carried out during pregnancy, in which a purse-string suture is placed around an incompetent cervix. This suture is removed before labour starts.

Spirometer An instrument used to measure the tidal and minute volumes of the lungs.

Stapedectomy Surgical removal of the stapes (a small bone in the middle ear) and its replacement with teflon or a vein graft.

Subcostal Below the rib.

Subdural Below the dura mater.

Sublingual Below the tongue.

Suboccipital Beneath the occiput, in the nape of the neck.

Supraorbital Above the orbit.

Suprapubic Above the pubis.

Synovectomy Excision of synovial membrane.

Tachypnoea An abnormally fast rate of respiration.

Tarsorrhaphy Suturing of the eyelids together (usually only partial)

Tetanus Disease caused by *Clostridium tetani*, classically following a puncture wound in the garden. These organisms are present in road dust and manure.

Tetany A condition in which muscles are hyperexcitable and mild stimuli produce cramps. It is seen in patients with a low serum calcium level.

Tetralogy of Fallot A congenital heart defect that consists of narrowing of the pulmonary artery, hypertrophy of the right ventricle, a septal defect between the ventricles and a displacement of the aorta to the right.

Thoracotomy Surgical exposure of the thoracic cavity.

Thyroglossal Relating to the thyroid gland and the back of the tongue.

Thyroidectomy Surgical removal of the thyroid gland.

Trabeculectomy An operation carried out for glaucoma. A channel is created through the trabecular meshwork from the canal of Schlemm to the angle of the anterior chamber of the eye.

Tympanoplasty A reconstructive operation carried out on the middle ear to improve hearing.

Ultrasonic Relating to mechanical vibrations of very high frequency (usually above 30 000 Hz).

Ureterolithotomy Surgical removal of a stone from a ureter.

Urethrocele Prolapse of the urethra, usually into the anterior vaginal wall.

Vagolytic A drug (e.g. atropine) that prevents the slow heart rate (bradycardia) that accompanies stimulation of the vagus nerve.

Vagotomy The surgical division of the vagus nerves carried out in association with pyloroplasty of the stomach in the treatment of peptic ulcer.

Valgus Displacement or angulation away from the midline of the body, an seen in, for example, hallux valgus.

Varicocele Varicosity of the veins of the spermatic cord.

Vasoconstrictor Any drug, for example methoxamine, that causes a narrowing of the lumen of blood vessels.

Vasodilator Any drug, for example sodium nitroprusside, that causes a widening of the lumen of blood vessels.

Volvulus A twisting of a section of bowel, thus occluding the lumen.

Xerostomia A dry mouth.

Yttrium[90] A substance emitting beta particles, with a half-life of 64 hours. Yttrium is implanted in the pituitary fossa after hypophysectomy for breast cancer.

Zygoma Cheek bone.

Index